DENTAL MANAGEMENT
OF THE MEDICALLY
COMPROMISED PATIENT

SECOND EDITION

JAMES W. LITTLE

DONALD A. FALACE

Dental management of the
medically compromised patient

DENTAL MANAGEMENT
OF THE MEDICALLY
COMPROMISED PATIENT

JAMES W. LITTLE, D.M.D., M.S.

Professor of Oral Diagnosis and Oral Medicine,
University of Minnesota School of Dentistry,
Minneapolis, Minnesota

DONALD A. FALACE, D.M.D.

Associate Professor of Oral Diagnosis and Oral Medicine,
The University of Kentucky College of Dentistry,
Lexington, Kentucky

SECOND EDITION

with 157 illustrations

The C. V. Mosby Company

ST. LOUIS • TORONTO • PRINCETON   1984

A TRADITION OF PUBLISHING EXCELLENCE

Editor: Samuel E. Harshberger
Assistant editor: Nancy B. Hughson
Manuscript editor: Timothy O'Brien
Design: Jeanne E. Bush
Production: Carol O'Leary, Barbara Merritt, Ginny Douglas

SECOND EDITION

The C.V. Mosby Company
11830 Westline Industrial Drive, St. Louis, Missouri 63146

Library of Congress Cataloging in Publication Data

Little, James W., 1934-
  Dental management of the medically compromised patient.

  Includes bibliographies and index.
    1. Sick—Dental care.   2.   Chronically ill—Dental care.
3. Oral manifestations of general diseases.   I.   Falace,
Donald A., 1945-   .   II.   Title.   [DNLM: 1. Dental Care.
2. Disease.   3. Oral Manifestations.   WU 29 L778d]
RK55.S53L57   1984   617.6   84-6949
ISBN 0-8016-3035-5

AC/VH/VH   9   8   7   6   5   4   02/A/266

FOREWORD

It is my privilege to prepare this foreword for the second edition of Dr. Little and Falace's book on the care of the medically compromised patient, as I did for the first edition. This is an area of growing interest and need for the clinician. I was afforded the unusual opportunity to note the numerous additions and expansions of the second edition.

Fortunately, the same format is used for this edition. In general, the text draws special attention to the cause and prevention of bacteremias associated with operative dental procedures. The authors also give special attention to surgery of the coronary and larger vessels. This is a type of surgery that is being used more and more widely today.

The patient with replacement of the larger joints (hip) is well covered. With the aging population, this becomes a more important subject to the dentist and his or her patient.

The hepatitis B section has been brought up to date, including the substantial risks to the dentist and to laboratory personnel. The dental management of patients with the history and carrier states of hepatitis is also discussed.

Patients in the end stages of renal disease and patients receiving long-term dialysis, peritoneal dialysis, and hemodialysis are well covered, as are patients receiving renal transplants and aggressive management of those receiving dental care.

The combination of cytotoxic drugs used for therapy and given to minimize bacteremia and avoid postoperative infection is well covered.

The section on sexually transmitted diseases and genital herpes has been enlarged and brought up to date, affording the clinician a current knowledge of this group of ever-increasing diseases.

The section on the dental management of the epileptic patient has been improved. These patients still present a problem in dental management.

The sections on benign and malignant bleeding disorders are equally well done.

It is obvious that this second edition has been thoroughly revised and the references made current.

Every dentist treating the medically compromised patient should find Little and Falace's book most informative and a real addition to his or her clinical library.

Lester W. Burket D.D.S., M.D.

PREFACE

The need for a second edition of *Dental Management of the Medically Compromised Patient* became apparent because of the ever-increasing flow of new knowledge and changing concepts in medicine and dentistry.

The purpose of the book remains to provide the dental practitioner with a concise, factual reference work describing the dental management of patients with selected medical problems. The more common medical disorders that may be encountered in a dental practice continue to be the focus. This book is not a comprehensive medical reference, but rather a book that contains only enough core information about each of the medical conditions covered to enable the reader to recognize the basis for various dental management recommendations. Where appropriate, medical problems are organized to provide a brief overview of the basic disease process, pathophysiology, signs and symptoms, laboratory findings, and currently accepted medical therapy of each disorder. This is followed by a detailed explanation and recommendations for specific dental management.

We have found that those who may benefit from reading this book include practicing dentists, practicing dental hygienists, dental and dental hygiene students, and dental graduate students in specialty programs or in general practice residencies.

Several major changes have been made in this second edition. New chapters on the management of the cancer patient and patients with surgically corrected cardiovascular lesions have been added as well as a separate chapter devoted to the management of patients with arthritis and joint disorders. The chapters on renal disease and disorders of the parathyroid glands and mineral homeostasis have been combined, as have the chapters on pulmonary disease and tuberculosis. The chapter on viral hepatitis has been expanded to include alcoholic liver disease. The focus of the chapter on neurologic disorders has been markedly changed, with the emphasis now on stroke and seizure disorders. A separate chapter has been devoted to infective endocarditis. A section on lactation and the nursing mother has been added to the pregnancy chapter, and a section on murmurs has been added to the chapter on rheumatic fever and rheumatic heart disease. Major updating and organization were done to the chapters on diabetes, allergy, hypertension, ischemic heart disease, and sexually transmitted diseases. The remaining chapters were updated where indicated.

Our sincere thanks and appreciation are extended to those many individuals who have contributed their time and expertise to the writing and revision of the text. Particular thanks is extended to Heloyse Anderson and Rebecca Turpin for typing and editing the drafts of the new chapters and revisions of old chapters.

James W. Little
Donald A. Falace

CONTENTS

Dental management of the medically compromised patient

DENTAL MANAGEMENT
A SUMMARY

This table, Dental Management: A Summary, summarizes the more important factors to be considered in the dental management of the medically compromised patient. Each medical problem is outlined according to the potential medical problems related to dental treatment, the prevention of these complications, the effect of these problems on dental treatment planning, oral changes that may be found associated with the medical condition, and modifications indicated when rendering emergency dental care for patients with the medical condition.

The information contained in this table will be more easily understood if the text has been read first. The table has been designed for use by the dentist or dental student as a convenient reference work for dental management of patients who have the medical diseases covered in this book.

Dental management: a summary

Medical problem	Potential problem relating to dental treatment	Prevention of medical complications

Rheumatic fever and rheumatic heart disease (pp. 53-63)	If rheumatic heart disease is present, patient is susceptible to infective endocarditis following dental procedures that may cause transient bacteremias	I. Medical consultation to confirm presence or absence of rheumatic heart disease
		II. Medical referral to evaluate patient for presence or absence of rheumatic heart disease
		  A. Electrocardiogram
		  B. Chest x-ray film
		  C. Physical examination of chest including auscultation for murmurs
		III. Patients with rheumatic heart disease require prophylactic antibiotic coverage for all dental procedures (including certain examination procedures)
		  A. In patients not allergic to penicillin
		    1. Give 1 million units of crystalline penicillin G mixed with 600,000 units of procaine penicillin G, IM, at least 30 minutes before dental procedure followed by 500 mg penicillin V, orally, every 6 hours for eight doses *or*
		    2. Give 2 g of penicilin V, orally, at least 30 minutes before dental procedure followed by 500 mg penicillin V, orally, every 6 hours for eight doses
		  B. In patients allergic to penicillin
		    Give 1 g erythromycin, orally, at least 1½ hours before dental procedure followed by 500 mg erythromycin, orally, every 6 hours for eight doses
		  C. In patients taking low daily oral dose of penicillin or monthly injections of penicillin to prevent recurrent attacks of rheumatic fever
		    1. Instruct patient to continue medication
		    2. Then add 1 g erythromycin, orally, at least 1½ hours before dental procedure followed by 500 mg erythromycin, orally, every 6 hours for eight doses

Artificial heart valve(s) (pp. 88-102)	1. Prosthetic valve endocarditis can occur following dental procedures that may cause transient bacteremias
	2. Prolonged bleeding may occur following scaling or surgical procedures in patients being treated with anticoagulants
		1. Medical consultation to determine patient's current status and presence of other medical problems and to confirm dental management plan
		2. Prophylactic antibiotic coverage to prevent prosthetic valve endocarditis—for all dental procedures
		  a. In patients not allergic to penicillin
		    Give 1 million units of crystalline penicillin G mixed with 600,000 units of procaine penicillin G, IM, at least 30 minutes before dental procedure and 1 g of streptomycin, IM, followed by 500 mg penicillin V, orally, every 6 hours for eight doses
		  b. In patients allergic to penicillin
		    Give 1 g of vancomycin, IV, over 30-minute period just before dental procedure followed by 500 mg erythromycin, orally, every 6 hours for eight doses
		3. In patients taking anticoagulant medication
		  If scaling or surgical procedures are planned, dosage of anticoagulant medication should be reduced by physician so that on day of procedure prothrombin time is twice normal or less

Treatment plan modifications	Oral complications	Emergency dental care

1. No dental procedures are contraindicated for asymptomatic patient with rheumatic heart disease
2. Management plan should include
  a. Carry out as much treatment as possible on first day of 3-day coverage period—no treatment on last 2 days
  b. Allow at least 1 week to elapse before starting a new coverage period to allow penicillin-resistant organisms to disappear from oral flora
  c. If multiple coverage periods are needed, antibiotic used can be alternated, first using penicillin and then erythromycin; at least 1 week must elapse between coverage periods
3. Length of coverage period may be extended to 5 to 7 days under certain *special* conditions
  a. Surgical procedures with sutures or surgical areas that are slow to heal
  b. Patients with very poor oral hygiene who will receive daily (4 to 5 days) scaling, brushing, and flossing procedures
  c. No treatment should occur on last 2 days of coverage period
  d. Erythromycin can be used for last 2 to 3 days to avoid possibility of bacteria developing resistance to penicillin
	Usually none	1. Patients with asymptomatic rheumatic heart disease need prophylactic antibiotic coverage for all emegency dental treatment
		2. Patients with history of rheumatic fever who have not been evaluated for presence or absence of rheumatic heart disease must be considered to have rheumatic heart disease until proved otherwise; give prophylactic antibiotic coverage to prevent infective endocarditis
		3. Patients with history of rheumatic fever who have been told they do not have rheumatic heart disease; once this has been confirmed antibiotic coverage is not needed

1. Patients allergic to penicillin
  a. Present special problem because most dental offices are not prepared to provide IV infusion of vancomycin—routine dental treatment must be done in hospital; patients with poor dental status should be counseled concerning problems and expense and directed toward complete dentures
  b. Patients should be given antibiotic coverage during extractions and at time of denture insertion until all overextended areas are identified and corrected
2. Patients not allergic to penicillin
  a. Can be managed on outpatient basis; no dental treatment is contraindicated, but patients with advanced periodontal disease should be encouraged to consider complete denture therapy rather than prolonged, complicated periodontal-restorative treatment
  b. As much dental treatment as possible should be done during each coverage period
  c. At least 1 week should elapse between coverage periods
  d. Coverage period may have to be extended in cases where healing is slow following surgical procedures, sutures have been placed, or an attempt is made to improve the patient's oral hygiene
	Usually none unless patient is receiving anticoagulation therapy; these patients may have areas of ecchymosis or gingival bleeding	Antibiotic coverage to prevent infective endocarditis needed for any dental treatment; conservative management of pain and infection if prothrombin time is greater than twice normal

Continued.

Medical problem	Potential problem relating to dental treatment	Prevention of medical complications
Murmurs (pp. 63-64)	1. No problem if murmur is functional in nature 2. If murmur is organic (pathologic) infective endocarditis must be prevented	1. Medical consultation to confirm nature of murmur 2. If organic murmur, management same as for patient with rheumatic heart disease

Congenital heart disease (pp. 65-72)	1. Infective endocarditis
	2. Infective endarteritis
	3. Prolonged bleeding following scaling or surgical procedures; bleeding problem may be present in patients with right-to-left shunting of blood caused by
	  a. Thrombocytopenia
	  b. Lack of coagulation factor as result of thrombosis occurring in small vessels
	  c. Antigoagulation medication to prevent thrombosis
	4. Congestive heart failure
	  a. Infection
	  b. Cardiac arrest
	  c. Cardiac dysrhythmias
	  d. Breathing difficulties (caused by pulmonary edema)
		1. Detection by history and examination findings
		2. Referral for medical diagnosis and treatment
		3. Consultation with physician before any dental treatment is performed
		4. Prophylactic antibiotic coverage before and after any dental procedure
		  a. For patients with congenital heart disease
		    Coverage same as for patient with rheumatic heart disease
		  b. For patients who have just had surgery to correct congenital heart defect
		    Coverage same as for patient with artificial heart valve
		  c. After consultation with physician many patients with treated defects that have healed will no longer need coverage
		5. Avoidance of dehydration in patients with oral infection
		6. Bleeding time and prothrombin time tested before any surgical procedures—consultation with physician if prolonged

Coronary atherosclerotic heart disease with history of brief pain (angina pectoris) (pp. 73-87)	1. Stress and anxiety related to dental visit may precipitate angina attack in dental office
	2. Myocardial infarction may occur when patient is in dental office
	3. Sudden death caused by disruption of cardiac rhythm or cardiac arrest without acute myocardial infarction may occur in dental office
		1. Detection of patient with history of angina pectoris
		2. Referral of patient thought to have untreated angina based on medical history for medical evaluation and treatment
		3. Patient under medical treatment for angina—during dental visit every attempt should be made to reduce stress
		  a. Concern and warm approach by staff and dentist
		  b. Make patient feel free to talk about fears
		  c. Morning appointments
		  d. Short appointments
		  e. Premedication—diazepam (Valium), 5 to 10 mg; prophylactic nitroglycerin, one tablet preoperatively
		  f. Nitrous oxide
		  g. Effective local anesthetic—epinephrine 1:100,000 can and should be used; aspirate; inject slowly
		4. Reinforce importance of risk factors that can be influenced by patient
		5. If patient develops chest pain during dental treatment, stop procedure and give patient nitroglycerin tablet sublingually
		  a. If pain continues longer than 2 or 3 minutes, monitor vital signs and give up to a total of 3 nitroglycerin tablets within 15 minutes; if pain persists and patient's condition is stable, transport patient to hospital emergency room and call physician; if unstable, call for medical aid and be prepared to render cardiopulmonary resuscitation
		  b. If patient has stable type of angina and pain is relieved within 2 or 3 minutes with nitroglycerin, dental treatment may be continued or terminated depending on circumstances
		  c. Patient with unstable angina whose pain is relieved with nitroglycerin within 2 or 3 minutes should have appointment terminated and physician informed of what happened
		6. Terminate appointment if patient becomes fatigued or develops change in pulse rate or rhythm

Treatment plan modifications	Oral complications	Emergency dental care
1. Patients with functional murmurs would be treated as normal patients 2. Patients with organic murmurs would be managed same as patients with rheumatic heart disease or congenital heart disease	Usually none	1. Patients with history of murmur during childhood or pregnancy that since has disappeared do not require prophylactic coverage unless history is not clear 2. Patients with murmur who require emergency dental care should be protected from infective endocarditis with prophylactic antibiotics; medical consultation by phone can be used in attempt to determine nature of murmur
Usually none unless congestive heart failure present (see p. 121)	1. Cyanosis— blue color 2. Polycythemia —ruddy color 3. Thrombocytopenia—small hemorrhages 4. Leukopenia— infection	1. Asymptomatic patient As indicated but protect agaisnt infective endocarditis or endarteritis 2. Symptomatic patient—congestive heart failure and/or polycythemia a. Consultation with physician before any treatment b. Analgesics for pain c. Antibiotics for infection d. Avoidance of dehydration in patient with acute infection e. Patient may have bleeding problem, in which case surgery should be avoided
1. Patients with stable form of angina Any routine dental care 2. Patients with unstable form of angina Only care needed to deal with or prevent dental pain or infection or both	Usually none; however, on rare occasions patients may have lower jaw pain of cardiac origin (referred pain); history of what initiates the pain and how it is relieved should provide clue to its cardiac origin	1. No restrictions for patient with stable angina 2. Conservative treatment, antibiotics for infection, and analgesics for pain control (consult with physician) 3. Patients with unstable form of angina Consult with physician; based on patient's status, emergency treatment may be as indicated or conservative, using antibiotics for infection and analgesics for pain

Continued.

Dental management: a summary—cont'd

Medical problem	Potential problem relating to dental treatment	Prevention of medical complications

Coronary atherosclerotic heart disease with history of brief pain (angina pectoris) (pp. 73-87)—cont'd		7. Avoid use of vasopressors except for epinephrine 1:100,000 in local anesthetic
		  a. Do not use vasopressors to control local bleeding
		  b. Do not use gingival packing material that contains vasopressor

Surgically corrected cardiovascular lesions (pp. 88-102)	1. Infective endocarditis 2. Infective endarteritis 3. Prolonged bleeding following scaling or surgical procedures because of anticoagulant medication	1. Antibiotic prophylaxis up to 6 months postoperatively using regimen B (medical consultation) 2. Patients with coronary bypass graft surgery usually are not considered susceptible 1 to 2 weeks after surgery; confirm by consultation and treat as normal patients 3. 6 months after surgery, most patients are no longer susceptible unless foreign material was used to correct cardiovascular problem; in cases where synthetic materials such as Dacron were used, patient is considered susceptible to infective endocarditis or endarteritis—coverage with regimen A and confirmation by consultation 4. Patients with artificial heart valves remain very susceptible; coverage with regimen B and confirmation by consultation
Myocardial infarction (pp. 81-86)	1. Cardiac arrest 2. Myocardial infarction 3. Angina pectoris 4. Congestive heart failure 5. Bleeding tendency secondary to anticoagulant 6. Infective endocarditis complicating implanted pacemaker 7. Electrical interference with pacemaker	1. No routine dental care until at least 6 months after infarction because of increased risk of new infarction 2. Consultation with patient's physician before starting routine dental care to confirm patient's current status and need for antibiotic prophylaxis for patients with transvenous pacemakers 3. Morning appointments 4. Short appointments 5. Termination of appointment if patient becomes fatigued or short of breath, develops change in pulse rate or rhythm, or develops chest pain—inform patient's physician 6. Use of local anesthetic with epinephrine 1:100,000 (no more than three cartridges); aspirate before injecting; inject slowly 7. Premedication before appointment to reduce stress associated with dental visit—diazepam, 5 to 10 mg 8. Anticoagulant medication—if surgery or scaling procedures are planned, physician should be contacted and dosage of anticoagulant reduced so that prothrombin time will be twice normal or less—will take 3 to 4 days; check to see if desired result was obtained day of procedure by having another prothrombin time done 9. Digitalis—patient more prone to nausea and vomiting; avoid stimulating gag reflex 10. Antisialagogues—atropine, methantheline—may cause tachycardia; check with patient's physician before using 11. Antiarrhythmic agents—quinidine, procainamide—nausea and vomiting may occur; hypotension may occur; oral ulceration may indicate agranulocytosis 12. Antihypertensive agents (see p. 110) 13. Avoidance of use of instruments such as Cavitron, electric cautery equipment, etc., with patients who have pacemaker

Treatment plan modifications	Oral complications	Emergency dental care

See sections on rheumatic heart disease (pp. 62-63), congenital heart disease (p. 72), and artificial heart valves (pp. 99-101)	Usually none unless patient is receiving anticoagulant medication	1. Patient with coronary bypass graft that has healed does not require antibiotic prophylaxis
		2. Patients for whom it has been at least 6 months since surgery
		  a. Foreign material used to correct defect—coverage indicated
		  b. Defect closed or corrected without use of foreign material—coverage not indicated
		3. Patients with artificial heart valve(s) must have coverage
		4. Surgical procedures should be avoided if possible for patients taking anticoagulant medication

1. Patients 6 months or more after infarction with no complications
Any routine dental care
2. If complications such as congestive heart failure are present
Dental treatment should be limited to immediate needs only
	Usually none except those related to drugs used to treat patient's medical problem	1. During first 6 months after infarction, emergency dental care only, after consultation with patient's physician; dental treatment should be as conservative as possible—drugs for pain control, antibiotics for infection, pulpotomy rather than extraction
		2. Patients more than 6 months after infarction
		  a. Patient with no complications can receive any treatment indicated
		  b. Patients with complications—medical consultation is indicated; treatment should be based on medical complication(s) present (refer to appropriate sections)

Continued.

Medical problem	Potential problem relating to dental treatment	Prevention of medical complications

Hypertensive disease (pp. 103-115)	1. Stress and anxiety related to dental visit may cause increase in blood pressure; in patient with already elevated blood pressure as a result of hypertensive disease, myocardial infarction or cerebrovascular accident may be precipitated
	2. If blood pressure is significantly elevated, excessive bleeding may occur following surgical or scaling procedures
	3. Patients being treated with antihypertensive agents may become nauseated and vomit, may become hypotensive, or may develop postural hypotension
	4. Excessive use of vasopressors will cause significant elevation of blood pressure, which in these patients may be very dangerous
	5. Many antihypertensive agents will potentiate sedative action of barbiturates
	6. Sedative medication used in patients taking certain antihypertensive agents may bring about hypotensive episode(s)
		1. Detection and referral of patients with marked elevation of blood pressure and those with moderate prolonged elevation of blood pressure for medical evaluation and treatment
		2. Patients being treated with antihypertensive agents
		  a. Reduce stress and anxiety of dental visit by premedication, short appointments, morning appointments, and open, concerned atmosphere by dentist and staff; let patient talk about fears and concerns related to dental visit; nitrous oxide can be used, but hypoxia must be avoided
		  b. If patient becomes stressed, terminate appointment
		  c. Avoid orthostatic hypotension by changing chair positions slowly and supporting patient when he gets out of chair
		  d. Avoid stimulating gag reflex—nausea
		  e. Select sedative medication and dosage based on consultation with patient's physician
		  f. Avoid excessive use of vasopressors
		3. Drug considerations
		  a. Use local anesthetics with small concentration of vasopressor (epinephrine 1 : 100,000) and no more than three cartridges; aspirate before injection and inject slowly
		  b. Do not use vasopressors to control local bleeding
		  c. Do not use gingival packing material that contains vasopressor
		  d. Reduce dosage of barbiturates and other sedatives whose actions are enhanced by many antihypertensive agents
		  e. Avoid use of general anesthesia, since severe hypotension can be precipitated in patients being treated with certain antihypertensive agents
		  f. Avoid use of central nervous system depressants—sedative/hypnotics and narcotics, etc.—in patients being treated with monoamine oxidase inhibitors
		  g. Epinephrine should not be used in any form in patient being treated with antihypertensive agent pargyline (Eutonyl) or any other monoamine oxidase inhibitor

Congestive heart failure (pp. 116-122)	1. If polycythemia is present, bleeding resulting from thrombocytopenia and depletion of fibronogen secondary to thrombosis occurring in small vessels may be present
	2. Sudden death resulting from cardiac arrest or dysrhythmia
	3. Myocardial infarction
	4. Cerebrovascular accident
	5. Infection
	6. Infective endocarditis if heart failure is caused by rheumatic heart disease, congenital heart disease, etc.
	7. Shortness of breath
		1. Detection and referral to physician
		2. No routine dental care until under good medical management
		3. Patients under good medical management
		Cause of heart failure and any other complications must be dealt with in dental management plan
		  a. Hypertension (p. 110)
		  b. Valvular disease (rheumatic heart disease) (p. 60)
		  c. Congenital heart disease (p. 71)
		  d. Myocardial infarction (p. 83)
		  e. Renal failure (p. 157)
		  f. Thyrotoxicosis (p. 222)
		4. Antibiotics to prevent postoperative infection
		5. Patient should be in upright position during treatment to decrease collection of fluid in lung
		6. Bleeding time and prothrombin time should be obtained before any surgical procedures; if abnormal, consult with physician
		7. Terminate appointment if patient becomes fatigued, etc.
		8. Drug considerations
		  a. Digitalis—patient more prone to nausea and vomiting
		  b. Anticoagulants—dosage should be reduced so that prothrombin time is twice normal value or less (takes 3 to 4 days)
		  c. Antidysrhythmic drugs (p. 85)
		  d. Antihypertensive agents (pp. 113 and 114)
		  e. Use of vasoconstrictors (p. 114)
		  f. Avoidance of general anesthesia

Treatment plan modifications	Oral complications	Emergency dental care
1. In uncontrolled hypertensive patient No routine dental care 2. In patients under good medical management with no complications such as renal failure or congestive heart failure Any indicated dental treatment 3. In patients with complications Refer to appropriate section	1. Excessive bleeding in uncontrolled hypertensive patient following surgical procedures 2. Xerostomia in patients overtreated with diuretic agents 3. Mercurial diuretics may cause oral ulceration or stomatitis as an allergic reaction to drug 4. Acetazolamide may cause facial paresthesia	1. No emergency dental treatment other than analgesics for pain control and antibiotics for infection for patients with marked elevation of blood pressure (diastolic, 115 mm Hg or higher) 2. Other patients can be treated as indicated
1. Cause of heart failure, presence of complications, and patient's current status must be considered 2. In some patients only urgent dental needs should be taken care of (by conservative methods) 3. In patients under good medical management with no complications Any indicated dental care	1. Infection 2. Bleeding 3. Petechiae 4. Ecchymoses	1. Conservative for patients with acute congestive failure—drugs for pain control and antibiotics for infection 2. As indicated for patients under good medical management—must deal with underlying cause and presence of any complications in dental management

Continued.

Dental management: a summary—cont'd

Medical problem	Potential problem relating to dental treatment	Prevention of medical complications

Asthma (pp. 123-126)	Precipitation of asthmatic attack	I. Identification of asthmatic patient by history
		II. Determination of character of asthma
		   A. Type (allergic or nonallergic)
		   B. Precipitating factors
		   C. Age at onset
		   D. Frequency and severity of attacks
		   E. How usually managed
		   F. Medications being taken
		   G. Necessity for past emergency care
		III. Avoidance of known precipitating factors
		IV. Consultation with physician for severe, active asthma
		V. Drug considerations
		   A. Regularly taken medications
		   B. Recent corticosteroid use may require supplementation—see Chapter 16
		   C. If inhaler is used, patient should bring it to appointment
		   D. Premedicate anxious patient (nitrous oxide or diazepam)
		   E. Avoid (if possible)
		     1. Antihistamines
		     2. Anticholinergics
		     3. Narcotics
		     4. Aspirin
		     5. Nonsteroidal antiinflammatory drugs
		     6. Penicillin
		VI. Provision of stress-free environment

Tuberculosis (pp. 126-131)	1. Tuberculosis may be contracted by dentist from actively infectious patient
	2. Patients and staff can be infected by dentist who is actively infectious
		I. In patients with active tuberculosis
		   A. Consultation with physician before treatment
		   B. Treatment limited to emergency care only (over age 6 years)
		   C. Treatment in hospital setting with proper isolation, sterilization, mask, gloves, gown, ventilation
		   D. Patient under age 6 years
		     Treatment as normal patient (noninfectious) after consultation
		   E. When patient produces consistently negative sputum and remains in chemotherapy
		     Treatment as normal outpatient
		II. In patients with past history of tuberculosis
		   A. Approach with caution; obtain good history of disease and its treatment (treatment of at least 9 to 18 months' duration); appropriate review of systems is mandatory
		   B. Should give history of periodic chest x-ray films and examination to rule out reactivation
		   C. Consult with physician and postpone treatment if
		     1. Questionable history of proper treatment
		     2. Lack of appropriate medical supervision since recovery
		     3. Signs or symptoms of relapse
		   D. If present status "free of active disease"
		     Treatment as normal patient
		III. In patients with recent conversion to positive skin test (PPD)
		   A. Should have been evaluated by physician to rule out active disease
		   B. May be receiving isoniazid (INH) for 1 year prophylactically
		   C. Treatment as normal patient
		IV. In patients with signs or symptoms of tuberculosis
		   A. Referral to physician and postpone treatment
		   B. If treatment necessary, treat as in category I

Treatment plan modifications	Oral complications	Emergency dental care
None required	None	Basic recommendations also apply for emergency care

None required	1. Oral ulceration, tongue most common
	2. Tuberculosis involvement of cervical and submandibular lymph nodes (scrofula)
		1. If active disease present:
		  a. Consultation with physician before treatment
		  b. Isolation of dental operatory (hospital)
		  c. Strict aseptic procedures
		  d. Gloves, gown, mask
		  e. Use of rubber dam when possible
		  f. Use of slow-speed handpiece when possible
		  g. Minimized use of air syringe
		  h. Only necessary work done
		  i. Scrubbing and sterilizing of all equipment after use
		2. If free of active disease
		Normal care provided as needed

Continued.

Dental management: a summary—cont'd

Medical problem	Potential problem relating to dental treatment	Prevention of medical complications

Viral hepatitis, type B, type NANB (pp. 138-148)	1. Hepatitis may be contracted by dentist from infectious patient (active or carrier of type B hepatitis)
	2. Patients or staff can be infected by dentist with active hepatitis or who is carrier of type B hepatitis
		Caveat: Since most carriers are undetectable by history, all patients should be treated with strict aseptic approach; much risk can be eliminated by use of hepatitis B vaccine
		I. Patients with active hepatitis
		  A. Consultation with physician
		  B. Treatment on emergency basis only
		II. Patients with history of hepatitis (selective screening will not reveal many carriers)
		  A. Consultation with physician
		  B. Probable type determination
		    1. Age at time of infection (type B uncommon under age 15 years)
		    2. Source of infection (if food or water, usually type A)
		    3. If type indeterminate, order RIA for HBsAg
		III. Patients in high-risk categories
		  Order a screening RIA for HBsAg
		IV. If HBsAg positive (carrier)
		  A. Consultation with physician
		  B. Strict aseptic technique
		  C. Rubber gloves, mask
		  D. Rubber dam
		  E. Minimize aerosol production
		  F. Scrub and sterilize all equipment after use
		  G. Minimize drugs metabolized by liver

Alcoholic liver disease (cirrhosis) (pp. 133-138)	1. Bleeding tendencies
	2. Impaired ability to metabolize certain drugs
		1. Detection of alcoholic patient
		  a. History by patient
		  b. Clinical examination
		  c. Repeated detection of odor on breath
		  d. Information from friends or relatives
		2. Consultation with physician to verify current status
		3. Laboratory screening
		  a. CBC
		  b. SGOT
		  c. Bleeding time
		  d. Thrombin time
		  e. Prothrombin time
		4. Minimize drugs metabolized by liver

End-stage renal disease (pp. 149-160)	1. Bleeding tendency 2. Hypertension 3. Anemia 4. Intolerance to nephrotoxic drugs or drugs metabolized by kidney	1. Consultation with physician 2. Pretreatment screening for bleeding disorder (bleeding time, prothrombin time, partial thromboplastin time) 3. Close monitoring of blood pressure before and during treatment 4. Avoidance of drugs metabolized by kidney or nephrotoxic drugs 5. Meticulous attention to good surgical technique to minimize chances of abnormal bleeding or infection
Hemodialysis (pp. 154-156)	1. Bleeding tendency 2. Hypertension 3. Anemia 4. Intolerance to nephrotoxic drugs or drugs metabolized by kidney 5. Bacterial arteritis of arteriovenous fistula secondary to bacteremia 6. Hepatitis (active or carrier of type B hepatitis)	1. Consultation with physician 2. No dental treatment until off dialysis machine for at least 4 hours (because of heparin); best on day following 3. Pretreatment screening for bleeding disorder (bleeding time, prothrombin time, partial thromboplastin time) 4. Avoidance of drugs metabolized by kidney or nephrotoxic drugs 5. Antibiotic prophylaxis for all dental work to minimize effects of bacteremia 6. Pretreatment screening for HBsAg

Treatment plan modifications	Oral complications	Emergency dental care
None required	Bleeding	1. If active disease a. Consult with physician b. Minimize drugs detoxified by liver c. If surgery necessary obtain prothrombin time and bleeding time before surgery d. Use strict aseptic technique e. Wear gloves, gown, and mask f. Isolate operatory g. Use rubber dam when possible h. Minimize aerosol production i. Scrub and sterilize all equipment j. Do only necessary work 2. If no active disease and not carrier Provide normal care as indicated
Since oral neglect is commonly seen in alcoholics, patients should be required to demonstrate interest in and ability to care for dentition before any significant treatment	1. Neglect 2. Bleeding 3. Ecchymoses 4. Petechiae	In addition to prior medical recommendations, abnormal laboratory values in surgical patients may suggest the use of antifibrinolytic agents, platelets, fresh frozen plasma, and vitamin K
1. Major emphasis on oral hygiene and optimum maintenance care to eliminate possible sources of infection 2. No contraindications for routine dental care but would discourage extensive reconstructive crown and bridge procedures	Oral ulcerations and candidosis	Follow same management recommendations as for routine dental care but consider hospitalization for severe infection or major procedures
1. Major emphasis on oral hygiene and optimum maintenance care to eliminate possible sources of infection 2. No contraindication for routine dental care but would discourage extensive procedures	Oral ulcerations and candidosis	Follow same management recommendations as for routine dental care but consider hospitalization for severe infection or major procedures

Dental management: a summary—cont'd

Medical problem	Potential problem relating to dental treatment	Prevention of medical complications
Renal transplant (pp. 159-160)	1. Inability to tolerate stress secondary to steroids 2. Susceptible to infection secondary to immunosuppressive drugs 3. Poor wound healing secondary to immunosuppressive drugs 4. Hepatitis (carrier of type B hepatitis) as a result of past experience with hemodialysis 5. Hypertension secondary to corticosteroids	1. Consultation with physician before treatment 2. Consideration of supplementing steroid dosage; however, many patients will already be receiving sufficient steroids to prevent untoward problems 3. Prophylactic antibiotic coverage to prevent oral infection in surgical patient 4. Aggressive treatment of orofacial infection 5. Meticulous attention to surgical technique and gentle tissue management 6. Screening for presence of HBsAg 7. Avoidance of nephrotoxic drugs

Gonorrhea (pp. 161-164, 174)	1. Gonorrhea may be contracted by dentist from actively infectious patient
	2. Patients or staff can be infected by dentist who has gonorrhea
		1. Patients currently receiving treatment for gonorrhea
		  a. Consultation with physician before treatment
		  b. Provide necessary care—use gloves
		  c. Oral lesions of gonorrhea are infectious—treat cautiously
		2. Patients with past history of gonorrhea
		  a. Approach with caution; obtain good history of disease and its treatment and follow-up culture
		  b. If no follow-up culture after treatment
		  Consult with physician before treatment
		  c. If free of disease
		  Treat as normal patient
		3. Patients with signs or symptoms suggestive of gonorrhea
		  a. Refer to physician for evaluation and postpone treatment
		  b. If treatment necessary, treat as in category I

Syphilis (pp. 164-169, 174)	1. Syphilis may be contracted by dentist from actively infectious patient
	2. Patients or staff may be infected by dentist who has syphilis
		1. Patients currently receiving treatment for syphilis
		  a. Consultation with physician before treatment
		  b. Emergency dental care only
		  c. Oral lesions of primary and secondary syphilis are infectious—treat cautiously
		2. Patients with past history of syphilis
		  a. Approach with caution; obtain good history of disease, its treatment, and negative STS test following therapy until negative
		  b. If no follow-up STS test
		  Order STS test or consult with physician before treatment
		  c. If free of disease
		  Treat as normal patient
		3. Patients with signs or symptoms suggestive of syphilis
		  a. Refer to physician and postpone treatment
		  b. May elect to order STS test before referral
		  c. If treatment necessary
		  Treat as in category I

Genital herpes (pp. 169-175)	Inoculation of oral cavity and potential transmission to dentist	1. Localized genital infection poses no problem; however, because of possibility of autoinoculation to oral cavity by patient, wear gloves 2. Oral infection of type 1 or type 2 Postpone elective dental care

Treatment plan modifications	Oral complications	Emergency dental care
1. Major emphasis on oral hygiene and optimum maintenance care to eliminate possible sources of infection 2. Advisable to remove teeth of questionable prognosis 3. No contraindication for routine simple dental procedures but would discourage any extensive procedures 4. In selected patients it may be best to consider complete dentures if it appears that patient cooperation will be poor	Oral infection and poor wound healing	Follow same management recommendations as for routine dental care but consider hospitalization for severe infection or major procedures

None required	Infrequent, but varied expression including pharyngitis, tonsillitis, generalized stomatitis, ulceration, and formation of pseudomembranous coating	1. If active oral disease present
		  a. Consult with physician before treatment
		  b. Use strict aseptic technique
		  c. Use gloves and mask
		  d. Use rubber dam when possible
		  e. Scrub and sterilize all equipment after use
		  f. Do only necessary work
		2. If free of disease
		  Provide normal care as indicated

None required	1. Chancre
	2. Mucous patch
	3. Gumma
	4. Interstitial glossitis
		1. If active disease present
		  a. Consult with physician before treatment
		  b. Use strict aseptic technique
		  c. Use gloves and mask
		  d. Use rubber dam when possible
		  e. Do only necessary work
		  f. Scrub and sterilize all equipment after use
		2. If free of disease
		  Provide normal care as indicated

None required	Autoinoculation of type 2 herpes to oral cavity	If oral herpetic lesions are present, use gloves and wear protective eyeglasses; do only necessary work

Continued.

Dental management: a summary—cont'd

Medical problem	Potential problem relating to dental treatment	Prevention of medical complications
Pregnancy (pp. 226-232)	1. Dental procedures can *potentially* cause harm to developing fetus via a. Radiation b. Drugs c. Stress 2. Supine hypotension in late pregnancy 3. Poor nutrition	1. Women of childbearing age a. Always use contemporary radiographic techniques including lead apron when performing radiographic examination b. Avoid prescribing drugs that are known to be harmful to fetus or whose effects are as yet unknown (Table 18-3) c. Encourage patients to maintain balanced, nutritious diet 2. Pregnant women a. Contact patient's physician to verify physical status, present management plan, and ask for suggestions regarding patient's treatment; obtain history of previous pregnancies b. Maintain optimum oral hygiene, including prophylaxis, throughout pregnancy c. Avoid elective dental care during first trimester and last half of third trimester; second trimester is best time for elective treatment d. Avoid radiographs during first trimester; thereafter take only those necessary for treatment, always using lead apron e. Avoid administration of drugs known to be harmful to fetus (Table 18-3) f. In advanced stages of pregnancy (third trimester), avoid placing patient in supine position for prolonged periods of time 3. Lactating mothers a. Most drugs are of no pharmacologic significance to lactation b. Avoid drugs known to be harmful (Table 18-4) c. Administer drugs just after breast-feeding
Rheumatoid arthritis (pp. 177-182)	1. Joint pain and immobility 2. Bleeding tendencies secondary to aspirin and nonsteroidal antiinflammatory drugs 3. Bone marrow suppression from gold salts or penicillamine resulting in anemia, agranulocytosis, or thrombocytopenia 4. Adrenal suppression secondary to steroids	1. Short appointments 2. Ensure physical comfort a. Position changes b. Comfortable chair position c. Physical supports 3. Management of drug complications a. Aspirin/nonsteroidal antiinflammatory drugs—obtain pretreatment bleeding time b. Gold salts/penicillamine—obtain complete blood count with differential and bleeding time c. Corticosteroids—discuss need for supplements with physician
Joint prosthesis (pp. 182-183)	Deep infection around joint prosthesis secondary to bacteremia from dental manipulation is thought to be possible problem	1. Obtain good history, including medications and surgery 2. Consult with physician, present plan of management, and ask for suggestions regarding need for prophylactic coverage; antibiotic to be used, dosage, and duration 3. Must minimize effects of bacteremia for all dental procedures by using antibiotic prophylaxis; same drugs and dosage schedule can be used as for prevention of infective endocarditis in patients with rheumatic heart disease; orthopedic surgeon often will have personal preference concerning drug, etc.

Treatment plan modifications	Oral complications	Emergency dental care

None, except that reconstructive procedures, crown and bridge fabrication, and significant surgical procedures are best delayed until after pregnancy	1. Exaggeration of periodontal disease
	  a. "Pregnancy gingivitis"
	  b. "Pregnancy tumor"
	2. Tooth mobility
		Essentially same as for routine care; be certain to consult physician before treatment

Dictated by severity of disability and temporomandibular joint involvement; if severe, extensive treatment not indicated; temporomandibular joint surgery may be helpful; encourage oral hygiene	1. Temporomandibular joint ankylosis 2. Stomatitis secondary to gold salts	Follow normal recommendations
None required	None	1. May need antibiotic prophylaxis before all dental care 2. Patients with acute oral infection must be treated aggressively by local and systemic means—cases have been reported in which acute oral infection has resulted in infection around prosthesis

Continued.

Medical problem	Potential problem relating to dental treatment	Prevention of medical complications

Stroke (pp. 190-196)	1. Dental treatment could precipitate stroke
	2. Bleeding secondary to drug therapy
		I. Identification of stroke-prone patient from history (hypertension, smoking, etc.)
		II. Reduce patient's risk factors for stroke
		III. For past history of stroke
		  A. For current TIAs—no elective care
		  B. Drug considerations
		    1. Aspirin/dipyridamole (Persantine)—obtain pretreatment bleeding time
		    2. Coumarin drugs—obtain prothrombin time under 28 seconds
		  C. Short, morning appointments
		  D. Monitor blood pressure
		  E. Avoid use of vasoconstrictor, or at least use sparingly
		  F. No epinephrine in retraction cord

Epilepsy (pp. 184-190)	1. Occurrence of grand mal seizure in dental office	1. Identification of epileptic patient by history
		  a. Type of seizure
		  b. Age at time of onset
		  c. Cause of seizures
		  d. Medications
		  e. Regularity of physician visits
		  f. Degree of control
		  g. Frequency of seizures
		  h. Last seizure
		  i. Precipitating factors
		  j. History of seizure-related injuries
		2. Well controlled—provide normal care
		3. Poorly controlled—consult with physician; may require medication change
		4. Be alert to adverse effects of anticonvulsants
		5. Patients taking valproic acid—obtain bleeding time
		6. Be prepared to manage a seizure

Diabetes mellitus (pp. 197-211)	1. In uncontrolled diabetic patient
	  a. Infection
	  b. Poor wound healing
	2. In patient treated with insulin
	  Insulin reaction
	3. In diabetic patient
	  Early onset of complications relating to cardiovascular system, eyes, kidney, and nervous system (angina, myocardial infarction, cerebrovascular accident, renal failure, peripheral neuropathy, blindness, hypertension, congestive heart failure)
		1. Detection by
		  a. History
		  b. Clinical findings
		  c. Screening blood sugar
		2. Referral for diagnosis and treatment
		3. Patient receiving insulin—prevent insulin reaction
		  a. Advise patient to eat normal meals before appointments
		  b. Schedule appointments in morning or midmorning
		  c. Advise patient to inform you of any symptoms of insulin reaction when they first occur
		  d. Have sugar in some form to give in case of insulin reaction
		4. Patients with diabetes being treated with insulin who develop oral infection may require increase in insulin dosage—consult with physician in addition to local and systemic aggressive management of infection
		5. Drug considerations
		  a. Insulin—insulin reaction
		  b. Hypoglycemic agents—on rare occasions aplastic anemia, etc.
		  c. In severe diabetics avoid general anesthesia

Adrenal insufficiency (pp. 212-217)	1. Inability to tolerate stress
	2. Delayed healing
	3. Susceptibility to infection
	4. Hypertension (Cushing syndrome)
		I. Patients currently receiving steroids
		  Obtain history or disease, time of treatment, dosage, and type of drug, then contact physician to verify patient's history, drugs, and status and to discuss planned management scheme based on following suggested guidelines
		  A. Patients receiving equivalent of normal daily output (20 mg hydrocortisone) or less for 1 month or longer; when uncertain, however, assume patient to have significant suppression and treat as in category B unless physician indicates otherwise

Treatment plan modifications	Oral complications	Emergency dental care
1. Dependent on physical impairment 2. All restorations should be easily cleansable 3. Modified oral hygiene aids may be needed	None	Follow normal recommendations
1. Maintenance of optimum oral hygiene 2. Surgical reducation of gingival hyperplasia if indicated 3. Replace missing teeth with fixed prostheses as opposed to removable 4. Choose metal over porcelain where possible	Gingival hyperplasia secondary to phenytoin (Dilantin)	Follow normal recommendations
In well-controlled diabetic patient No alteration of treatment plan is indicated unless complication of diabetes present such as 1. Hypertension (p. 110) 2. Congestive heart failure (p. 121) 3. Myocardial infarction (p. 86) 4. Angina (p. 86) 5. Renal failure (p. 158)	1. Accelerated periodontal disease 2. Periodontal abscesses 3. Oral ulcerations	1. In patient with infection Have physician increase insulin dosage in patient being treated with drug 2. In patient with diabetes not under medical treatment Referral and consultation are necessary so that diabetes can be brought under control 3. In general Other emergency problems can be dealt with as in normal patients
None required	1. Primary—pigmentation of oral mucous membranes 2. Delayed healing 3. Infection	1. In patients taking equivalent of 40 mg of hydrocortisone daily or less Administer 100 mg hydrocortisone, IM, 1 hour before procedure then double normal oral dose following day 2. In patients taking equivalent of greater than 40 mg hydrocortisone daily Provide care in normal manner

Continued.

Medical problem	Potential problem relating to dental treatment	Prevention of medical complications

Adrenal insufficiency (pp. 212-217)— cont'd		B. Patients receiving equivalent of up to two times normal daily output (20 to 40 mg hydrocortisone) for 1 month or longer
		  1. Routine dental care—double normal dose day of procedure
		  2. Major dental procedures—consider hospitalization and parenteral steroids
		C. Patients taking greater than equivalent of twice normal daily output (40 mg hydrocortisone)
		  Probably adequate coverage with their normal medication and would not require additional supplementation
		D. Patients using topical steroids
		  Supplementation may be required if applied to large, inflamed areas and occlusive dressings used; physician should make determination
		II. Patients with history of steroid use
		  A. If no steroids taken in past 12 months and doing well
		    No steroids required
		  B. If steroids taken within past 12 months
		    Treat under appropriate dosage category

Hyperthyroidism (thyrotoxicosis) (pp. 218-225)	1. Thyrotoxic crisis (thyroid storm) may be precipitated in untreated or incompletely treated patient with thyrotoxicosis by
	  a. Infection
	  b. Trauma
	  c. Surgical procedures
	  d. Stress
	2. Patients with untreated or incompletely treated thyrotoxicosis may be very sensitive to actions of epinephrine and other pressor amines; thus these agents must not be used. Once patient is well managed from medical standpoint these agents can be resumed.
		1. Detection of patient with thyrotoxicosis by history and examination findings
		2. Referral for medical evaluation and treatment
		3. Avoidance of any dental treatment for patient with thyrotoxicosis until under good medical control; however, any acute oral infection will have to be dealt with by antibiotic therapy and other conservative measures to prevent development of thyrotoxic crisis; suggest consultation with patient's physician during management of acute oral infection
		4. Avoidance of epinephrine and other pressor amines in untreated or incompletely treated patient

Hypothyroidism (pp. 218-225)	1. Untreated patients with severe hypothyroidism exposed to stressful situations such as trauma, surgical procedures, or infection may develop hypothyroid coma 2. Untreated hypothyroid patients may be very sensitive to actions of narcotics, barbiturates, and tranquilizers	1. Detection and referral of patients suspected of being hypothyroid for medical evaluation and treatment 2. Avoidance of use of narcotics, barbiturates, and tranquilizers in untreated hypothyroid patients

Urticaria (angioneurotic edema) (pp. 243-244)	1. Nonemergency
	Edematous swelling of lips, cheek, etc. following contact with antigen
	2. Emergency
	Edematous swelling of tongue, pharynx, and larynx with obstruction of airway
		I. Identify patients who have had allergic reactions by history and what drug or materials caused reaction
		II. Avoid use of antigen in allergic persons
		III. If patients develop allergic reaction to drug or material to which they gave no indication of being allergic
		  A. Nonemergency reaction
		    No further contact with agent—administer oral diphenhydramine, 50 mg, qid or IM
		  B. Emergency reaction
		    Supine position, patent airway, oxygen, inject 0.5 ml of epinephrine 1:1000, IM, support respiration if necessary, check pulse, obtain medical assistance
		IV. Local anesthetics
		  A. Most patients who say they are allergic to local anesthetic on questioning will describe fainting episode or toxic reaction
		  B. If allergic reaction occurred, identify kind of anesthetic used and select one from different chemical group

Treatment plan modifications	Oral complications	Emergency dental care
1. Once under good medical management patient may receive any indicated dental treatment 2. If acute infection should occur, patient's physician should be consulted concerning management	1. Osteoporosis may occur 2. Periodontal disease may be more progressive 3. Dental caries may be more extensive 4. Premature loss of deciduous teeth and early eruption of permanent teeth 5. Early jaw development	1. In thyrotoxic patient Conservative treatment—antibiotics for infection, analgesics for pain, and consultation with patient's physician 2. In patients under good medical management Emergency dental care as indicated; however, if problem involves acute infection, consult with patient's physician
1. Hypothyroid patient under good medical management Any indicated dental treatment 2. Patients with congenital form of disease with severe mental retardation May need assistance with hygiene procedures	1. Increase in tongue size 2. Delayed eruption of teeth 3. Malocclusion	1. In untreated hypothyroid patient a. Control of pain with nonnarcotic analgesics b. Avoidance of precipitation of hypothyroid coma in patients with severe hypothyroidism; thus avoid surgical procedures and treat acute oral infection by conservative measures 2. In patients under good medical management Render whatever emergency care is indicated
1. Avoidance of drug or material to which patient is allergic 2. In rare patient who is allergic to many local anesthetics Diphenhydramine (Benadryl) can be used as local anesthetic or refer to allergist for provocative dose testing	Soft tissue swelling	As indicated; avoid any agent patient is allergic to; diphenhydramine can be used as local anesthetic for patients allergic to more than one local anesthetic or who had allergic reaction to local anesthetic but cannot identify what agent was used

Continued.

Dental management: a summary—cont'd

Medical problem	Potential problem relating to dental treatment	Prevention of medical complications

Urticaria (angioneurotic edema) (pp. 243-244)—cont'd		C. Inject 1 drop (aspirate first) of alternate anesthetic; wait 5 minutes; if no reaction, proceed with injection of remaining anesthetic
		D. If anesthetic that patient reacted to cannot be identified
		  1. Refer to allergist for provocative dose testing
		  2. Use diphenhydramine (Benadryl) with epinephrine 1:100,000 as local anesthetic—1% solution, 1 to 4 ml
		V. Penicillin
		  A. In allergic individual alternate choice would be erythromycin
		  B. In nonallergic person administer by oral route whenever possible—lowest incidence of sensitization
		  C. Do not use in topical form

Bleeding problems as suggested by examination and history findings but no clues as to underlying cause (pp. 254-255)	Excessive blood loss following surgical procedures, scaling, etc.	1. Screen patient with following (if one or more are abnormal, refer patient for diagnosis and medical treatment)
		  a. Prothrombin time
		  b. Partial thromboplastin time
		  c. Tourniquet test
		  d. Bleeding time
		  e. Platelet count
		2. Avoid use of aspirin

Vascular wall alterations (scurvy, infection, chemical, allergic, autoimmune, others) (p. 255)	Prolonged bleeding following surgical procedures or any insult to integrity of oral mucosa	1. Identification of patient
		  a. History
		  b. Clinical findings
		  c. Screening tests—tourniquet test, bleeding time
		2. Consultation with hematologist
		3. Splint
		4. Local measures to control blood loss
		5. Prophylactic antibiotic in surgical case to avoid postoperative infection
		6. If allergy involved in etiology, antigen must be avoided if it has been identified

Thrombocytopenia (primary, secondary, chemical, radiation, leukemia) (pp. 255-256)	1. Prolonged bleeding
	2. Infection in patients with bone marrow replacement or destruction
	3. In patient being treated with steroids, stress may lead to serious medical emergency
		1. Identification of patient
		  a. History
		  b. Examination findings
		  c. Screening tests—bleeding time, platelet count
		2. Referral and consultation with hematologist
		3. Correction of underlying problem or replacement therapy before surgery
		4. Local measures to control blood loss—splint, thrombosis, etc.
		5. Prophylactic antibiotics in surgical cases to prevent postoperative infection
		6. Additional steroids for patients being treated with steroids

Disorders of platelet function (genetic defect, aspirin, allergic, autoimmune diseases, von Willebrand disease, others) (pp. 255-256)	Prolonged bleeding following scaling, surgical procedures, or any insult to integrity of soft tissues of oral cavity	1. Identification of problem
		  a. History
		  b. Clinical findings
		  c. Screening laboratory tests, platelet count, bleeding time
		2. Consultation with hematologist
		  a. Correction of problem
		  b. Replacement therapy
		  c. In severe cases hospitalization
		3. Construction of splint
		4. Local measures to control blood loss
		5. Prophylactic antibiotics to prevent postsurgical infection that would complicate control of blood loss
		6. If allergy involved in etiology, antigen must be avoided if it has been identified

Treatment plan modifications	Oral complications	Emergency dental care
None unless test(s) abnormal, then manage based on nature of underlying problem once diagnosis established by physician	Excessive bleeding following dental procedures	Conservative—antibiotics and analgesics, but avoid use of aspirin
Surgical procedures must be avoided in these patients unless underlying problem has been corrected or patient has been prepared for surgery by hematologist and dentist is prepared to control excessive loss of blood by local measures	1. Excessive bleeding following scaling and surgical procedures 2. Petechiae 3. Hematomas	Conservative management of infection and pain
No dental procedures unless replacement of platelets is done before procedures or unless underlying problem has been taken care of	1. Spontaneous bleeding 2. Prolonged bleeding following certain dental procedures 3. Petechiae 4. Hematomas	Conservative management of infection and pain
Routine surgical procedures must be avoided in patients with platelet disorder unless underlying condition has been corrected or replacement therapy has been performed	1. Excessive bleeding following surgical procedures, scaling, etc. 2. Spontaneous bleeding 3. Petechiae 4. Hematomas	Conservative, nonsurgical treatment for pain, etc.

Continued.

Medical problem	Potential problem relating to dental treatment	Prevention of medical complications

Congenital disorders of coagulation (hemophilia, Christmas disease, von Willebrand disease, others) (pp. 255-258)	Excessive bleeding following dental procedures	1. Identification of patient
		  a. History
		  b. Examination findings
		  c. Screening tests—prothrombin time, partial thromboplastin time
		2. Consultation and referral for diagnosis and treatment and for preparation before dental procedures
		3. May be treated on outpatient basis depending on results of consultation
		4. Local measures for control of bleeding—splints, thrombin, etc.
		5. Prophylactic antibiotics to prevent postoperative infection in surgical cases

Acquired disorders of coagulation (liver disease, broad-spectrum antibiotics, malabsorption syndrome, biliary tract obstruction, heparin, coumarin drugs, other) (pp. 255-258)	Excessive bleeding following dental procedures that result in soft tissue or osseous injury	1. Identification of patient with disorder
		  a. History
		  b. Examination findings
		  c. Screening laboratory tests—prothrombin time, bleeding time (liver disease)
		2. Consultation and referral
		3. Preparation before dental procedure
		4. Local measures to control blood loss
		5. Prophylactic antibiotics
		6. Reduction of anticoagulant so that prothrombin time is twice normal or less
		7. In patients with liver disease; avoidance of drugs metabolized by liver or reduction in dosage

Agranulocytosis (p. 263)	Infection	1. Referral for medical diagnosis and treatment 2. Drug considerations—avoidance of use of chloramphenicol for control of oral infection because of high incidence of agranulocytosis
Cyclic neutropenia (p. 263)	Infection	1. Antibiotics to avoid infection 2. Serial white blood cell count to pick time in cycle when count is closest to normal level
Hereditary spherocytosis (pp. 260 and 266)	Accelerated hemolysis of red blood cells	1. Control infection 2. Avoid drugs containing phenacetin 3. These patients often have increased frequency of drug sensitivity to sulfa drugs, aspirin, and chloramphenicol
Iron deficiency anemia (pp. 260-261)	1. Usually none 2. In rare cases severe leukopenia and thrombocytopenia may result in problems with infection and excessive loss of blood	1. Detection and referral for diagnosis and treatment 2. In females most cases will be caused by physiologic process—menstruation or pregnancy 3. In males most cases will be secondary to underlying disease such as peptic ulcer, carcinoma of colon, etc.

Treatment plan modifications	Oral complications	Emergency dental care
No dental procedures unless patient has been prepared based on consultation with hematologist	1. Spontaneous bleeding 2. Prolonged bleeding following dental procedures that injure soft tissue or bone 3. Petechiae 4. Hematomas	Conservative management of infection and pain, if possible; otherwise, patient must be prepared
No dental procedures unless patient prepared based on consultation with hematologist	1. Excessive bleeding 2. Spontaneous bleeding 3. Petechiae 4. Hematomas	1. Conservative 2. Vitamin K injection can be given if surgical procedure is necessary
No dental treatment except emergency care and supportive therapy for oral lesions	1. Oral ulcerrations 2. Periodontitis 3. Necrotic tissue	Conservative pain control and control of infection
Depending on severity of disease may limit to disease control and maintenance procedures	1. Periodontal disease 2. Oral infection 3. Oral ulceration similar to aphthous stomatitis	As indicated; if white blood cell count depressed severely, antibiotics to avoid postoperative infection
Usually none unless anemia severe, then only urgent dental needs	Usually none	As indicated unless patient is having hemolytic crisis; then conservative control of pain and infection
Usually none	1. Paresthesias 2. Loss of papilla from tongue 3. In rare cases infection and bleeding complications 4. Patients with dysphagia seem to have increased incidence of carcinoma of oral and pharyngeal area (Plummer-Vinson syndrome)	Usually as indicated (white blood cell count and platelet status should be checked)

Continued.

Medical problem	Potential problem relating to dental treatment	Prevention of medical complications
Leukemia (pp. 264-270)	1. Prolonged bleeding 2. Infection 3. Delayed healing	1. Detection and referral for diagnosis and treatment 2. Determination of platelet status day of any surgical procedure, including scaling of teeth. If bleeding time is within normal range, proceed; if not, postpone procedure (platelet count less than 80,000 mm³ 3. Avoidance of postoperative infection by prophylactic use of antibiotics
Pernicious anemia (p. 261)	1. Infection 2. Bleeding 3. Delayed healing	Detection and medical treatment (early detection and treatment can prevent permanent neurologic damage)
Sickle cell anemia (pp. 261-262)	Sickle cell crisis	1. Avoidance of any procedure that would produce hypoxia 2. Drug considerations Usually none but must avoid hypoxia; thus general anesthesia should not be used in these patients 3. Nitrous oxide may be used, provided 50% oxygen is supplied at all times; critical to avoid diffusion hypoxia at termination of nitrous oxide administration
Head and neck cancer (pp. 271-287)	1. Patients treated by surgery Usually none 2. Patients treated by radiation a. Osteoradionecrosis b. Infection c. Poor healing 3. Patients treated by chemotherapy a. Bleeding b. Infection c. Poor healing 4. Patients with "generalized" disease with bone marrow involvement a. Bleeding b. Infection c. Poor healing	1. Radiation patients a. Perform needed dental repair before radiation therapy, including extraction of all questionable teeth b. Initiate preventive measures before radiation therapy, including daily application of fluoride gel c. Avoid trauma to oral mucosa—use salivary substitute such as Xero-Lube 2. Chemotherapy patients and/or patients with "generalized" disease with bone marrow involvement a. Avoid surgical procedures b. When surgery is required use local measures to control bleeding and platelet replacement when indicated c. Use prophylactic antibiotics for all invasive dental procedures

Treatment plan modifications	Oral complications	Emergency dental care
1. During acute stages of disease avoidance of dental care of any kind if at all possible 2. When patient is in state of remission all active dental disease should be treated and patient placed on good hygiene maintenance program 3. Avoidance of long, drawn-out dental procedures	1. Infection 2. Ulceration 3. Gingival bleeding 4. Ecchymosis 5. Petechiae 6. Gingival hyperplasia 7. Soft tissue and osseous lesions 8. Paresthesias—numbness, burning, tingling	1. As indicated during remission 2. Conservative otherwise 3. Drainage through pulp chamber, etc.
None once patient under medical care	1. Paresthesia of oral tissues (burning, tingling, numbness) 2. Delayed healing (severe cases), infection, red tongue, angular cheilosis 3. Petechial hemorrhages	Usually can be rendered without complications; in patient suspected of having pernicious anemia, suggest conservative treatment until medical diagnosis and therapy established
Usually none unless symptoms of severe anemia present—only urgent dental needs should be met under this condition	1. Osteoporosis 2. Loss of trabecular pattern	As indicated unless crisis present, then conservative control of pain with drugs and of infection with antibiotics

1. Surgery patients
  a. Extract all questionable teeth before surgery
  b. Plan for prosthetic replacement before surgery; make casts, consult with maxillofacial prosthodontist whenever possible
2. Radiation patients
  a. Extract all questionable teeth before radiation therapy
  b. Perform endodontics rather than extractions whenever possible in patients who have had radiation
  c. Plan preventive measures, including daily fluoride gels to prevent radiation caries
  d. Avoid denture construction until oral mucosa has returned to normal
3. Chemotherapy patients and/or patients with disease involving bone marrow
  a. Extract all questionable teeth before chemotherapy starts if possible
  b. In general, plan only maintenance dental care because of poor prognosis
  c. Avoid invasive dental procedures when thrombocytopenia and leukopenia are present (screening with platelet count and WBC count)
	1. Surgery patients
	  a. Functional complications
	  b. Esthetics
	2. Radiation patients
	  a. Mucositis
	  b. Xerostomia
	  c. Muscular dysfunction
	  d. Radiation caries
	  e. Osteoradionecrosis
	3. Chemotherapy patients/bone marrow involvement
	  a. Mucositis
	  b. Bleeding
	  c. Infection
	  d. Petechiae, ecchymoses, and hematomas
		1. Surgery patient
		  As needed
		2. Radiation patient
		  a. Avoid invasive dental procedures if at all possible
		  b. Antibiotics for infection
		  c. Drugs for pain control
		  d. Endodontics rather than extractions whenever possible
		  e. Consultation with physician
		3. Chemotherapy patient and/or patient with disease involving bone marrow
		  a. Consultation with physician
		  b. Avoidance of invasive dental procedures
		  c. Antibiotics for infection
		  d. Drugs for pain control

1

INTERRELATIONSHIPS OF MEDICINE AND DENTISTRY

The practice of dentistry today is not what it was as recently as 10 years ago. The patients treated today are often very different from those treated in the past. Advances in the medical sciences have led to better forms of medical and surgical treatment for many chronic illnesses that in the past claimed their victims at an early age. For example, damaged heart valves are now replaced, blocked coronary arteries are being bypassed, patients have transplanted kidneys, medicine is available to control hypertension, and many patients are being treated with antimetabolites and radiation to control leukemia and other forms of cancer. The ability of the dentist to treat oral conditions has improved at a rapid rate. This is because of advances in dental sciences and incorporation of basic science material in the education of the dentist. The dentist is involved in patient care concerning the management of soft-tissue and bone changes using techniques of periodontal surgery, pulp therapy, minor tooth movement, and gingival contouring as part of restorative dentistry. The dentist no longer treats "teeth in patients" but "patients who have teeth." It is now most important for the safety of the patient and the success of treatment for the dentist to identify patients with systemic illness.

The purpose of this chapter is to provide an overview of the significance and applications of medicine in dentistry. It is not intended to be all-inclusive but rather to provide some insight and appreciation for medical problems. The following chapters will provide details of specific problems and dental management recommendations.

The following are some major reasons why a dentist should incorporate physical evaluation, including medical history, physical examination, and screening laboratory tests, into dental practice:

1. To identify patients with undetected systemic disease that could be a serious threat to the life of the patient or that could be complicated by dental treatment
2. To identify patients who are taking drugs or medicine that could be potentiated by drugs prescribed, complicate therapy planned, or serve as a clue to an underlying systemic disease that the patient has failed to mention
3. To allow the dentist to modify the treatment plan for the patient in light of the systemic disease or drugs the patient may be taking
4. To protect the dentist from a medical-dental-legal standpoint
5. To better enable the dentist to communicate effectively with medical consultants concerning the patient's systemic problems
6. To help establish a good patient-dentist relationship by demonstrating to patients that the dentist is interested in them as individuals and is concerned about their overall health and well-being

HEALTH HISTORY

It is mandatory that a medical history be taken on every patient who is to receive dental treatment. There are a number of techniques that may be used to obtain the medical history, ranging from an interview, in which the questioner records the patient's responses on a blank sheet, to a printed questionnaire that the patient fills out himself. The latter is most commonly used in dental practice. There are many types of questionnaires commercially available today. The American Dental Association has, for example, two types of forms available, a long form and a short form. Both are excellent, the only difference being the degree of information obtained. It is also feasible to develop a questionnaire of your own to meet the specific needs of your practice. Fig. 1-1 is the health questionnaire that is used at the University of Kentucky College of Dentistry. It provides a comprehensive review of a patient's dental and medical history and review of systems. One of the most effective history methods is a questionnaire followed by a pertinent interview by the dentist.

The extent and detail of the history are somewhat dependent on personal preference and type of services to be rendered. For example, a detailed medical history may not be indicated for a patient who is seen only for recementation of a crown. On the other hand, if a patient is to have comprehensive dental care, a complete health history is necessary.

Regardless of the format used to obtain a health history or the type of services a patient may require, there is a certain amount of essential health information that should be known about every patient before examination procedures or treatment is undertaken. This essential information is not all-inclusive by any means but does serve a screening function. Although it does not replace a comprehensive health history, thorough answers to these questions can be a good basis from which to begin evaluating a patient's health status and may be used in an emergency situation as a method of rapid screening or in isolated treatment situations (Table 1-1).

1. *Are you under the care of a physician?* If the patient answers yes, information should then be sought regarding why the patient requires medical care, diagnoses made, and treatment being received. If the reason for seeing a physician was for a physical examination only, the patient should be asked if any abnormalities were discovered and the date of the examination. The name, address, and phone number of the patient's physician should be recorded for future reference.

The patient who answers no to this question may need a more cautious approach than the person who has had regular checkups. This is especially true for the patient who has not seen a physician in several years. The patient may be perfectly healthy; however, he could also have an undetected problem. The response to this question may also provide insight into the priorities that the person assigns to health care.

2. *Have you ever been hospitalized or had any operations?* A history of hospitalizations can give a good record of past serious illnesses that may have current significance to the present treatment. For example, a patient may have been hospitalized for cardiac catheterization during which time a congenital septal defect was discovered. Another example would be a patient hospitalized for hepatitis. Both of these patients might never have had medical follow-up for these problems, and the response to this question might be the only indication of these past problems. It is essential to learn as much as possible about the various hospitalizations, such as diagnosis, treatment, duration of stay, and complications.

In addition to past hospitalizations, it is important to know what kind of operations the patient has had, the reason for the procedures, and any untoward events associated with them, such as anesthetic emergencies, unusual postoperative bleeding, or infections.

3. *Are you taking any drugs, medicines, or pills of any kind?* Medications being taken for an illness may be the only clue to the patient's disorder. The patient may not have believed that it was important to mention a problem but may include it in an answer to this question. An example might be the patient with long-standing stable angina pectoris who takes nitroglycerin but has not seen a physician recently.

Drugs may also cause untoward reactions during dental treatment; thus dentists should identify the various drugs that patients may be taking and should become familiar with their actions and possible side-effects and drug interactions. The dentist must be cautious not to administer any drug or medication that may interact adversely with the patient's medications. The *Physicians' Desk Ref-*

Albert B. Chandler Medical Center
College of Dentistry

Health questionnaire

Name	□ Adult □ Child	Child's nickname

1. Why did you come to our clinic? _____

2. The date of your last visit to a dentist was: _____

3. Name and address of previous dentist: _____

4. Date of last full-month x-ray: _____

5. How often do you brush your teeth? _____

6. What other aids do you use in cleaning your teeth? _____

7. Do the following apply to you?

	Yes	No		YES	NO
Fear of dentist	□	□	Bleeding gums	□	□
Pain in jaw, face, mouth	□	□	Jaw joint sounds or pain	□	□
Pain in ear	□	□	Pain when you open wide (or take a big bite)	□	□
Frequent headaches	□	□	Difficulty in opening mouth	□	□
Discolored teeth	□	□	Poorly functioning teeth	□	□
Crooked teeth	□	□	Complications with extraction	□	□
Bad breath	□	□	Clenching or grinding teeth	□	□
Teeth sensitive to heat	□	□	Food wedging between teeth	□	□
Teeth sensitive to cold	□	□	Inability to floss between teeth	□	□
Lump or swelling in mouth	□	□	Poorly fitting dentures or appliance	□	□
Dry mouth	□	□			
Pain or discomfort with denture appliance	□	□			

1. In general, my health is: _____

2. Has there been any change in your general health within the last year? □ Yes □ No

3. Are you presently under the care of a physician? If so, for what condition? □ Yes □ No

4. The name and address of your physician is: _____

5. My last physical exam was on: _____

6. At that examination was anything unusual or abnormal found? If yes, what? □ Yes □ No

FIG. 1-1. University of Kentucky College of Dentistry health questionnaire.

		Yes	No
7. Have you ever been hospitalized or had a serious illness? If yes, what was the problem?		☐	☐
8. Have you ever had any operations or surgery? If yes, for what?		☐	☐
9. Have you ever required a blood transfusion? If yes, what were the circumstances?		☐	☐
10. Are you taking any medicine, drugs, or pills of any kind? If yes, what kind?		☐	☐
11. Do you have any allergies? If yes, to what and how do you react?		☐	☐

12. Have you ever had an unusual reaction to a dental anesthetic?_____

13. Have you ever had any of the following disorders?

	Yes	No		Yes	No
Rheumatic fever	☐	☐	Tuberculosis	☐	☐
Rheumatic heart disease	☐	☐	Asthma	☐	☐
Congenital heart lesions	☐	☐	Jaundice	☐	☐
Heart attack	☐	☐	Hepatitis	☐	☐
Stroke	☐	☐	Venereal disease	☐	☐
High blood pressure	☐	☐	Blood disorder	☐	☐
Diabetes (sugar disease)	☐	☐	Heart murmur	☐	☐

	Yes	No
14. Do you urinate more than six times a day?	☐	☐
15. Are you thirsty much of the time?	☐	☐
16. Does hot weather bother you more than it does other people?	☐	☐
17. Have you ever had abnormal bleeding associated with surgery, injuries, or extractions?	☐	☐
18. Have you ever had surgery or x-ray treatment for a tumor, growth or other condition in your mouth or on your lips?	☐	☐

19. Are you frequently bothered by any of the following?

	Yes	No		Yes	No
Severe headaches	☐	☐	Nose bleeds	☐	☐
Dizziness or fainting	☐	☐	Sore throat	☐	☐
Convulsions or fits	☐	☐	Chest pain on exertion	☐	☐
Ear problems	☐	☐	Shortness of breath	☐	☐
Eye problems	☐	☐	Swollen ankles	☐	☐
Sinus problems	☐	☐	Cough blood	☐	☐
Persistent cough	☐	☐	Vomiting	☐	☐
Swallowing problems	☐	☐	Vomit blood	☐	☐
Kidney problems	☐	☐	Excessive nervousness	☐	☐
Bruise easily	☐	☐	Frequent colds	☐	☐
Tire easily	☐	☐	Speech problems	☐	☐

	Yes	No
20. (women) Are you pregnant at the present time?	☐	☐
21. (child) Does your child need any immunizations?	☐	☐
22. (child) Has your child ever been treated in an emergency room?	☐	☐
23. (child) Does your child have emotional, mental or nervous disorders?	☐	☐
24. (child) Will your child be an uncooperative dental patient?	☐	☐
25. (child) Has your child ever sucked his thumb or fingers?	☐	☐
26. (child) Has your child inherited any family dental characteristics?	☐	☐
27. (child) Does your child receive any form of fluoride?	☐	☐

28. (child) School: _____ Grade: _____

29. (child) Names and ages of brothers and sisters:_____

Date _____   Signature _____

FIG. 1-1, cont'd. University of Kentucky College of Dentistry health questionnaire.

TABLE 1-1. Screening health history

1. Are you under the care of a physician?
2. Have you ever been hospitalized or had any operations?
3. Are you taking any drugs, medicines, or pills of any kind?
4. Do you have any allergies?
5. Have you ever had any type of heart disease, high blood pressure, or rheumatic fever?
6. Do you have diabetes?
7. Have you ever had tuberculosis or any other lung disease?
8. Have you ever had hepatitis or other liver disease?
9. Have you ever had a kidney disease?
10. Have you ever had any bleeding problems or blood disorders?
11. Have you ever had a sexually transmitted disease?
12. (Women) Are you pregnant?

erence (PDR) and *Accepted Dental Therapeutics* are useful sources to aid in the identification of drugs and their actions.

One drug that has important consequences if taken within the past year for an extended period is a corticosteroid. If a patient has taken steroids for a prolonged period (more than 1 month), the adrenal glands may be suppressed and the patient may not be able to cope physiologically with stress. Thus the dentist should strive to identify drug history over the past year.

It is important to stress "drugs, medicine, or pills *of any kind*," since frequently people will not consider over-the-counter drugs as being legitimate medicine. It is not unusual for a patient who is taking several aspirin tablets a day for arthritis to answer "none" to this question.

4. *Do you have any allergies?* This question should not be limited to allergies to medications, since it is conceivable that the patient could be exposed to other allergens in the dental office, such as cements, tape, stains, or iodine. Also, a person may be identified as an "allergic" individual because of existing allergies to numerous substances and as such would be at risk to be or to become allergic to other medications or substances used in dentistry.

If a person responds that he is "allergic" to something, it is mandatory to find out what kind of

reaction the patient had to the substance. It is not uncommon for a patient to label simple syncope following an injection of a local anesthetic as an allergy. Another common manifestation of a non-allergy is upset stomach following oral usage of codeine or other narcotics. This is, in fact, a side effect of the drug and not an allergy. A true allergy is usually manifested by skin rash (urticaria), rhinorrhea, angioneurotic edema, or respiratory difficulty. If an allergic history lacks one or more of these signs or symptoms, it is probably not a true allergy.

In response to this question, a history of asthma is often obtained. If a person does have asthma, the dentist should inquire about causative agents, frequency of episodes, severity of episodes, and type of treatment usually required. It is informative to find out if it has ever been necessary for the patient to go to an emergency room for treatment of asthma, since this would indicate asthma of a more severe degree. Also, persons with severe asthma may be receiving steroids for control of their disease.

5. *Have you ever had any type of heart disease, high blood pressure, or rheumatic fever?* This is a particularly important question, since people with various forms of heart disease are very susceptible to physical or emotional insults that may be encountered during dental treatment.

A history of myocardial infarction within the past 6 months precludes elective dental care, since during this immediate postinfarction period the patient is more susceptible to another infarction than is the healthy individual. These patients may also be receiving various medications including vasodilators, anticoagulants, beta blockers, and digitalis, some of which may affect the dental management of these patients. Efforts should be made to find out as much as possible about the myocardial infarction, such as severity, length of hospital stay, complicating factors, present medications, and the physician's recommendations for limitations of activity.

Patients with hypertension should be identified at this time. It is important to find out if there has *ever* been a finding of high blood pressure, since it is not infrequent that patients fail to continue treatment or monitoring or decide to stop taking their medications. Current blood pressure readings should be noted as should any symptoms and present medications. Some medications for blood pressure control may require special consideration during dental treatment.

Heart failure, regardless of etiology, may cause management problems for the dentist. The cause of the failure, degree of compensations, and medications that the patient may be taking should be investigated.

Patients may frequently admit to various forms of dysrhythmias and should be questioned further as to type, severity, and type of treatment.

The patient with a history of rheumatic fever is of special interest to the dentist. It is essential to determine if a patient has evidence of rheumatic heart disease as a result of the rheumatic fever. Patients who do have rheumatic heart disease are susceptible to infective endocarditis from bacteremias that can result from dental procedures. The physician is the person who must make the evaluation of rheumatic heart disease; this is done using the history, physical examination, electrocardiogram, and chest x-ray film, in addition to other diagnostic aids. The most common sign of rheumatic heart disease is a murmur. It should be kept in mind that about two thirds of patients with a history of a single episode of rheumatic fever will have rheumatic heart disease. These patients must be given prophylactic antibiotics during all dental care. (See Tables 2-2 and 2-3 for specific dose schedules.) Patients with most types of congenital cardiac defects are also susceptible to infective endocarditis and should be afforded the same antibiotic protection as patients with rheumatic heart disease.

6. *Do you have diabetes?* For the person who is a diagnosed diabetic, the severity of the disease, age at time of diagnosis, and type of treatment received should be determined. If the patient is insulin dependent, the dose, type of insulin, degree of control, and time of injections are important to determine when dental treatment should best be rendered. It should be kept in mind that diabetic persons may be slow healers and may demonstrate exaggerated responses to infection. Also, periodontal disease seems to be accelerated in diabetic persons.

7. *Have you ever had tuberculosis or any other lung disease?* If a patient has a past history of tuberculosis, he also should give an account of treatment lasting usually a minimum of 9 to 18 months. It may be that only a few weeks of this time were spent in a hospital. In most cases the patient is able to resume employment and public contact in a few months at most. It is important that these patients have had periodic postrecovery examinations, including chest x-ray films, approximately every year to minimize the chances of unrecognized reactivation of the disease.

When a person has a positive tuberculin test (one that converts from negative to positive), this is an indication that the person has been infected with tuberculosis. This does not necessarily mean that the person is infectious. When a person converts to positive and there is no demonstrable clinical or radiographic evidence of active disease, the usual course is to place the patient on chemotherapy, usually isoniazid (INH), for 1 year as a preventive measure. This patient needs no special precautions during dental treatment.

Other pulmonary diseases such as emphysema, bronchitis, or asthma also may be noted in response to this question. Information on severity, treatment, and restriction of activity should be obtained.

8. *Have you ever had hepatitis or other liver disease?* Since the identification of carriers of hepatitis B is extremely important, it would be valuable to be able to identify what type of hepatitis a patient has had. Unfortunately, this is difficult, since (1) more than 50% of carriers give no history of previous hepatitis infection and (2) patients with a positive history of hepatitis are only 50% reliable as to what type they had. Questions regarding age at time of infection and causative agent, such as food or water, may be of value in distinguishing type A from type B. If type B is identified, laboratory screening with a radioimmunoassay for hepatitis B surface antigen (HBsAg) is indicated to identify a potential carrier. Finally, it is recommended that all dental personnel receive the hepatitis B vaccine, which markedly reduces or effectively eliminates the possibility of contracting hepatitis B.

Other liver disease, in general, may adversely affect the patient's dental treatment through bleeding problems or drug intolerance. It also is appropriate to question the patient about his alcohol intake if alcoholism is suspected, since chronic alcoholism is associated with liver disease.

9. *Have you ever had a kidney disease?* The purpose of this question is to identify the patient with renal failure who may be receiving dialysis treatments or the patient who has had a renal transplant. Problems encountered in these patients include inability to detoxify certain drugs, anemia, bleeding problems, infection, hepatitis, hypertension, and poor stress response.

10. *Have you ever had any bleeding problems or blood disorders?* If the patient relates that he had a "bleeding problem," he should be questioned about circumstances, type of injury, length of time he bled, and what, if any, treatment was required. Also, he should be asked whether he bleeds excessively when cut shaving or by similar injury. A family history of bleeding tendencies should be elicited. A good clue is to ask if any problems were encountered following tooth extractions. Laboratory screening tests should be ordered for any patient suspected of having a bleeding problem.

Other blood disorders might include anemia, white cell deficiencies, malignancies, or immune deficiencies. Follow-up information should be obtained if the patient has any of these problems.

11. *Have you ever had a sexually transmitted disease?* If the patient answers yes, it is important to learn the diagnosis and what the treatment was. The patient should have been followed up after treatment with cultures or serum tests to ensure a cure. An affimative answer should also clue the dentist to look for any suspicious skin or mucosal lesions that may result from reinfection or an inadequately treated primary infection and also to question the patient as to whether he may have active disease at present. Also, the fact that a patient has had a sexually transmitted disease places him in a group at high risk to contract the disease again, and he should be approached with caution.

12. *(Women) Are you pregnant?* If a patient is pregnant or thinks she may be, elective dental care should be postponed until the second trimester. As a general rule, emergency care only should be provided during the first trimester. It is helpful to obtain a history about any previous pregnancies regarding complications. The patient's obstetrician should be consulted before any dental care.

Review of systems

In addition to a past medical history, a review of signs or symptoms may indicate an undiagnosed medical problem and should be included in a comprehensive health history. For example, a patient may complain of rapid, unintentional weight loss, fatigue, blood-tinged sputum, and chest pain. Based on these symptoms, which strongly suggest malignancy, this patient should be referred for immediate medical evaluation and treatment. The importance of the medical history cannot be overemphasized. If done well, it will allow the dentist to avoid rendering care that may be detrimental to the patient's health and well-being, will allow identification of the presence of an undetected systemic condition, and will provide a written record in the event of an unwarranted malpractice action.

Dental history

A thorough dental history is also very important for any patient who is to be treated from a comprehensive standpoint. It is important to know what has been done in the past, when it was done, and the outcome of the previous treatment. This would include restorative procedures, prosthetic devices, surgical procedures, orthodontic treatment, endodontic therapy, periodontal treatment, and radiographs. Any complications with the treatment, anesthetic, or medications prescribed should be noted. It is also helpful to learn how the patient feels about dentists and what the patient expects from you. Also, dental problems may occasionally serve as a clue to an underlying systemic disease. For example, a patient with severe progressive periodontal disease may be found to have diabetes or leukemia.

PHYSICAL EXAMINATION

In addition to a comprehensive health history, the dental patient should be afforded the benefits of a simple abbreviated physical examination, which should include at least assessment of general appearance, pulse rate, blood pressure, respiratory rate, and body temperature (if appropriate) as well as a head and neck examination.

General survey

The general survey requires a purposeful but tactful visual inspection of the patient. Careful observation will lead to awareness and recognition of abnormal or unusual conditions that may exist.

From a patient's general appearance or affect, one can notice sex, age, build, nutritional state, alertness, anxiety, speech, hygiene, and neatness. Deviations from "normal" may have significant implications. For example, early identification of fear and anxiety can lead to more appropriate management approaches. Also, obvious disregard of body cleanliness and neatness may indicate a patient's disregard for oral health measures.

Vital signs

The benefits of measuring vital signs during an initial examination are twofold. First, the establishment of *baseline normal values* ensures a standard of comparison in the event an emergency occurs during treatment. If an emergency did occur, it would be necessary to know what was "normal" for that particular patient to determine the severity of the problem. For example, if a patient lost consciousness unexpectedly and the blood pressure obtained was 90/50 mm Hg, the concern would be entirely different for a patient whose blood pressure was normally 110/65 mm Hg than it would be for the hypertensive patient whose blood pressure normally was 180/100 mm Hg. In the first patient one would probably be working with simple syncope as opposed to a shock state in the second patient.

The second benefit of obtaining vital signs during an examination is one of *screening* to identify patients with medical abnormalities, either diagnosed or undiagnosed. The adage of "never treat a stranger" has good foundation. For example, if a person with severe, long-standing hypertension was not identified and was treated with no management alteration, the consequences could be fatal. It should be kept in mind that the purpose of this examination is merely detection of an abnormality and not diagnosis. This is the responsibility of the physician. If it is determined that the abnormal finding is significant, the patient should then be referred to a physician for further evaluation.

PULSE

In examining the pulse, the standard procedure is to palpate either the carotid artery (at the side of

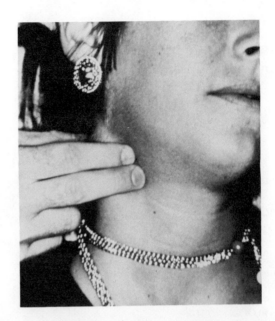

FIG. 1-2. Palpation of carotid pulse.

the trachea) or the radial artery (on the thumb side of the wrist). However, it is recommended that the carotid artery be used routinely for monitoring the pulse (Fig. 1-2) for three reasons. The carotid pulse is most accessible, since the dentist is already working in the head and neck area. It is most reliable, since it is a central artery supplying the brain; therefore, in emergency situations it may remain palpable when peripheral arteries are not. It is easily found since it is a large artery and easily palpated.

The carotid pulse can be palpated along the anterior border of the sternocleidomastoid muscle at approximately the level of the superior aspect of the thyroid cartilage. Displacing the sternocleidomastoid muscle slightly posteriorly will allow palpation of the pulse with the first and middle finger. The thumb should not be used to examine the pulse. The pulse should be monitored for a full minute to detect irregular patterns.

Rate. The average rate of the pulse in normal adults is 60 to 90 beats per minute.

Rhythm. The normal pulse is a series of rhythmic beats that follow each other at regular intervals. When the beats follow each other at irregular

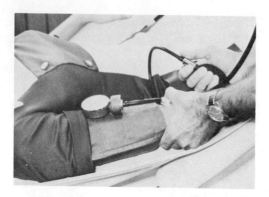

FIG. 1-3. Blood pressure cuff and stethoscope in place.

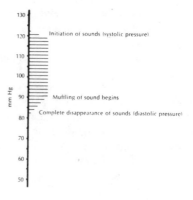

FIG. 1-4. Typical sound pattern obtained when recording blood pressure of normotensive adult.

intervals, the pulse is termed *irregular* or *dysrhythmic.*

BLOOD PRESSURE

Blood pressure is usually determined indirectly in the upper extremities by employing a blood pressure cuff and stethoscope (Fig. 1-3).

The auscultation method of obtaining blood pressure has gained universal acceptance. The cuff should be placed above the elbow in a snug fashion with the lower border about an inch above the antecubital fossa. The standard cuff has arrows designating the area of the brachial artery (at the medial aspect of the tendon of the biceps). Applying the cuff too loosely will give falsely elevated values. No clothing should be left under the cuff since this too may yield incorrect readings. Discrepancies may exist between the relative cuff size and limb size. Using a standard size cuff, the relatively obese arm yields falsely elevated values, whereas an emaciated arm or the arm of a child may give falsely depressed values.

It is possible to fail to recognize an "auscultatory gap." Sounds may disappear between the systolic and diastolic pressures and then reappear. If the cuff pressure is raised only to the range of the gap, the systolic reading will be falsely low. This error is eliminated by first determining the systolic level by the palpatory method.

The cuff is inflated until the radial pulse disappears. The stethoscope is then placed over the brachial artery at the bend of the elbow in the antecubital fossa (not under the cuff), and nothing should be heard.

The pressure is then slowly released, and as the needle falls a point is reached when beats become audible. This is recorded as the systolic pressure.

As the needle continues to fall, the sound of the beats becomes louder, then gradually diminishes until a point is reached at which there is a sudden marked diminution in intensity. The weakened beats are heard for a few moments and then, at a point 5 to 10 mm lower, disappear altogether (Fig. 1-4). The most reliable index of diastolic pressure is the point at which there is complete disappearance of sound.

In the average, normal, healthy adult the normal systolic range varies from 90 to 140 mm Hg, generally increasing with age. The normal diastolic range is from 60 to 90 mm Hg. Pulse pressure is the difference between the systolic and diastolic pressure.

The anxious patient may have a falsely elevated blood pressure, therefore the dentist should never be satisfied with a single high reading. The cuff should be left in place and the pressure rechecked at periodic intervals.

RESPIRATION

The rate and depth of respirations should be monitored by carefully observing the movement of the chest and abdomen in the quietly breathing patient. The respiratory rate in a normal resting adult is approximately 12 to 16 breaths per minute.

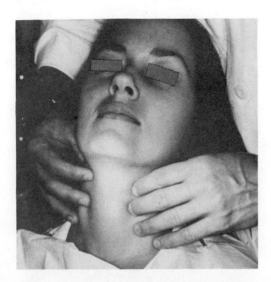

FIG. 1-5. Bimanual palpation of anterior neck.

The respiratory rate in infants may be double that of an adult.

Notice should be made of patients with labored breathing, rapid breathing, or irregular breathing patterns, since all may be signs of systemic problems, especially cardiopulmonary disease.

One common finding in apprehensive patients is hyperventilation (rapid, prolonged, deep breathing or sighing) that results in lowered carbon dioxide levels and may cause disturbing symptoms, including perioral numbness, tingling in the fingers and toes, nausea, a "sick" feeling, and carpopedal spasms.

TEMPERATURE

Temperature is not usually recorded during a normal examination but rather when a patient has febrile signs or symptoms. Normal oral temperature is 98.6° F (37° C) but may vary as much as 1° F plus or minus over the course of a day. Rectal temperature is about 1° F higher than oral, and axillary temperature is about 1° lower than oral.

WEIGHT

The patient should be questioned about any recent unintentional gain or loss of weight. A rapid loss of weight may be caused by malignancy or other wasting disease, while a rapid weight gain could be caused by heart failure.

Head and neck examination

The examination of the head and neck region may vary in its comprehensiveness but should at least include inspection and palpation of the soft tissues of the oral cavity, maxillofacial region, and neck (Fig. 1-5).

Additional areas of examination may include eyes, ears, nose, and cranial nerves; however, the extent of these examinations will vary with the training of the individual dentist.

CLINICAL LABORATORY

Laboratory evaluation for screening purposes is the final phase in the determination of a patient's health status. Obviously, not every patient requires laboratory screening; however, for those patients who do require it, it can be a very useful tool. The dentist should know the indications for certain clinical laboratory procedures, how to perform some of these tests, how to order others from a clinical laboratory, and how to interpret the results of the tests.

It is important that clinical laboratory tests be performed when indicated. Cancerous lesions can be diagnosed and the patient treated early in the course of the disease, thus increasing the chances for a cure. As a case finder, the dentist can screen for and identify patients with serious medical conditions such as diabetes mellitus, anemia, and leukemia and refer these patients for medical diagnosis and treatment. Serious complications in dental treatment such as infection, delayed healing, and bleeding in patients with systemic disease can be avoided by the use of clinical laboratory procedures. The diagnosis of many oral diseases may be established and thus provide a sound basis for the rational management of the problems.

The following illustrations are examples of when patients should have screening tests. First, if a patient has classic signs and symptoms of a disease, it is a waste of time and money to order laboratory tests. That patient should be referred directly to a physician for diagnosis and treatment.

CASE 1. A 13-year-old female had a chief complaint of very tender and swollen gums that bled spontaneously. The symptoms had begun about 3 weeks previously and progressively worsened. She also complained of weakness and weight loss. Examination revealed a very pale, fragile 13-year-old girl with red, swollen gingiva, numerous small petechial hemorrhages of the skin and oral mucosa, and generalized lymphadenopathy. In view of the sudden onset of symptoms and the clinical findings, the impression was acute leukemia and the patient was referred immediately to a physician for diagnosis and treatment. Evaluation by the physician confirmed the initial impression. Nothing would have been gained by having laboratory tests done by the dentist in this case.

A patient who has signs and symptoms that are only suggestive of an underlying disease is the classic patient on whom laboratory screening tests should be performed to decide if medical referral is necessary.

CASE 2. A 38-year-old male was going to be treated for a periodontal condition that would require surgery. During the history he mentioned that when he had had a tooth extracted about 3 years earlier he had bled for several days following the extraction. He had gone to a physician, who had given him an injection of vitamin K, after which the bleeding stopped. Before the periodontal surgery this patient was screened for a possible bleeding condition through a commercial laboratory. A bleeding time, prothrombin time and partial thromboplastin time were ordered. These tests were necessary, since there was no real insight into the possible cause of the bleeding problem, if indeed the patient had one. The possibilities to be ruled out included coagulation disorders, platelet deficiency, and vascular wall defects. The screening tests for this patient were all normal, and he was treated with no complications.

Finally, patients who have no signs, symptoms, or history of a systemic illness but are in a high-risk group for a certain disease because of heredity, life-style, or occupation may also be screened.

CASE 3. A 40-year-old male who had advanced periodontitis stated during the medical history that his mother had diabetes. This placed the patient in a high-risk group for diabetes. A fasting glucose test was ordered for this patient, and the results were 100 mg/100 ml. (This procedure can easily be done in the office by the dentist, using a Dextrostix indicator and a drop of blood from a finger stick.) (Fig. 1-6) This result was normal, but it was recommended to the patient that he be checked once a year in a similar manner.

The question invariably arises as to who should actually perform laboratory tests. Unless the test is rapid, inexpensive, and simple, such as the Dex-

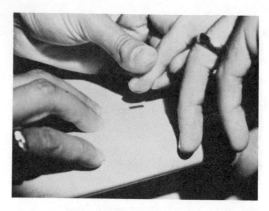

FIG. 1-6. Transferral of drop of blood from patient's finger to Dextrostix.

trostix test, the dentist should not be expected to perform most of the tests but rather should rely on a commercial laboratory. In dealing with a commercial laboratory, the dentist should take the time to visit the laboratory facilities and meet the physician in charge. At this time the dentist should find out what tests of interest to him or her are performed by the laboratory, what the cost of these tests are, and what the normal ranges of results for these tests are. Copies of the order sheets for these tests should also be obtained. If the patient is sent to the laboratory for collection of the sample to be tested (blood), the laboratory will send the results directly to the dentist for his or her interpretation and will bill the patient. The dentist should have informed the patient what the cost would be before sending him to the laboratory.

If the dentist does not want to become involved with using a laboratory facility, then patients should be referred directly to a physician for medical screening.

REFERRAL TO PHYSICIAN OR CONSULTATION

Based on the past medical history, physical examination, or results of laboratory screening, it may be necessary to contact the patient's physician for consultation or referral purposes. The usual methods are by phone, personal contact, or letter. Personal contact is very common, particularly in a small community where physicians and dentists may socialize frequently and may informally discuss a mutual patient. The main drawback to this type of "sidewalk consultation" is its lack of formality and a legal record of the transaction. Mistakes or misunderstandings are not uncommon. If this method is employed, a letter should be sent to confirm the conversation as soon as possible. A phone conversation also should have this type of formal follow-up and confirmation. The principal advantage of the conversational approach is one of immediate information and the chance to gain additional information to questions that may not have been included in a letter. If a patient needs work without delay, a phone call to find out the pertinent information from the physician will allow the dentist to proceed with the work; however, this should be followed immediately with a chart entry and a letter to the physician stating the dentist's understanding of the conversation and requesting confirmation in writing. This should then be attached to the patient's chart, and it becomes a part of the legal document.

A letter to a physician should be kept concise and to the point; only pertinent information should be included, and questions or the reasons why the patient was referred should be specific. It should be kept in mind that physicians are busy and will appreciate a brief, specific request. The following are examples of letters to physicians for various reasons.

The dentist should expect a formal response from the physician summarizing the findings and indicating agreement with the planned management scheme or making additional suggestions. The sample letter on the bottom of p. 41 is a copy of a letter from a physician to whom a patient was referred by a dental student based on a history of excessive bleeding following an extraction and an abnormal partial thromboplastin time (PTT) from a screening laboratory test series. The patient also gave a history of a heart murmur of unknown cause.

An additional approach to the referral/consultation request is the printed form. Fig. 1-7 is the "Request for Medical Consultation" form in use at the University of Kentucky College of Dentistry. The advantage of this approach is one of simplicity both for the dentist and physician as well as standardization of procedure.

REFERRAL TO VERIFY THE PRESENCE OF RHEUMATIC HEART DISEASE

Re: Patient's name
Chart number

Dear Dr. ——————————— :

Mr. A. Smith, a 37-year-old white male, has reported to my office for comprehensive dental care. He reports a history of rheumatic fever at age 8 years but is unaware of any residual damage to his heart that would predispose to infective endocarditis. He denies any symptoms associated with heart disease and is a well-developed, well-nourished, athletic individual. We are planning to provide comprehensive dental care for Mr. Smith.

The purpose of this referral is to request an evaluation of his cardiac status to rule out the presence of rheumatic heart disease and the need for prophylactic antibiotics to prevent infective endocarditis or any additional medical problems of which I should be aware. If, in your opinion antibiotics are required, I would plan to follow the current recommendations of the American Heart Association.

I would appreciate receiving a summary of your findings at your earliest convenience. Thank you for seeing this patient.

Sincerely,

———————————————, D.M.D.

REFERRAL BECAUSE OF UNCONTROLLED HYPERTENSION

Re: Patient's name
Chart number

Dear Dr. _____ :

Mrs. A. Jones, a 50-year-old obese black female, has reported to my office for dental care. During the examination and history she reported frequent headaches and dizzy spells in addition to her "eyes bothering her." She has not seen a physician for several years but remembers taking a "water pill" for blood pressure at one time. In my office today her blood pressure was 215/125 mm Hg, right arm, sitting, at the beginning of the appointment and 210/125 mm Hg at the termination of the appointment. At this point I have elected to discontinue any further dental work and have advised her to seek an immediate medical evaluation from you.

I would appreciate a summary of your findings and treatment of this patient, and I will plan to resume treatment when you believe that her condition has stabilized.

Thank you for seeing this patient.

Sincerely,

_____, D.M.D.

REFERRAL FOR EVALUATION OF SCREENING TEST RESULTS

Re: Patient's name
Chart number

Dear Dr. _____ :

Mr. A. Johnson, a 42-year-old white male, has reported to my office for comprehensive dental treatment. His past medical history is unremarkable except that both of his parents had non-insulin-dependent diabetes. Mr. Johnson is asymptomatic and appears to be in good health.

Based on the familial history of diabetes, we elected to run a fasting blood glucose screening test using a Dextrostrix strip with capillary blood. The result was 250 mg/100 ml.

Because of the family history and the elevated blood glucose screening test, I am referring Mr. Johnson to you for further evaluation. I would appreciate a summary of your findings.

Thank you for seeing this patient.

Sincerely,

_____, D.M.D.

REQUEST FOR WRITTEN CONFIRMATION OF PHONE CONSULTATION

Re: Patient's name
Chart number

Dear Dr. _____ :

   This letter is to confirm our phone conversation of 2/1/85, concerning our mutual patient, Mr. A. Bett, during which time you indicated that you do not believe that Mr. Bett's heart murmur is significant and therefore would not require prophylactic antibiotic coverage during dental work.

   If you are in agreement with this, I would appreciate receiving a short summary of your opinion to include in the patient's record.

   Thank you for your concern.

Sincerely,

_____, M.D.

PHYSICIAN'S SUMMARY OF REFERRAL FINDINGS

Re: Patient's name

Dear Dr. _____ :

   A patient by the name of Mrs. _____ was seen by me after a referral by a dental student, _____, for an evaluation of a bleeding disorder and a heart murmur.

   I can summarize Mrs. _____ findings by indicating that she has very mild von Willebrand disease. I do not believe that this will be a major problem in her dental extractions, and I would not routinely give her any therapy for it. She will need no treatment at the time of her extraction but probably will bleed slightly more than normal. I do not believe, however, that it will be enough to cause any significant problems.

   She does have a mild heart murmur, which I consider a functional murmur, probably related to her mild pectus excavatum, and I do not believe that it requires antibiotic prophylaxis for dental work.

   I appreciate your referral of this patient, and if I may be of any service to you please contact me.

Sincerely,

_____, M.D.

Albert B. Chandler Medical Center
College of Dentistry
Lexington, Kentucky
Department of Oral Diagnosis/Oral Medicine
Phone (606) 233-5950
Medical consultation

Patient name:

Number:

Referred to

Patient's address

Student

Date

Age

Sex

Attending dentist

Family physician

Patient history

Planned dental treatment

Reason for referral

Report of medical consultant

Date

Signature of consultant

FIG. 1-7. "Request for Medical Consultation" form in use at University of Kentucky College of Dentistry. (From Halpern, I.L.: Medical consultation: essential in today's dental practice, Dent. Surv. **55**(2):26-29, 1979. Copyright © 1979 Harcourt Brace Jovanovich, Inc.)

2

INFECTIVE ENDOCARDITIS

Infective endocarditis is a disease caused by microbial infection of the heart valves or endocardium, most often in proximity to congenital or acquired cardiac defects. A similar disease, infective endarteritis, may occur involving a patent ductus arteriosus, a coarctation of the aorta, surgical grafts of major vessels, and surgical arteriovenous shunts. These diseases are most often caused by bacteria; however, in recent years fungi and other microorganisms have been identified as causative agents.

The dentist must make every attempt to identify patients who have cardiovascular defects, congenital or acquired, before any dental manipulations are performed that could produce a transient bacteremia. In these patients the bacteremia could result in endocarditis or endarteritis. These infections were essentially 100% fatal before the antibiotic era. Even with the best of medical treatment these diseases have about a 17% to 65% mortality.[10,16] It appears that endocarditis and endarteritis can be prevented in most cases in the susceptible patient by adequate prophylactic antibiotic therapy. This chapter will deal primarily with endocarditis and its prevention. However, the same principles of prevention would apply to endarteritis.

GENERAL DESCRIPTION
Incidence

The incidence of endocarditis is not known. A study by Porgrel and Welsby[22] in Scotland found 83 cases of endocarditis over a 15-year period from a population of about 500,000 people served by the Aberdeen Royal Infirmary. This would suggest an incidence much lower than 1%. Mostaghim and Millard[16] reported 64 cases of endocarditis treated at the University of Michigan Hospital over a 10-year period. Based on hospital admissions during that period, the incidence was again much lower than 1%. Falace and Ferguson[10] reported 49 patients admitted to the University of Kentucky's Teaching Hospital for endocarditis between 1963 and 1975. During this time there were 142,082 admissions to the hospital; again, the incidence was much lower than 1% (0.034%). The incidence of endocarditis appears to be between 0.3 to 3.0 cases per 1000 hospital admissions. From this standpoint it is clear that endocarditis is a rare or relatively rare disease in the population as a whole.

However, when only the more susceptible portion of the population is considered, endocarditis becomes a much more common problem. The Bland and Jones study[2] of rheumatic fever in 1951 found that 10% of the deaths were caused by endocarditis. Considering the total study, 30 patients out of 1000 died of endocarditis. No mention was made of the number of patients who developed the disease and lived. Thus the true incidence of endocarditis is still not known; however, it appears to be very low in the general population and to increase sharply in susceptible individuals.

Certain features of endocarditis have changed during the past 20 years. For example, it is now more common in men (2:1 ratio), the median age has increased from 30 to 50 years, and there has been an increase in the number of acute cases. Also, the number of cases caused by fungi and gram-negative bacteria has increased.[7]

The use of prophylactic antibiotics does not appear to have reduced the number of cases of endocarditis reported.[7] This may be because fewer than 1 in 5 cases of subacute endocarditis have been associated with medical or dental procedures, and very few of the acute cases are reported to be associated with medical or dental procedures.[7]

More than 200 cases of streptococcal endocarditis that followed dental and genitourinary tract procedures have been reported in the literature. In the vast majority of these cases, symptoms of the disease occurred within 2 weeks of the procedure.[7]

Etiology

Endocarditis occurs when bacteria enter the bloodstream and infect damaged endocardium or endothelial tissue located near high-flow shunts between arterial and venous channels. Other microorganisms such as fungi may rarely infect these sites. Other host factors must be important in the development of this disease. For example, a number of patients with congenital or acquired heart lesions have had dental extractions without antibiotic protection and have not developed endocarditis. The report by Mostaghim and Millard[16] suggested that drug addicts, with or without cardiac lesions, may be much more susceptible to the disease. Recent reports have confirmed the increased risk of endocarditis in drug addicts.[5,7,15,21] Bacteria are released directly into the bloodstream because of the use of nonsterile needles, or an infection develops at the injection site and then bacteria gain access to the bloodstream. Over 50% of cases of endocarditis in drug addicts are caused by *Staphylococcus aureus,* and about 66% of the cases involve the right side of the heart, usually the tricuspid valve.[7] Septic pulmonary infarcts are a common finding in these patients.

Endocarditis may occur in other patients who do not have cardiac defects. The disease has been reported to involve young children under the age of 2 years who had no cardiac defects.[18] Most studies reporting endocarditis will show that 60% to 80% of the patients have some type of predisposing heart or arterial disease.[18] The remainder of the patients will have no known predisposing cardiovascular defects. About 37% to 76% of cases of endocarditis occur in patients with rheumatic heart disease, and 6% to 24% occur in patients with congenital heart disease.[18]

Streptococci and staphylococci are responsible for about 80% of cases of endocarditis.[7,15,21] However, the number of cases caused by streptococci is going down. During the 1960s gram-negative bacteria accounted for about 1.7% of cases of endocarditis. These organisms now cause about 7% of cases of endocarditis.[4]

The risk of endocarditis occurring in a patient after a dental procedure is not known. The risk has been reported to vary from zero to as high as 1 in 533.[18,22] The number of patients considered to be susceptible to endocarditis has been estimated to be as high as 5% of the general population.[22] This included individuals with rheumatic heart disease, congenital heart disease, prosthetic heart valves, etc.

Pathophysiology and complications

The lesions of endocarditis are divided into three groups—cardiac, embolic and general. The cardiac lesions are usually valvular. The mitral valve is most often affected. Infection of the pulmonary valve is rare. Vegetative lesions occur on line of contact of the damaged valve cusps and cover the valve. The vegetations consist of an amorphous mass of fused platelets, fibrin, and bacteria (Fig. 2-1).

Embolic lesions are common, since the vegetations are friable and easily detached. Petechial hemorrhages on skin and mucous membranes may result from these emboli (Fig. 2-2). Osler nodes (small, raised, tender, vascular lesions) involving the skin may arise from emboli or may represent a reaction to bacterial endotoxins. Emboli may affect the kidney, brain, eyes, and other tissues.

Other conditions that may occur in patients with endocarditis include cardiac failure, liver disease, and anemia. These effects may be a result of a toxemia resulting from the infection.

As stated earlier, patients with endocarditis who do not receive antibiotic treatment have a mortality of 100%. The mortality for treated patients varies from about 17% to 65%.[10,16] The morbidity of this disease is significant. The average hospital stay is 4 to 6 weeks. Patients who recover are still faced with many potential complications, including reinfection, congestive heart failure, renal disease, and cerebrovascular accident. Early, effective treatment decreases the death rate and the number of complications.

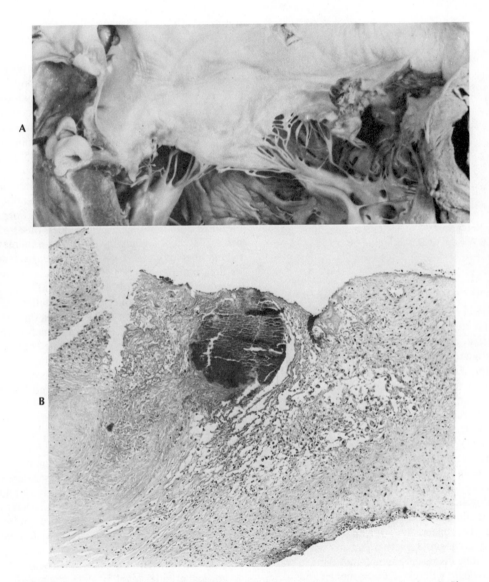

FIG. 2-1, A, Gross appearance of vegetations of infective endocarditis of mitral valve. **B,** Photomicrograph of vegetations of infective endocarditis of mitral valve. (Courtesy J. E. Edwards, M.D., St. Paul, Minn.)

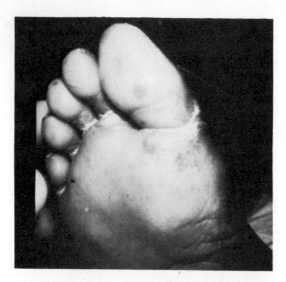

FIG. 2-2. Septic emboli of bacterial endocarditis. (Courtesy H.D. Wilson, M.D., Lexington, Ky.)

CLINICAL PRESENTATION
Signs and symptoms

The onset of endocarditis is often insidious. The patient is often unable to pinpoint when the disease first started. Symptoms include weakness, weight loss, fatigue, fever, night sweats, anorexia, and arthralgia. Emboli may produce paralysis, chest pain, abdominal pain, blindness, and hematuria. The fever may spike, with peaks often being noted in the afternoon or evening. Petechiae may be found on the skin or mucosal tissues. Linear hemorrhages may be found under the nails, and Osler nodes may be found in various subcutaneous areas. In long-standing endocarditis, clubbing of the fingers may be found. Heart findings are related to the underlying heart disease, which is usually valvular. Thus almost all of these patients will have a murmur. The spleen and liver may be enlarged.

Highly pathogenic microorganisms will cause a sudden appearance of symptoms, and a rapid course to death will result unless medical measures are taken. The more fulminating infections often involve otherwise normal hearts. Severe suppurative infections often precede the onset of this type of endocarditis. The study by Mostaghim and Millard[16] suggested that the number of cases of this type of endocarditis may be increasing.

Laboratory findings

Laboratory tests for the presence of active infection are usually positive in the patient who has endocarditis. Leukocytosis with neutrophilia is common. The erythrocyte sedimentation rate is increased. The C-reactive protein is positive. Serum immunoglobin levels may be increased.

Blood for culture and antibiotic sensitivity testing is usually taken before specific therapy for the infection is begun. Patients who have been receiving penicillin to prevent recurrent attacks of rheumatic fever and who develop endocarditis may not show a positive blood culture for 7 or more days. The blood culture is positive in over 85% of the patients who have endocarditis.

Streptococcus viridans is the most common microorganism responsible for the form of endocarditis that has a slow onset. *Staphylococcus aureus* is the most common cause of a sudden onset of the disease. Recent studies have shown an increase in the number of cases caused by *S. aureus* and a reduction in the number caused by *S. viridans*.

Penicillin is the current drug of choice for prophylaxis of endocarditis. However, antibiotic sensitivity data reported in recent studies on this disease suggest that erythromycin is much more effective in vitro than penicillin.[16] Whether this will be true clinically remains to be investigated. Penicillin remains the foundation for treatment of endocarditis and is the drug of choice for antibiotic prophylaxis in patients susceptible to this disease.

MEDICAL MANAGEMENT

The basic principles for the treatment of patients with endocarditis are (1) treat as early as possible; (2) base therapy on culture and sensitivity findings whenever possible; (3) treat with bactericidal agents; (4) treat with adequate doses of antibiotics; (5) administer antibiotics IV; and (6) continue treatment for a long enough time.

Along with cultures and sensitivity tests, a serum bactericidal level is sometimes performed. This is an in vitro study in which the patient's serum, which contains the administered antibiotic, is titered against the causative organism. If the serum is bactericidal for the causative organism at 1:8 dilution or greater, the antibiotic dosage is thought to be adequate.

Penicillin is the drug of choice for most cases of endocarditis caused by *S. viridans*. Ten million units a day IV is usually an adequate starting dose for endocarditis caused by *S. viridans*. One gram of streptomycin may be given twice a day IM in addition to the penicillin.[12,24]

For infections caused by *S. aureus* found to be sensitive to penicillin, the starting dose of penicillin is 16 to 24 million units per day IV. For penicillinase-producing organisms, 12 to 24 g of methicillin given daily IV is the usual starting dose. Vancomycin, cephalothin, lincomycin, and oxacillin are other drugs that may have to be considered, depending on culture and sensitivity findings.

Mycotic infections are usually treated with large doses of amphotericin B. The length of treatment is usually 4 to 6 weeks. Therapy for mycotic infections may be extended from 4 to 12 weeks. The prognosis is poor with mycotic endocarditis, and patients who do not respond to amphotericin B may require surgery to remove the infected valve.

Patients who have a history of mild allergic reactions to penicillin may still be given this drug following desensitization. Corticosteroids may be given before starting the penicillin therapy. The penicillin is started by giving small (5-unit) subcutaneous injections and increasing the dose every 90 minutes (to 10, 100, 1000, 10,000, 50,000 units). If no serious reaction occurs after these injections, the IV dosage is started. Another technique is to infuse 1 unit of aqueous penicillin in 250 ml of 5% glucose and water. If no immediate reaction occurs, the penicillin dosage is increased by sixfold to tenfold every 20 minutes until therapeutic levels are reached.[12,24]

Surgical correction of infected valves is indicated when (1) severe, intractable heart failure is present; (2) systemic emboli recur; (3) the infecting organism is a fungus and the patient does not respond to medical therapy; or (4) endocarditis is superimposed on an artificial valve. Patients who have congenital heart defects and endocarditis are best managed by corrective surgery following successful medical treatment of the endocarditis (Fig. 2-3). However, if the infection cannot be controlled, surgical repair may be attempted.

Dacron and other prosthetic materials used in cardiovascular surgery to correct congenital or acquired lesions may become infected. Often under

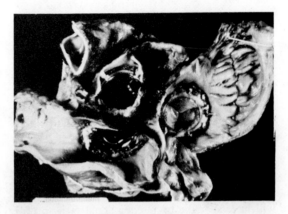

FIG. 2-3. Postmortem specimen from patient with rheumatic heart disease who had surgical replacement of three valves. (Courtesy W. O'Conner, M.D., Lexington, Ky.)

these circumstances a cure can be obtained only by removing the infected graft and replacing it.

The surgical risk is high for the preceding procedures in patients who have endocarditis, but the alternative is a very high mortality.

Patients who have exteriorized transvenous cardiac pacemakers have on occasion developed an infection that resembles endocarditis. For this condition the pacemaker and wire are replaced and moved to another location. The removed wire is cultured, and sensitivity tests are made from the cultured microorganisms. The patient is then treated as if he had endocarditis.

DENTAL MANAGEMENT
Medical considerations

The dentist's goal is to prevent endocarditis from occurring in susceptible dental patients. Any dental procedure that causes injury to the soft tissue or bone can produce a transient bacteremia that, in the susceptible patient, can result in endocarditis. Even minor dental manipulations such as the cleaning of teeth or the placement of a matrix band can result in a transient bacteremia. In normal patients the body's defenses handle these bacteremias, and usually no serious problem develops. However, in the patient with a heart defect such as rheumatic heart disease, the anatomy and function of the affected valve are altered because of the scarring that follows the acute rheumatic fever attack.[27] During bacteremias the altered valvular tissue provides an ideal location for attachment and growth of bacteria. Thus in the patient who has rheumatic heart disease or patients who have other types of cardiovascular defects (see Table 2-1) there is a very real threat of endocarditis during each and every one of these periods of bacteremia.

The risk of producing a transient bacteremia has been estimated to be up to about 85% when teeth are extracted, 88% with periodontal surgery, 40% with tooth brushing, 50% with oral irrigation, and 50% when chewing paraffin.[18] Normal patients will have sporadic bacteremia about 60% to 80% of the time. It is clear that transient bacteremias are common following many dental procedures; yet the incidence of endocarditis is very, very low. The number of bacteria released, the duration of the bacteremia, and the type of bacteria involved appear to be important factors in determining the risk level of the susceptible patient in developing endocarditis.

The prevention of endocarditis involves the following concepts or procedures. The first, at the broadest level, is the prevention of the diseases that produce cardiac defects. This involves giving vaccines to prevent certain infections that may cause congenital heart defects and avoiding drugs that could cause cardiac defects in the fetus when taken by the pregnant female. In some situations hygiene measures can be taken at the site of an injury following a medical or dental procedure to reduce the number of bacteria released into the bloodstream. Also, antibiotic prophylaxis can be given just before the medical or dental procedure to protect the patient.[5]

From the dental viewpoint the only effective measures available at this time to provide protection to the susceptible patient are antibiotic prophylaxis and, in certain cases, oral hygiene procedures. Attempts to "clear" the mouth by using topical agents before performing a dental procedure have had some effect on the degree or duration of the bacteremia. A study of Scopp[25] showed that rinsing and irrigation with povidone-iodine (Betadine) mouthwash before performing invasive dental procedures reduced the incidence of bacteremia from 56% in the control group to 28% in the rinse group.

TABLE 2-1. Degree of risk for infective endocarditis and suggested regimen for prophylaxis

High degree of risk (regimen B)
Prosthetic valves
Recent surgical repair of cardiovascular defect
Previous infective endocarditis

High to moderate degree of risk (regimen A or B)
Arteriovenous fistulae
Patent ductus arteriosus
Ventricular septal defect
Aortic valve disease
Intravenous catheter (ventriculojugular shunt)
Coarctation of aorta
Tetralogy of Fallot
Marfan syndrome
Mitral insufficiency

Moderate degree of risk (usually regimen A)
Mitral valve prolapse
Tricuspid valve disease
Pulmonary valve disease
Pure mitral stenosis
Idiopathic hypertrophic subaortic stenosis
Large atrial septal defect
Surgically corrected cardiovascular lesion with synthetic prosthetic implant (greater than 6 months postoperatively)

Low to negligible degree of risk (usually no coverage or regimen A)
Arteriosclerotic plaques
Coronary sclerosis
Small atrial septal defect
Cardiac pacemaker
Surgically corrected cardiovascular lesion with no prosthetic implant (greater than 6 months postoperatively)
Syphilitic aortitis

Prevention of medical complications

To prevent endocarditis from occurring, the susceptible patient must be identified and high doses of antibiotics administered just before, during, and after dental manipulation. The bacteremia itself will not be prevented, but the possibility of bacteria growing on damaged endothelial surfaces is greatly reduced. Endocarditis is a disease that must be prevented whenever possible because of its high mortality even with the best medical treatment.

Several important general principles are involved with antibiotic prophylaxis.[19] The specific oganism involved should be known. An antibiotic effective against that organism should be selected. The proper dosage of the antibiotic should be used. The antibiotic should be given just before the procedure to provide maximum blood levels at the time of the injury. The antibiotic should be continued as long as bacteria could be released. The benefit to risk ratio must be considered for each procedure; in other words, the dentist must consider whether the risk of developing a problem outweighs the risks involved by the use of the antibiotic. General agreement exists for the use of antibiotic prophylaxis for the following: organ transplant patients, patients with impaired host defenses such as blood dyscrasias, patients undergoing chemotherapy and radiation therapy, patients susceptible to endocarditis, and patients who are about to have certain surgical procedures such as total hip prosthesis and prosthetic heart valve placement.[5,15,18]

It has been estimated that 25% to 50% of antibiotic use in hospitals is for prophylaxis. The complications associated with antibiotic use include toxicity, allergy, superinfections, resistant bacteria, high costs, and in some cases careless surgery. The problem with allergy alone is very significant. About 5% to 10% of patients who take penicillin will have an allergic reaction.[23] A small number of these patients (0.04%) will develop an anaphylactic reaction, and 10% of these individuals will die. Anaphylactic deaths caused by penicillin account for over 300 deaths per year in the United States.[23]

There are several problems with the current use of antibiotic prophylaxis against endocarditis. The risk of developing the disease in the susceptible patient is not known. A number of different microorganisms are found to cause endocarditis, therefore no one antibiotic is effective in preventing the disease. The duration of coverage is not known for oral wounds that heal by second intention. Bacterial resistance during a coverage period is becoming a problem as is the presence of resistant strains in the oral flora before the initiation of antibiotic prophylaxis. The last major problem relates to patients who were given antibiotic prophylaxis but still developed endocarditis.

In 1981 the American Heart Association formed a national registry to report prophylaxis failures for endocarditis.[1,7] There have been 52 cases reported involving recent development of endocarditis in patients given antibiotic prophylaxis. Most of these patients had cardiac lesions, and 10 had prosthetic heart valves. They had been given either penicillin or erythromycin prophylaxis. However, only 6 of the 52 cases reported had received one of the standard regimens recommended by the American Heart Association.[7] These data are interesting from two aspects. First, the majority of these failures received improper coverage. Second, 6 cases involved patients who were given coverage as recommended and still developed the disease. A number of questions remain unanswered concerning this topic. To find the answers and determine the real value of antibiotic prophylaxis it has been estimated that a double-blind placebo study involving 6000 at-risk patients would be needed.[18] This of course will not be done because of the serious nature of the disease and the moral and ethical problems involved in such a study. Thus current practice involves the identification of the at-risk patient and the use of antibiotic prophylaxis before dental procedures, using the recommendation of the American Heart Association.[5,7,21]

Regimen A (Table 2-2) is recommended for patients with rheumatic heart disease,[14] congenital heart disease, prolapse of the mitral valve, syphilitic heart disease, calcific nodular aortic stenosis, idiopathic hypertrophic subaortic stenosis, and calcified mitral anulus and for hemodialysis patients with arteriovenous shunts, intravenous catheters, and ventriculojugular shunts. Regimen A can be used in the patient for whom it has been at least 6 months since surgery for the repair of a cardiac or vascular defect using synthetic materials such as Dacron. Some physicians will suggest regimen A for patients with transvenous pacemakers; others will recommend that no prophylaxis be used.

Regimen B (Table 2-3) is recommended for patients who have prosthetic heart valves and patients who have had commissurotomy for a diseased valve. It is also recommended during the healing stage following coronary bypass operation, closure of atrial or ventricular septal defects, closure of

TABLE 2-2. Regimen A—prophylactic antibiotic coverage to prevent infective endocarditis in adult dental patients

---

I. Patients not allergic to penicillin
   A. 1 million units of aqueous crystalline penicillin G mixed with 600,000 units of procaine penicillin G, IM, administered at least 30 minutes before dental procedure followed by 500 mg penicillin V, orally, every 6 hours for eight doses *or*
   B. 2 g of penicillin V, orally, at least 30 minutes before dental procedure, followed by 500 mg penicillin V, orally, every 6 hours for eight doses
II. Patients allergic to penicillin or who are receiving low penicillin dosage to prevent recurrent attacks of rheumatic fever
   1 g of erythromycin, orally, at least 1½ to 2 hours before dental procedure followed by 500 mg erythromycin, orally, every 6 hours for eight doses

---

Recommended by the American Heart Association for control of subacute bacterial endocarditis following dental procedures. From Kaplan, E.L.: Prevention of bacterial endocarditis, Circulation **56:**139A-143A, 1977. By permission of the American Heart Association, Inc.

TABLE 2-3. Regimen B—prophylactic antibiotic coverage to prevent infective endocarditis in high-risk adult dental patients.

A. Patients not allergic to penicillin
   1 million units of aqueous crystalline penicillin G mixed with 600,000 units of procaine pencillin G, IM, administered at least 30 minutes before dental procedure and 1 g streptomycin, IM, followed by 500 mg penicillin V, orally, every 6 hours for eight doses
B. Patients allergic to penicillin
   1 g of vancomycin, IV, 30 minutes to 1 hour before dental procedure, followed by 500 mg erythromycin, orally, every 6 hours for eight doses

---

Recommended by the American Heart Association for control of subacute bacterial endocarditis following dental procedures. From Kaplan, E.L.: Prevention of bacterial endocarditis, Circulation **56:**139A-143A, 1977. By permission of the American Heart Association, Inc.

ductus arteriosus, or placement of arterial grafts. Recent findings suggest that gentamicin may replace streptomycin in Regimen B.[17] Patients whose cardiovascular defect has been corrected using autogenous tissue will not require prophylaxis 6 months after their surgery. Regimen B is also recommended for patients who have already had endocarditis.

The dentist is given a choice with regimen A of using the parenteral route or the oral route for the initial loading dose. Whenever possible the oral route should be selected. When penicillin is given by injection, about 1% to 2% of patients will develop an allergy to the drug. When penicillin is given orally, this incidence is reduced to about 0.1% to 0.2%. Hence with reliable patients the oral regimen is recommended (Chapter 19). Penicillin V should be used rather than penicillin G; high blood levels are obtained within ½ to 1 hour using penicillin V, while inadequate blood levels are noted with penicillin G.

Recent studies in animals have demonstrated that the high loading dose is necessary to prevent endocarditis.[5,7,8] The dental procedures planned during a given coverage period should be performed after the loading dose is given. It would appear that procedures performed by extending the coverage period to 5 to 7 days, for example, would carry increased risk to the patient, because the longer the patient is receiving antibiotic prophylaxis, the greater the risk of releasing resistant strains of bacteria.*

Based on these considerations we recommend that all routine dental procedures be performed during the first 1 to 3 hours of the standard coverage period. If additional coverage periods are needed, at least 1 week should elapse before another coverage period is initiated. This will allow the oral flora to return to normal. There is some confusion on this point. Several studies have suggested that resistant bacteria may remain as long as 6 months after the use of penicillin.[26] In contrast, other studies have shown that penicillin V and ampicillin had no effect on the oral, throat, and fecal flora.[11,13] In one study the agents were given for 10 days and the various flora examined each day and for 9 days following termination of the

---

*References 3, 6, 9, 17, 20, 26.

antibiotics. No resistant strains were found; both aerobic and anaerobic testing was done.[11]

If one is concerned about the presence of resistant bacteria, the next coverage period could use erythromycin rather than penicillin. In our opinion this is not necessary if at least 1 week has elapsed before the next coverage period is started.[3]

Another problem that often comes up is how to deal with the surgery patient in whom the tissues are healing by second intention. The standard duration of coverage may not be adequate, particularly if secondary infection develops in the wound area. The only option in this situation is to extend the coverage period using 500 mg of penicillin V four times a day during the extended period. If the coverage must be extended further, erythromycin could be used.

Patients who are having orthodontic bands adjusted do not require prophylactic coverage, and patients who are undergoing exfoliation of their deciduous teeth do not appear to need coverage.

Treatment planning consideration

The treatment planning considerations for patients susceptible to endocarditis are covered in the chapters on rheumatic heart disease and dental management of patients with surgically corrected cardiovascular disease (Chapters 3 and 6).

Oral complications

There are no specific oral complications associated with endocarditis.

Emergency dental care

Susceptible patients must be identified and given antibiotic prophylaxis before any emergency dental treatment is performed.

REFERENCES

1. Bisno, A.L., et al.: Failure of prophylaxis for bacterial endocarditis: American Heart Association Registry, J. Fam. Pract. **19**:16-20, 1980.
2. Bland, E.F., and Jones, T.D.: Rheumatic fever and rheumatic heart disease, Circulation **4**:836-843, 1951.
3. Bornfield, M.: Bacterial endocarditis, J. Am. Dent. Assoc. **96**:27-29, 1978.
4. Cohen, P.S., Maguire, J.H., and Weinstein, L.: Infective endocarditis caused by Gram-negative bacteria: a review of the literature, 1945-1977, Prog. Cardiovasc. Dis. **22**:205-242, 1979.
5. Dascomb, H.E.: The current status of prophylaxis against infective endocarditis, J. La. State Med. Soc. **132**:91-99, 1980.
6. Drucker, D.B., and Jolly, M.: Sensitivity of oral microorganisms to antibiotics, Br. Dent. J. **131**:442-444, 1971.
7. Durack, D.T.: Infective and non-infective endocarditis. In Hurst, J.W., editor: The heart, ed. 5, New York, 1983, McGraw-Hill Book Co., pp. 1250-78.
8. Durack, D.T., and Petersdorf, R.G.: Changes in the epidemiology of endocarditis. In Kaplan, E.L., and Taranta, A.V., editors: American Heart Association Monograph No. 52: infective endocarditis, 1977, pp. 3-8.
9. Elliot, R.H., and Dunbar, J.M.: Antibiotic sensitivity of oral alpha hemolytic Streptococcus from children with congenital and acquired cardiac disease, Br. Dent. J. **142**:283-285, 1977.
10. Falace, D., and Ferguson, T.: Bacterial endocarditis, Oral Surg. **40**:189-195, 1976.
11. Hermdahl, A., Nord, C.E., and Weilander, K.: Effect of phenoxymethylpenicillin, bacampicillin and clindamycin on the oral, throat and colon microflora of man, Swed. Dent. J. **4**:39-52, 1980.
12. Hurst, J.W.: The heart arteries and veins, ed. 4, New York, 1978, The McGraw-Hill Book Co., pp. 981-1092.
13. Istre, G.R., et al.: Susceptibility of group A beta-hemolytic Streptococcus isolates to penicillin and erythromycin, Antimicrob. Agents Chemother. **20**:244-246, 1981.
14. Kaplowitz, G.J., and Reifler, J.R.: Compliance with AHA guidelines for preventing bacterial endocarditis: report of a study, J. Acad. Gen. Dent. **31**:56-59, 1983.
15. Kaye, D.: Infective endocarditis. In Rose, L.F., and Kaye, D., editors: Internal medicine for dentistry, St. Louis, 1983, The C.V. Mosby Co., pp. 178-186.
16. Mostaghim, D., and Millard, H.O.: Bacterial endocarditis: a restrospective study, Oral Surg. **40**:219-234, 1975.
17. Oill, P.A., et al.: Choice of antibiotics for prophylaxis for treatment of group D streptoccal endocarditis, N. Engl. J. Med. **305**:101, July 1981.
18. Pallasch, T.J.: Principles of antibiotic therapy: prevention of infective endocarditis, Dent. Drug Serv. Newsletter **4**:1, January 1983.
19. Pallasch, T.J.: Principles of antibiotics therapy; principles of antimicrobal chemoprophylaxis, Dent. Drug. Serv. Newsletter **3**:12, December 1982.
20. Parillo, J.E., et al.: Endocarditis due to resistant viridans Streptococci during oral penicillin chemoprophylaxis, New Engl. J. Med. **300**:269-300, 1979.
21. Pelletier, L.L., Jr., and Petersdorf, R.G.: Infective endocarditis. In Petersdorf, R.G., et al., editors: Harrison's principles of internal medicine, ed. 10, New York, 1983, McGraw-Hill Book Co., pp. 1418-23.
22. Porgrel, M.A., and Welsby, P.D.: The dentist and prevention of infective endocarditis, Br. Dent. J. **139**:12-16, 1975.
23. Requa-Clark, B., and Holroyd, S.V.: Antimicrobial agents. In Holroyd, S.V., and Wynn, R.L., editors: Clinical pharmacology in dental practice, ed. 3, St. Louis, 1982, The C.V. Mosby Co., pp. 245-278.

24. Scheld, W.M., and Sande, M.A.: Endocarditis and intravascular infections. In Mandell, G.L., et al. editors: Principles and practice of infectious disease, New York, 1979, John Wiley & Sons, Inc.
25. Scopp, I.W.: Gingival degerming, bacteremia reduction in dental procedures. In Kaplen, E.L., and Taranta, A.V., editors: American Heart Association Monograph No. 52: infective endocarditis, 1977, p. 51.
26. Sprunt, K.: Role of antibiotic resistance in bacterial endocarditis. In Kaplen, E.L., and Taranta, A.V., editors: American Heart Association Monograph No. 52: infective endocarditis, 1977, pp. 17-19.
27. Stollerman, G.H.: Rheumatic fever. In Thorm, G.W., et al., editors: Harrison's principles of internal medicine, ed. 8, New York, 1977, McGraw-Hill Book Co., pp. 1237-1243.

3

RHEUMATIC FEVER AND RHEUMATIC HEART DISEASE

Patients who have a history of rheumatic fever may have residual cardiac damage and rheumatic heart disease. These patients need to be given prophylactic antibiotic therapy during dental treatment to prevent infective endocarditis. For patients who have a history of rheumatic fever but no evidence of rheumatic heart disease there is no need for prophylactic antibiotics, since these patients are not susceptible to infective endocarditis.

For the dentist to be able to detect and manage the patient who has rheumatic heart disease, he or she must be aware of the basic pathogenesis and clinical manifestations of rheumatic fever and rheumatic heart disease. Because of the close relationship of these two diseases in the clinical situation that most commonly confronts the dentist, they are covered in sequence in this chapter. Other conditions that render the patient susceptible to infective endocarditis or endarteritis are discussed in Chapters 2, 4, and 6.

Rheumatic fever

Rheumatic fever is an acute inflammatory condition that develops in some individuals as a complication following group A streptococcal infections. It is thought to arise as a result of an autoimmune reaction between "normal" tissues that have been altered by products of the bacteria and antibodies that have been produced by the host in response to these altered tissues.[9]

GENERAL DESCRIPTION
Incidence

Acute rheumatic fever is a sequela of group A streptococcal infection. The rheumatic fever attack rate in patients with proved streptococcal infection varies from 0.5% to 3.0% and is related to the virulence of the strain causing the infection.[10,11,12]

Rheumatic fever is principally a childhood disease; about 75% of the cases occur before the age of 20 years. Rheumatic fever and its sequela account for about 95% of all cases of heart disease in children.[10,11,12]

The incidence and severity of rheumatic fever attacks have been decreasing in developed countries. About 100,000 cases are still being reported per year in the United States. In addition, the incidence of carditis associated with recent attacks of rheumatic fever has been decreasing.[6] Rheumatic fever is rare before the age of 3 and is most common between the ages of 5 and 15.[6,10]

Rheumatic fever is found at the rate of 0.7 cases for 1000 schoolchildren and 6 to 9 cases per 1000 college freshmen.[6,10,12]

It is estimated that 1% to 6% of the population of the United States exhibits specific valvular defects of the heart.[10] This may give some clue to the real incidence of rheumatic fever in this country.

Many cases of rheumatic fever are probably unrecognized but leave behind the residual of a damaged heart valve. To support this concept, various studies have shown that only about 60% of the patients with mitral valve disease give a history of having had acute rheumatic fever.

Age does not alter susceptibility to rheumatic fever. However, streptococcal infections are much less likely to be acquired in adult life, thus the lower incidence of rheumatic fever in adults.

Etiology

The clinical sequence of events usually starts with a sore throat that, if cultured, often will reveal group A streptococci (Fig. 3-1). The presence of a streptococcal infection, however, must be established by detecting an increase in antibody titer to one of the various antigens found on the bacteria, because group A streptococcus can be cultured from throats of individuals who do not have streptococcal infection.

The most important clinical finding that supports the diagnosis of rheumatic fever is an elevated titer of antibodies, which confirms a recent streptococcal infection. Bacterial cultures of the throat may even be negative in some of these patients.[10,11,12]

Not all patients who develop rheumatic fever will have complained of a sore throat. Also, all patients with sore throats do not have streptococcal infection, since any number of other bacteria or viruses may cause this symptom.

About 3% of individuals who have a symptomatic exudative streptococcal pharyngitis will develop rheumatic fever. This incidence falls to about 0.5% in persons who have a less severe streptococcal pharyngitis.[11] The incidence of rheumatic fever following streptococcal pharyngitis increases to 5% to 50% in the patient with a history of rheumatic fever.[10,11]

In individuals who develop rheumatic fever following a streptococcal infection, a latent period of 2 weeks to as long as 6 months occurs. Once an attack of rheumatic fever has developed, the patient is much more susceptible to recurrent attacks than is the rest of the population to a first attack.

Since the streptococcal organisms do not directly invade the heart or joints, rheumatic fever is not an infectious disease from that standpoint. The group A streptococcal throat infection is believed

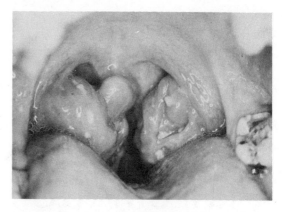

FIG. 3-1. Hypertrophied tonsils with areas of purulent exudate.

to sensitize the tissues of the heart, joints, etc. by prosthetic groups from the organism that unite with connective tissue protein to form an antigen. The prosthetic groups may be endotoxins or exotoxins. The antigen complex then stimulates the production of specific antibodies. Once these antibodies are in circulation, they combine with the antigens at the various tissue locations and cause an allergic necrosis that is accompanied by a characteristic cellular response to the allergic reaction.

Accessory factors also play an important part in the etiology of rheumatic fever. Overcrowded, poor, undernourished populations who live in cold, damp climates appear to be much more susceptible to rheumatic fever. This may be explained on the basis that streptococcal throat infections also are much more frequent under these circumstances or that certain vitamin deficiencies are important factors in themselves in determining susceptibility to rheumatic fever. The reduced frequency of severe streptococcal throat infections in developed countries explains their reduced incidence of rheumatic fever.[10,11,12]

Pathophysiology and complications

Rheumatic fever, as mentioned previously, is an immune-related disease associated with group A streptococcal throat infections. Products from the bacteria sensitize connective tissue, forming antigens that stimulate antibody production. Antigen-antibody combinations then occur and produce local tissue necrosis and an inflammatory reaction. The connective tissue of the heart, including the valves, is very susceptible to the disease. In addition, the connective tissue of the larger joints and the lungs and the subcutaneous tissues are very susceptible.

Thus the major manifestations of the disease, from a clinical standpoint, are signs and symptoms relating to the inflammatory reactions that take place in the heart, larger joints, and skin. Pulmonary involvement may be an important part of the clinical picture in some patients.

The acute attack of rheumatic fever leaves no permanent skin or joint damage or functional impairment. The primary complication of the disease relates to its cardiac and pulmonary effects. The patient may develop congestive heart failure and die during the acute attack, or the heart may be damaged so that complications occur following the acute attack. These complications include constrictive pericarditis, valve damage resulting from scarring, and congestive heart failure. In addition, the patient with damaged valves is susceptible to endocarditis. In a few cases, lung involvement during the acute attack may be so severe that the patient dies.

CLINICAL PRESENTATION
Signs and symptoms

The major manifestations of rheumatic fever are arthritis, carditis, chorea, erythema marginatum, and subcutaneous nodules. Minor manifestations include fever, arthralgia, abnormal erythrocyte sedimentation rate, and possibly electrocardiogram changes.

The diagnosis of rheumatic fever is based on the presence of at least two major and one minor manifestations or one major and two minor manifestations and a history of presiding throat infection with nonelevation of the antistreptolysin O (ASO) titer.[10,11,12]

The arthritis associated with rheumatic fever develops rapidly and lasts for about 2 to 3 weeks. The large joints of the knees and ankles are commonly affected. The small joints of the hands and feet are uncommonly involved. Pain is the first symptom, followed by redness, heat, and then swelling of the joint. Joint involvement is transient and migratory, and usually no permanent deformi-

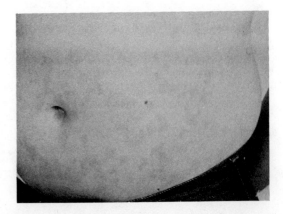

FIG. 3-2. Erythema marginatum as manifestation of rheumatic fever. (Courtesy C. Cottrill, M.D., Lexington, Ky.)

ties result. Severe joint involvement is much more common in adults than in children.

Chorea is a spasmodic, nonrepetitive motion involving voluntary muscles that does not occur when the patient is asleep. The onset of chorea is variable and may be several months after the streptococcal infection.

Erythema marginatum is a nonpruritic, flat skin rash that occurs in about 5% of patients who have rheumatic fever (Fig. 3-2). It usually coexists with arthritis, chorea, or carditis. When it occurs, it lasts for about 2 to 3 days.[11,12]

Subcutaneous nodules are firm, painless, colorless subcutaneous swellings that occur in about 5% of patients with rheumatic fever (Fig. 3-3). They usually coexist with carditis. They occur most commonly on the skin over the elbows and persist for about 1 or 2 weeks.[11,12]

The carditis associated with rheumatic fever reveals itself clinically as an abnormal murmur, pericardial rub, cardiac enlargement, congestive heart failure, or a combination of these. The murmur results from dilation of the valvular ring, destruction of the valvular substance, or contraction of chordae tendineae. The mitral valve is affected most often, followed by the aortic valve. Pericardial rub is caused by an acute inflammatory pericarditis. Congestive heart failure, when present, develops rapidly. The patient will have dyspnea with rales. An ache in the upper right quadrant of

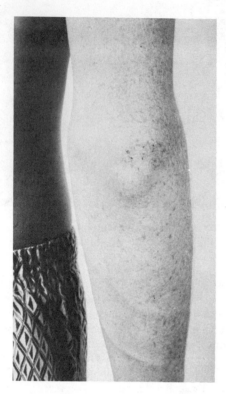

FIG. 3-3. Subcutaneous nodules as manifestation of rheumatic fever. (Courtesy C. Cottrill, M.D., Lexington, Ky.)

tack of rheumatic fever varies from 30% to 80% of cases. In recent years there has been a decline in the severity of rheumatic fever attacks, incidence of associated carditis, and frequency of residual cardiac disease.[3,10,11,12]

Patients who develop an abnormal heart murmur during the initial attack of rheumatic fever must be considered to have rheumatic heart disease until proved otherwise. Patients who have both an abnormal murmur and congestive heart failure during the initial attack will have significant rheumatic heart disease. About 20% of them will die within 10 years after the initial rheumatic fever attack.[3] In general, the susceptibility to recurrent attacks of rheumatic fever is in direct relation to the severity of heart damage, and susceptibility decreases as the patient becomes older. During the first rheumatic fever attack, carditis is often not detected because of its own clinical manifestations but is found by the physician because the patient seeks medical attention for arthritis, chorea, or fever.

Laboratory findings

The urine is usually normal in rheumatic fever, although trace amounts of albumin may be found during the febrile period. If the acute attack of rheumatic fever is prolonged, anemia as well as leukocytosis may be present. The sedimentation rate of the blood usually increases during the acute phase of the disease. As clinical improvement is made, the sedimentation rate decreases and usually returns to normal. The C-reactive protein content of the blood is measured. Its appearance and increase in amount correlate with the presence of a bacterial infection and are not specific for rheumatic fever. The C-reactive protein level is very useful for judging the degree of rheumatic activity. A high ASO titer that falls during the convalescent period is an important finding that confirms the presence of a previous group A streptococcal infection. Throat culture for group A streptococcal organisms also is helpful. However, as mentioned previously, a negative culture does not rule out the presence of rheumatic fever. No single laboratory test establishes the diagnosis of rheumatic fever. The most important factors in establishing the diagnosis of rheumatic fever are the presence of various combinations of the following clinical manifestations of rheumatic fever: polyarthritis,

the abdomen may develop as a result of liver congestion and distention of the hepatic capsule. Pulmonary congestion may cause a nonproductive cough. Swelling of the ankles and distention of neck veins may occur. About 5% to 10% of the patients may have epistaxis secondary to cardiac involvement.

Definite evidence of carditis occurs in about half of the patients having their first attack of rheumatic fever. Patients who have carditis during the first attack are much more prone to develop recurrent attacks of rheumatic fever than those with no carditis. Patients who do not develop carditis during the first attack usually remain free of rheumatic heart disease thereafter unless they suffer additional attacks of rheumatic fever.

The incidence of significant cardiac damage (rheumatic heart disease) following the initial at-

carditis, chorea, erythema marginatum, subcutaneous nodules, and recurrent attacks supported by positive laboratory tests (increased sedimentation rate, presence of C-reactive protein, and ASO titer above 100.

MEDICAL MANAGEMENT

Medical treatment of rheumatic fever usually starts with a large dose of penicillin G benzathine given by injection to eradicate group A streptococcal bacteria from the throat, even if these have not been cultured (increased antibody titer to one or more of the antigens found on the bacteria, however, would have been demonstrated). Bed rest has no proved value and in many cases may be psychologically deleterious. Patients with very severe cardiac involvement will, in general, limit their own activity.[10,11,12]

Patients without carditis are treated by codeine or salicylates if they have symptoms of arthritis. Patients with evidence of carditis are treated with large doses of either salicylates or corticosteroids. Some physicians will start with salicylates and, if symptoms do not improve, change to corticosteroids. Other physicians begin directly with the steroids.

Many physicians will place all of their patients who have rheumatic fever on an antibiotic regimen for a minimum of 5 years to prevent recurrent attacks of streptococcal infections. Many physicians also will continue this prophylactic coverage until the patient is 25 years of age. They will then discontinue this coverage for patients who have had no sign or symptoms of carditis, but continue it indefinitely for those who have had cardiac involvement. Patients who have their first attack at age 20 years or later will usually be given coverage for a 5-year period. In cases in which there is evidence of cardiac involvement, this coverage period would be extended.

The prophylactic regimen used to prevent recurrent streptococcal infection in patients who have had a recent attack of rheumatic fever consists of one or the following:

1. Penicillin G benzathine, 1.2 million units
2. Oral sulfadiazine, 1 g per day
3. Oral penicillin (penicillin G potassium or penicillin V), 500 mg per day

These dose levels, however, are not sufficient to prevent endocarditis in patients who have cardiac damage resulting from a rheumatic fever attack. These patients will require additional antibiotics during dental manipulations to protect them from infective endocarditis.

Rheumatic heart disease

The cardiac damage that results from an acute attack of rheumatic fever is called rheumatic heart disease. It usually involves damage of the mitral or aortic valve. The scarring and calcification that occur in the affected valve may result in stenosis or regurgitation.

GENERAL DESCRIPTION
Incidence

Bland and Jones[3] give one of the best insights into the incidence of rheumatic heart disease following acute rheumatic fever attacks. In this study 1000 patients were followed up for at least 20 years or until they died. These patients were admitted to the Good Samaritan Hospital in Boston with acute rheumatic fever. The study was started in 1921, and the last new patient was added in 1931. The study was concluded in 1951.

The most common symptom of rheumatic fever found in these patients was carditis, followed by chorea, arthritis, arthralgia, subcutaneous nodules, and erythema marginatum. By the end of the study 301 patients were dead. The most common causes of death were congestive heart failure (231 patients) and infective endocarditis (30 patients).

Patients who had symptoms of either an enlarged heart or congestive heart failure during the acute attack of rheumatic fever had the poorest prognosis. Of the 70 patients who had heart enlargement, 56 were dead within 10 years and 57 within 20 years. Of the 207 patients who had initial congestive heart failure, 148 were dead within 10 years and 152 within 20 years.

However, patients who developed chorea during the acute attack had a much better prognosis. Only 63 of the 518 patients who had this symptom were dead by the end of 20 years.

Following the initial acute rheumatic fever attack, 653 patients showed clinical evidence of rheumatic heart disease. In contrast, 347 patients showed no early evidence of rheumatic heart disease, but by the end of the study 154 of these showed clinical evidence of the disease. An interesting observation was that chorea was a prominent feature in most of these 154 patients.

Thus by the end of the study 301 patients were free of any clinical evidence of rheumatic heart disease; 193 of these patients never developed any clinical evidence of the disease, and 108 had clinical evidence at one time but by the end of the study showed no evidence of the disease. Depending on how one looks at these data, the incidence of rheumatic heart disease could be said to be as low as 69% (based on patient status at the end of the study) or as high as 81% (based on presence of rheumatic heart disease at any time during the study).

Another interesting question that these data raise is whether there is significant scarring in the heart valves of those patients who lost any clinical evidence of rheumatic heart disease. In other words, would these individuals be susceptible later to infective endocarditis even though they showed no clinical evidence of rheumatic heart disease?

Etiology

Rheumatic heart disease develops as a sequela to acute rheumatic fever. The primary lesion in rheumatic heart disease is valvular deformity with associated compensatory changes in the size of the cardiac chambers and the thickness of their walls. Primary myocardial lesions occur but usually are of no clinical significance. A history of an acute attack of rheumatic fever is not obtained from all patients who have rheumatic heart disease. This may be explained by subclinical attacks that some patients may experience or by missed diagnosis of the rheumatic fever episode.

Pathophysiology and complications

The basic lesions in rheumatic heart disease consist of valvular changes, myocardial changes, and pericardial changes. Rheumatic nodules may involve just the endocardium of the valve or its entire thickness. The eventual outcome of the valve disease is accumulation of scar tissue and deformity of the valve. This interferes with function and, if the interference is significant, can lead

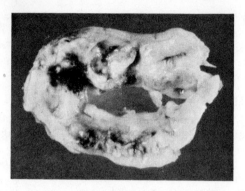

FIG. 3-4. Stenosis of mitral valve as result of rheumatic fever. (Courtesy W. O'Conner, M.D., Lexington, Ky.)

to congestive heart failure. The edges of valve cusps may be fused together with resulting stenosis of the valve opening (Fig. 3-4). All four heart valves may show microscopic evidence of rheumatic activity, however, functional impairment is most common in the mitral valve, followed by the aortic valve, and, much less commonly, the tricuspid valve. Calcification of the injured cusps is common.[2,4,8]

The most common valvular defect resulting from rheumatic fever is mitral stenosis. Incompetence of the aortic valve is the next most common. Aortic stenosis is less common. Lesions of the valves are more severe on the left side of the heart because of the greater strain placed on these valves. Mitral valve lesions are more common in women, and aortic valve lesions are more common in men. The damaged valves are susceptible to infective endocarditis.

The typical myocardial lesion is the Aschoff nodule (a focus of fibrinoid degeneration surrounded by a granulomatous inflammatory response) (Fig. 3-5). Depending on the amount of inflammation during the attack of rheumatic fever, there will be varying degrees of myocardial destruction. If inflammation is great, myocardial destruction will be great and congestive heart failure may develop. If destruction is less, the damage will be repaired by fibrous connective tissue.

Rheumatic fever is the commonest cause of acute pericarditis, which is serofibrinous inflam-

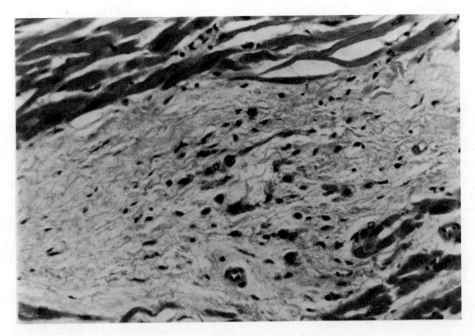

FIG. 3-5. Photomicrograph of Aschoff nodule. (Courtesy J.E. Edwards, M.D., St. Paul, Minn.)

mation of the pericardium. If the reaction is severe, a chronic, adherent pericarditis may develop.

CLINICAL PRESENTATION
Signs and symptoms

The clinical signs and symptoms found in patients who have rheumatic heart disease are usually associated with the valve disease and its effect on the heart. A murmur may be heard if the valve disease is sufficient to alter the function of the valve. This may be the only sign of rheumatic heart disease for a number of years. As the compensatory ability of the heart is exceeded, chamber dilation and hypertrophy may occur. Exertional dyspnea, angina pectoris, epistaxis, blood in the sputum, and congestive heart failure may then occur[2,4,8] (Table 3-1).

Laboratory findings

The diagnosis of rheumatic heart disease is made at two levels. At the first is the patient who is asymptomatic but has a murmur that indicates valvular damage. This type of patient also may show cardiac enlargement on chest radiograms and

TABLE 3-1. Signs and symptoms of rheumatic heart disease

Exertional dyspnea
Angina pectoris
Congestive heart failure
Epistaxis
Blood in sputum
Murmur
Electrocardiogram changes
Enlarged heart

electrocardiogram changes that suggest hypertrophy of the left ventricular wall. This type of patient may or may not give a history of rheumatic fever. The second type of patient has clinical symptoms of rheumatic heart disease and is usually much easier to identify.

Any patient with a history of rheumatic fever needs to be evaluated for the presence of rheumatic heart disease before dental treatment is begun. This evaluation may consist of communication with the physician who has followed up the patient since the rheumatic fever attack or evaluation by a physician to whom the patient is now going or would like to be referred. The presence or absence of rheumatic heart disease in the patient who has a history of rheumatic fever is best established by (1) history of symptoms, (2) chest x-ray films, (3) electrocardiogram, and (4) good physical evaluation, including auscultation of the heart.

MEDICAL MANAGEMENT

The patient who has asymptomatic rheumatic heart disease requires no medical treatment other than prevention of recurrent attacks of rheumatic fever and prevention of infective endocarditis. The patient who has congestive heart failure is managed as described in the section on congestive heart failure (see p. 120). This patient may be treated by the surgical removal of the damaged valve and the placement of an artificial valve.

DENTAL MANAGEMENT
Medical considerations

The basic problem that confronts the dentist when he or she is dealing with patients who have a history of rheumatic fever is whether or not rheumatic heart disease is present. If the patient has rheumatic heart disease, antibiotic prophylaxis is indicated to prevent infective endocarditis. If rheumatic heart disease is not present, the patient is not considered to be susceptible to endocarditis and does not require antibiotic prophylaxis.

Detection of patients with rheumatic heart disease

A medical history should be obtained from each patient before any dental manipulations are performed. Patients are asked if they are under the care of a physician at the present time. If they are, the nature of the problem being treated and the way it is being treated are established. Patients are asked if they have ever had rheumatic fever, rheumatic heart disease, or a heart murmur. The medical history is reviewed to see, among other things, if the patient has ever had a condition suggestive of rheumatic fever for which medical attention was not sought. An inquiry is made concerning the presence of signs or symptoms suggestive of rheumatic fever, rheumatic heart disease, and congestive heart failure.

The patient's physician's name, address, and phone number are recorded in the dental record. Any medications the patient is taking or has taken during the last year also are recorded. Of particular interest is the patient who may be taking prophylactic antibiotics to prevent recurrent upper respiratory streptococcal infections and thereby reduce the risk of recurrent rheumatic fever attacks.

The dentist is not qualified by training to examine a patient for many of the signs of rheumatic heart disease other than the gross signs associated with congestive heart failure—distention of neck veins and swelling of the ankles. These signs, however, usually do not develop until later in the course of this disease. Therefore, in general, the physical examination will be of very little aid to the dentist in identifying the patient with rheumatic heart disease.

Grouping of patients according to risk of rheumatic heart disease

Based on the findings of the medical history interview and, to a limited extent, the physical examination, four separate groups of patients can be identified who have or may have had rheumatic heart disease. These patients will require additional attention before examination or treatment procedures are begun. These four groups are listed here and summarized in Table 3-2.

Group I Patients with history of illness that could have been rheumatic fever, but physician was not sought at time of illness.

Subgroup 1A At least 20 years* have passed since illness, and patient has been free of any clinical evidence of rheumatic heart disease.

ACTION: Treat as normal patient and continue with examination and treatment.

Subgroup 1B Less than 20 years have passed since illness.

ACTION: Refer for medical evaluation concerning presence of rheumatic heart disease. If found, patient should be administered prophylactic antibiotics before further examination procedures and treatment are performed. If no evidence is found, patient would be managed as normal patient.

---

*This is an arbitrary time interval that has taken into account the probability of the original disease having been rheumatic fever and a significant period of time having elapsed with the patient remaining free of symptoms.

TABLE 3-2. Management of the dental patient with a history of rheumatic fever

Group 1 Patients with history of illness that could have been rheumatic fever, but physician was not sought at time of illness.

Twenty years since—if no evidence of rheumatic heart disease, no coverage.

Less than 20 years—if no evidence of rheumatic heart disease, refer for medical evaluation; if rheumatic heart disease is found, give coverage.

Current signs and symptoms of rheumatic heart disease—refer and give coverage.

Group 2 Patient gives history of having heart murmur but does not know cause.

Confirm presence and nature of murmur by consultation with patient's physician.

Refer to establish presence and nature of murmur.

Give coverage to all patients who have murmurs thought to be pathologic.

Group 3 Patient with history of illness that was diagnosed by physician as rheumatic fever.

No medical follow-up for rheumatic heart disease—refer, give coverage if rheumatic heart disease is found.

Medical follow-up and reported free of rheumatic heart disease—confirm with physician.

Medical follow-up and reported to have rheumatic heart disease (asymptomatic)—confirm with physician, then give coverage.

Group 4 Patients who have been treated for symptoms of rheumatic heart disease by physician.

Congestive heart failure caused by rheumatic heart disease—consult and give coverage.

Rheumatic heart disease with possible subacute infective endocarditis—consult and give coverage.

Open heart surgery—if valve replacement, consult and give coverage.

Subgroup 1C History of possible rheumatic fever and current signs and symptoms suggesting rheumatic heart disease.

ACTION: Refer for medical evaluation and treatment. Afterwards, patient returns for dental treatment and is given antibiotic coverage during all examination and treatment procedures. Patient's physician should be consulted before development of final dental treatment plan so that patient's current medical status can be taken into account.

Group II Patient gives history of having heart murmur but does not know cause.

ACTION: Refer for medical consultation. If murmur is confirmed and *thought to be pathologic*, patient must be given antibiotic coverage just before and after any dental treatment.

Group III Patient with history of illness that was diagnosed by physician as rheumatic fever.

Subgroup IIIA No medical follow-up since original illness: presence or absence of rheumatic heart disease not known.

ACTION: Refer to physician for evaluation. Patients found to have rheumatic heart disease would be given antibiotic coverage before further examination or treatment procedures. If for some reason medical evaluation cannot be obtained, these patients are considered to have rheumatic heart disease until proved otherwise and should be placed on prophylactic antibiotic coverage during the day of dental treatment and 2 days following.

Subgroup IIIB Patients who have been followed up by physician since rheumatic fever attack and are free of any evidence of rheumatic heart disease.

ACTION: To confirm this, call or write physician concerning medical history, diagnosis, absence of rheumatic heart disease, and his or her opinion concerning need for antibiotic coverage during dental manipulations. If no evidence of rheumatic heart disease is present, most physicians would not recommend antibiotic protection.

Subgroup IIIC Patients who have been followed up since rheumatic fever attack and have been found by physician to have asymptomatic rheumatic heart disease.

ACTION: Write or call physician to confirm presence of rheumatic heart disease and suggest antibiotic coverage during all examination and treatment procedures. Ask for comments concerning medical status and management.

Group IV Patients who have been treated for symptoms of rheumatic heart disease by physician.

Subgroup IVA Patients who have received medical treatment for congestive heart failure caused by rheumatic heart disease.

ACTION: Contact patient's physician to establish patient's current medical status. If congestive failure is under control and physician agrees with antibiotic coverage plan suggested, proceed with antibiotic regimen and examination and treatment procedures. Patients who, according to their physician, are not under good medical control should not be treated until their medical status improves or physician requests completion of dental treatment before open heart surgery.

Subgroup IVB Patients with rheumatic heart disease who have had infective endocarditis.

ACTION: Contact patient's physician to establish patient's current medical status and need for antibiotic coverage. Again, patients not under good medical control should not be treated until their medical status improves or physician requests completion of dental treatment before open heart surgery.

Subgroup IVC Patients who have had open heart surgery to replace damaged heart valve with artificial one.

ACTION: More vigorous steps are needed to protect these patients. If infective endocarditis does develop around artificial heart valve it most likely will be fatal, because necrotic tissue cannot retain sutures that hold artificial valve in place.

Specific dental management

No dental examination or treatment procedures should be performed on patients suspected of having rheumatic heart disease without antibiotic coverage or until they have been determined to be free of the disease by medical consultation or referral. Dental procedures should not be performed on patients with rheumatic heart disease who show signs and symptoms of congestive heart failure until consultation with a physician.

Once the need for prophylactic antibiotics has been determined, and the patient is free of significant evidence of congestive heart failure, regimen A is recommended for patients receiving either routine or emergency dental care (see Chapter 8).

In general, we suggest that the oral route of administration for the antibiotic be selected whenever possible because of its lower incidence of causing allergic sensitivity[13] (see Chapter 19).

Treatment planning modifications

Patients with rheumatic heart disease who show no evidence of congestive heart failure can receive any indicated dental care as long as they are protected by antibiotics against infective endocarditis. The usual coverage period is 3 days, and dental treatment is rendered only on the first day of the coverage period (see Chapter 2). The dentist should plan to do as much treatment as possible on the first day so that the patient's dental treatment will not be spread out over too long a time and the number of necessary coverage periods can be kept to a minimum.

The patient should receive prophylactic antibiotic coverage for all dental procedures, including certain examination procedures such as periodontal probing.

Certain types of dental treatment do not fit very well into a 3-day coverage program, for example, surgical procedures in which sutures have been placed, crown and bridge construction, orthodontic banding, and surgical procedures in areas in which healing has been delayed for some reason.

We would suggest that for cases in which sutures have been placed the coverage period be extended by several days. The patient can be seen on the fifth or sixth day after surgery, while he is still receiving prophylactic antibiotics, for suture removal. In cases in which surgical wounds are not healing in a normal manner, the coverage period should be extended.

With proper planning, crowns and bridges can be constructed for patients with rheumatic heart disease. During one coverage period the preparations can be made, impressions taken, and temporaries placed. Then a new coverage period can be used for the insertion of the crowns or bridges.

Orthodontic patients who have rheumatic heart disease should be given antibiotic coverage during the placement and removal of bands. However, they do not need coverage when wearing the bands.

Children with rheumatic heart disease who are in the process of losing deciduous teeth in a natural way are not given antibiotic coverage. They are given coverage if the teeth are being extracted.

Patients with rheumatic heart disease who have poor oral hygiene may be started on a concentrated 5- to 7-day program for improving their oral status. The patient should be given antibiotic coverage and gross calculus removal should be performed on the first day, followed by brushing and flossing instructions. If the patient has made good progress and the oral hygiene has improved, the risk of serious problems associated with hygiene procedures will be greatly reduced. It is impractical to provide antibiotic coverage for such individuals all the time, but it does seem reasonable to do so for 5 to 7 days in an attempt to get rid of gross calculus and gingival inflammation. If patients fail to demonstrate the interest or ability or both to maintain good oral hygiene, they should be encouraged to consider dentures.

If the coverage period is extended to 5 to 7 days and penicillin is being used as the antibiotic, the dentist can switch to erythromycin halfway through the coverage period to avoid the potential problem of penicillin-resistant bacteria being released into the bloodstream. However, under usual circumstances this would not appear to be indicated (Chapter 2). This modification was not mentioned in the 1977 report of the American Heart Association.

Edentulous patients who have rheumatic heart disease should be given antibiotic coverage during surgical procedures needed to prepare the mouth for dentures and at the time of insertion of the dentures. Overextended areas should be corrected and sore spots allowed to heal while the patient is receiving antibiotic coverage.

Emergency dental care

Patients with rheumatic heart disease who are free of congestive heart failure can receive any indicated emergency dental care as long as they are administered antibiotic therapy to protect them from infective endocarditis.

Heart murmurs

One of the more confusing problems that can face a dentist is evaluating a patient who has a history of a heart murmur and deciding when antibiotic prophylaxis is necessary. Dentists for the most part are not trained to detect or evaluate heart murmurs; therefore it is necessary to rely on our physician colleagues to perform these tasks. To enhance understanding of what murmurs are and to facilitate communication with physicians on the subject, the following information is presented.

Murmurs are nothing more than sounds caused by turbulence in the circulation through the valves and chambers of the heart. Turbulence in flow is usually the result of an increased flow rate, a change in viscosity, stenotic or narrowed valves or vessels, dilated valves or vessels, or a vibration of membranous structures such as the valve leaflets.[1] Innocent or functional murmurs are sounds caused by turbulence in the absence of any cardiac abnormality and do not require antibiotic prophylaxis. Organic murmurs are sounds caused by a pathologic abnormality in the heart and do require antibiotic prophylaxis.

Murmurs are described on the basis of their occurrence during the cardiac cycle (systole, diastole, or continuous), their loudness or intensity on a scale of I to VI, the location on the chest wall in which they are best heard, and whether they radiate or are localized. Therefore a common description of a functional murmur would be a grade II/VI (read "two over six") systolic ejection murmur best heard at the pulmonic area that does not radiate.

Interpretation of murmurs is not always easy for physicians. A combination of history, physical examination, chest x-ray films, electrocardiogram, and laboratory tests may be needed to make a final judgment. Diastolic murmurs are almost always organic in nature and therefore pathologic. Systolic murmurs may be organic or functional.[1] The physician must make that judgment.

Two examples of common innocent or functional murmurs that require no antibiotic prophylaxis are murmurs that occur during childhood and murmurs that occur during pregnancy. Murmurs discovered during childhood are extremely common, and in fact almost every child will have one at some time. These murmurs are usually detected between the ages of 3 and 7 years and subsequently disappear by adolescence.[5,7] It is felt that these murmurs probably result from an increase in flow rate combined with a thin chest wall that enhances normal flow sounds.

Pregnant women commonly develop a murmur that is probably caused by the significant increase in blood volume and resulting cardiac output. These murmurs disappear shortly after delivery as the cardiovascular system returns to its normal status.

In both the cases of a childhood murmur and a murmur during pregnancy, an innocent murmur is classically reported only during that period with disappearance on subsequent examinations. Pre-existing murmurs or murmurs that have persisted (into adulthood or after pregnancy) may be organic and require premedication.

Whenever a patient reports a history of heart murmur, it is recommended that the physician (preferably a cardiologist) be consulted for a definitive judgment, even in cases of murmurs that are probably innocent.

REFERENCES

1. American Heart Association Publication #51-014, A: innocent heart murmurs in children, 1969.
2. Barrett, M.J.: Valvular heart disease. In Rose, L.F., and Kaye, D., editors: Internal medicine for dentistry, St. Louis, 1983, The C.V. Mosby Co., pp. 510-516.
3. Bland, E.F., and Jones, T.D.: Rheumatic fever and rheumatic heart disease, Circulation **4:**836-843, 1951.
4. Braunwald, E.: Valvular heart disease. In Petersdorf, R.G., et al., editors: Harrison's principles of internal medicine, ed. 10, New York, 1983, McGraw-Hill Book Co., pp. 1402-1418.
5. Delp, M.H., and Manning, R.T.: Major's physical diagnosis: an introduction to the clinical process, ed. 9, Philadelphia, 1981, W.B. Saunders Co.
6. Kannel, W.B.: Incidence, prevalence, and mortality of cardiovascular disease. In Hurst, J.W., editor: The heart, ed. 5, New York, 1983, McGraw-Hill Book Co., pp. 621-629.
7. Kulangara, R.J., et al.: Differential diagnosis of heart murmurs in children, Postgrad. Med. **72:**219-228, 1982.
8. Rackley, C.E.: Valvular disease. In Hurst, J.W., editor: The heart, ed. 5, New York, 1983, McGraw-Hill Book Co., pp. 863-935.
9. Rose, L.F., Godfrey, P., and Steinberg, B.J.: Dental correlations. In Rose, L.F., and Kaye, D., editors: Internal medicine for dentistry, St. Louis, 1983, The C.V. Mosby Co., pp. 571-586.
10. Santoro, J.: Streptococcal infections and rheumatic fever. In Rose, L.F., and Kaye, D., editors: Internal medicine for dentistry, St. Louis, 1983, The C.V. Mosby Co., pp. 222-228.
11. Stollerman, G.H.: Rheumatic fever. In Petersdorf, R.G., et al., editors: Harrison's principles of internal medicine, ed. 10, New York, 1983, McGraw-Hill Book Co., pp. 1397-1402.
12. Stollerman, G.H.: Acute rheumatic fever and its management. In Hurst, J.W., editor: The heart, ed. 5, 1983, New York, McGraw-Hill Book Co., pp. 854-863.
13. Weinstein, L.: Chemotherapy of microbial diseases. In Goodman, L.S., and Gilman, A., editors: The pharmacological basis of therapeutics, ed. 5, New York, 1975, Macmillan Publishing Co., Inc., pp. 1090-1224.

4

CONGENITAL HEART DISEASE

There are three major types of congenital heart malformation. One type includes malformations with initial left-to-right shunting of blood—atrial septal defect, ventricular septal defect, and patent ductus arteriosus. The second group consists of malformations of the heart with initial right-to-left shunting of blood—transposition of great vessels, persistent truncus arteriosus, and tetralogy of Fallot. The third includes malformations that obstruct blood flow—pulmonary stenosis and coarctation of the aorta.[1,2,5]

In general, lesions that shunt blood from left to right do not result in clinical evidence of cyanosis unless myocardial failure or pulmonary hypertension develops.[1,2] Conditions that shunt blood from right to left will cause significant cyanosis. Thus it is important to differentiate between cyanosis that has been present since birth and cyanosis that developed following cardiac failure or pulmonary hypertension.

The prime concern of the dentist when dealing with a patient with congenital heart disease is the prevention of infective endocarditis and endarteritis, because many of the defects are susceptible to these complications. Patients with polycythemia may be thrombocytopenic and have depleted plasma coagulation factors as a result of thrombosis in small vessels. They may have significant bleeding problems following scaling or surgical procedures and must be identified and receive special attention before any dental treatment. In addition, the patient with congenital heart disease should be evaluated for the presence of pulmonary edema and cardiac failure, and, if these are present, the patient should be referred to a physician.

GENERAL DESCRIPTION
Incidence

Congenital heart disease occurs in about 0.5% of all live births. The incidence increases to about 1.0% in newborns, if stillborn infants and those with multiple defects who do not survive the first month are included.[1-3] Congenital heart disease constitutes 1% to 3% of all cases of heart disease after infancy.[2] When the complexity of the development of the heart and great vessels is considered, it is a wonder that the incidence of abnormal development is so low.

There are approximately 4 to 5 million live births per year in the United States and about 25,000 new cases of clinical congenital heart disease per year.[1,5]

The most common defect that causes cyanosis at birth and in infancy is tetralogy of Fallot, which consists of a high ventricular septal defect, pulmonary stenosis, dextroposed aorta, and right ventricular hypertrophy. About 70% of blue babies have tetralogy of Fallot.[2,5]

Patency of the foramen ovale is the most common and clinically least important of all congenital cardiac anomalies. The foramen ovale, an embryonic opening in the atrial septum, remains patent in about 25% of people, but in most cases the opening is very small and oblique, thus little blood is allowed to flow through the opening.[2,5] Large defects are much more rare and are found in females about four times more often than in males.

Over 90% of the patients who have congenital heart disease fall into one of the following groups. The most common significant anomaly is septal defect, followed by coarctation of the aorta, patent

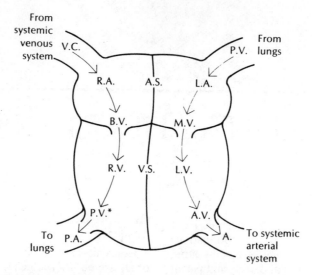

FIG. 4-1. Normal blood flow through the chambers of the heart, valves, and great vessels. *VC,* Vena cava; *RA,* right atrium; *BV,* bicuspid valve; *RV,* right ventricle; *PV*,* pulmonary valve; *PA,* pulmonary artery; *PV,* pulmonary vein; *LA,* left atrium; *MV,* mitral valve; *LV,* left ventricle; *AV,* aortic valve; *A,* aorta; *AS,* atrial septum; *VS,* ventricular septum.

ductus arteriosus (an embryonic channel from the pulmonary artery to the aorta), and tetralogy of Fallot.

Etiology

The cause of congenital heart disease generally is unknown.[1-4] The effect of rubella in the mother during early development of the embryo is well known as a cause of abnormal cardiac development. However, less than 2% of patients with congenital heart disease have this history. Fetal hypoxia, fetal endocarditis, immunologic abnormalities, and vitamin deficiencies have all been suggested as causes of congenital heart defects.[1-3] In addition, drugs taken by the mother during pregnancy may have some influence on congenital heart disease that develops in the fetus. For example, some of the thalidomide babies developed heart defects.

With few exceptions, patients with congenital heart disease have a negative familial history for congenital cardiac malformations. However, patent ductus arteriosus has been reported to occur in successive generations.[2]

Defects of the atrial septum and patency of the ductus arteriosus are more common in females.

Pulmonary stenosis and ventricular septal defects show little sex predilection. Coarctation of the aorta and congenital aortic stenosis are much more common in males.

Pathophysiology and complications

The physiologic effects of most of the congenital cardiac defects are a result of the shunting of blood. Left-to-right shunts result in the recirculation of blood that has flowed through the lungs. The blood that reaches the systemic capillaries is saturated with oxygen; thus cyanosis is not present. Under these conditions the pulmonary blood flow is about 12 to 15 liters per minute and the systemic flow about 4 to 5 liters per minute. The ratio of pulmonary to systemic flow can reach as high as 20:1 with large left-to-right shunts (Figs. 4-1 and 4-2).

When the shunt is at the atrial or ventricular level the right ventricle must work much harder, and this may lead to ventricular dilation and hypertrophy. If the shunt is at the pulmonary artery level, as with patent ductus arteriosus (without pulmonary hypertension), the left ventricle must work harder and will eventually undergo dilation and hypertrophy. If pulmonary hypertension de-

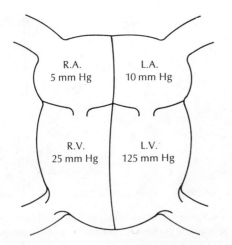

FIG. 4-2. Normal atrial and ventricular pressures.

TABLE 4-1. Complications of congenital heart disease

Infective endocarditis (or endarteritis)
Pulmonary edema
Cardiac failure
Decreased oxygen content of arterial blood
Thrombosis
Bleeding, fibrinogen depletion, thrombocytopenia
Brain abscesses

velops, right ventricular dilation and hypertrophy may also develop.

When venous blood from the systemic circulation enters the left heart chambers before passing through the lung, as in the right-to-left shunt, the functional effect is to reduce the partial pressure of oxygen in the arterial systemic blood. This leads to a need for greater blood flow and increases the work of both ventricles. The clinical results of right-to-left shunting of blood are primarily caused by the undersaturation with oxygen of the arterial blood.

If the arterial blood contains 5 g/100 ml or more of unsaturated hemoglobin, cyanosis will be present. In congenital heart disease early cyanosis indicates right-to-left shunting of blood.

The body attempts to compensate for the low oxygen content in the arterial system by polycythemia (increased numbers of red blood cells) and increased blood flow. The polycythemia may result in a hematocrit of 50% to 80% and increases the total blood volume and viscosity. This leads to increased work for the heart. Patients with severe polycythemia are most prone to thromboses and must avoid dehydration. The thromboses may cause infarctions in vital organs. Red blood cell precursors may replace platelet precursors in the bone marrow, thus leading to thrombocytopenia. The thromboses can lead to depletion of the fibrin-

ogen level; therefore the patient may have bleeding tendencies as a result of either or both of these effects, thrombocytopenia and hypofibrinogenemia.

Many patients with long-standing right-to-left shunts develop clubbing of the fingers and, in some cases, the toes. The etiology of the clubbing is unknown but may be caused by the increased blood flow in patients with cyanotic congenital heart disease. The terminal phalanges and nail beds are affected.

Pulmonary hypertension may develop in patients with congenital heart disease because of increased pulmonary blood flow or increased pulmonary arteriolar resistance. In left-to-right shunts pulmonary flow may increase more than five times the normal amount. The significance of pulmonary hypertension depends on the duration, site, and size of the cardiovascular defect and the amount of vasoconstriction present in the lung fields.

Pulmonary hypertension can lead to right ventricular hypertrophy, enlargement of the pulmonary artery, and development of cyanosis in patients with shunts that were initially left to right but changed to right to left because of the increased pulmonary resistance or myocardial failure or both.

The complications of congenital heart disease are many and significant[1,2,5] (Table 4-1). Patients tend to have a lowered resistance to infection. Of all cases of infective endocarditis, 10% are found in patients with congenital heart disease. Patients with ventricular septal defects and deformities of the aortic valve are most prone to endocarditis. Patients with patent ductus arteriosus and coarctation of the aorta are prone to endarteritis, which carries the same grave prognosis as endocarditis.

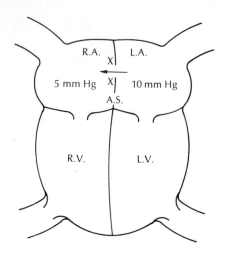

FIG. 4-3. Atrial septal defect resulting in left-to-right shunt; x indicates area most prone to infective endocarditis.

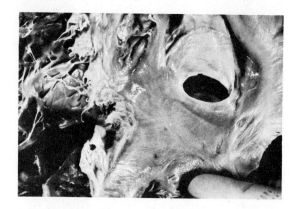

FIG. 4-4. Postmortem specimen of heart with large atrial septal defect. (Courtesy W. O'Conner, M.D., Lexington, Ky.)

Patients with small atrial septal defects do not appear to be prone to develop endocarditis.

Patients with right-to-left shunting of blood are prone to develop thromboses and may have bleeding tendencies, as indicated previously. They also are susceptible to increased frequency of brain abscesses, because infectious materials are not filtered by the lung. Any congenital heart disease patient who develops unexplained fever with headaches should be evaluated for a possible brain abscess.

Specific congenital heart defects
ATRIAL SEPTAL DEFECTS

Atrial septal defects, which include patent foramen ovale, are the most common congenital lesions of the heart (Figs. 4-3 and 4-4). The clinical effects depend on the size of the defect and the volume of blood shunted. Growth and development of the affected person usually are normal. Cyanosis and pulmonary hypertension develop only late in the course of the disease, if at all. Early symptoms are dyspnea, fatigue, and paroxysmal atrial tachycardia. Blood is usually shunted from left to right with this defect. The right atrium and ventricle may become enlarged, and right ventricular hypertrophy may develop. The pulmonary artery may become dilated.

VENTRICULAR SEPTAL DEFECT

Ventricular septal defect is the second most common congenital heart lesion (Fig. 4-5). Nine out of every ten patients with a ventricular septal defect will have some other cardiac anomaly. This most commonly is pulmonary stenosis. Blood is usually shunted from left to right unless pulmonary hypertension, pulmonary stenosis, or myocardial failure is present.

PATENT DUCTUS ARTERIOSUS

The fetal connection between the pulmonary artery and aorta that allows the fetal blood to bypass the lungs usually closes by the age of 2 years. This connection arises at the bifurcation of the pulmonary artery and ends in the aorta, usually just beyond the opening of the left subclavian artery.

If the ductus arteriosus remains patent, left-to-right shunting occurs (Fig. 4-6). A temporary reversal of blood flow may occur because of crying or violent physical activity. If pulmonary hypertension or heart failure develops, right-to-left shunting occurs, with the development of cyanosis.

TRANSPOSITION OF GREAT VESSELS

In transposition of great vessels the aortic root opens into the right ventricle and the pulmonary artery into the left ventricle. If no other anomaly is present to allow for blood flow from one circula-

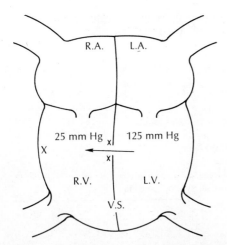

FIG. 4-5. Ventricular septal defect resulting in left-to-right shunt; x indicates area most prone to infective endocarditis.

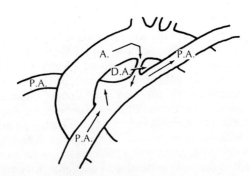

FIG. 4-6. Patent ductus arteriosus. *DA,* Ductus arteriosus—connection between aorta, *A,* and pulmonary artery, *PA,* resulting in blood flow from aorta into pulmonary artery.

tion to the other, this condition is not compatible with life.

PERSISTENT TRUNCUS ARTERIOSUS

In persistent truncus arteriosus a high ventricular septal defect is present, with blood flowing from both ventricles into a common trunk. The pulmonary artery branches from the common trunk. Patients with this defect will be cyanotic from birth.

TETRALOGY OF FALLOT

As mentioned earlier, tetralogy of Fallot consists of pulmonary stenosis, ventricular septal defect, dextroposition of the aorta, and right ventricular hypertrophy (Fig. 4-7). With extreme pulmonary stenosis, the ductus arteriosus must remain patent for life. If not, the Blalock-Taussig operation can be performed to bypass the obstructive lesion of pulmonary stenosis by making an artificial ductus arteriosus. The preferred treatment, when possible, is to correct the ventricular septal defect and pulmonary stenosis.

PULMONARY STENOSIS

Pure pulmonary stenosis reduces the pulmonary blood flow and leads to right ventricular dilation and hypertrophy and eventually to myocardial fail-

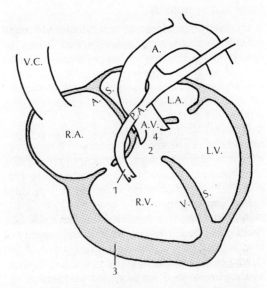

FIG. 4-7. Anatomic relationships in tetralogy of Fallot. *1,* Pulmonary stenosis; *2,* high ventricular septal defect; *3,* hypertrophied right ventricle; *4,* dextropositioned aorta (over the septum).

ure. Exertional dyspnea usually precedes the appearance of cyanosis in the patient. Once cyanosis has appeared, the entire symptom complex becomes much more severe.

COARCTATION OF AORTA

Coarctation of the aorta consists of a narrowing of the aorta in the region where it is joined by the ductus arteriosus. Two types of coarctation are found. In the infantile type, which usually is not compatible with life, the aortic constriction is proximal to the ductus arteriosus (between the ductus and left subclavian artery). In the adult type the constriction is at or distal to the ductus, which is usually obliterated. The adult type of coarctation leads to severe hypertension in the upper body and may lead to cardiac failure or cerebral hemorrhage. Endarteritis may develop at the site of coarctation. Aneurysms may form near the coarctation, and the aorta may rupture. The lower body obtains its blood flow by way of a greatly dilated collateral system. One half of patients with the adult form of coarctation will be dead by the age of 40 years unless they have surgery.

CLINICAL PRESENTATION
Signs and symptoms

Dyspnea is the most common symptom found in patients with congenital heart disease. It may be caused by overloading of the pulmonary circulation, as occurs in large atrial septal defects, or by the large amount of unoxygenated blood shunted into the systemic circulation in anomalies with right-to-left shunts.

Cyanosis occurs late in the lesions that produce initial left-to-right shunting of blood. When it occurs, it results either from pulmonary hypertension or myocardial failure. Lesions that initially produce right-to-left shunting of blood will produce cyanosis as an early sign.

Polycythemia is a condition that develops as a result of the decreased oxygen-carrying capacity of blood that has been shunted from right to left and thus has not passed through the pulmonary system. This causes a need for increased numbers of red blood cells to compensate for the decreased oxygen content.

Cerebral symptoms are common and consist of

TABLE 4-2. Signs and symptoms of congenital heart disease

Dyspnea
Cyanosis
Ruddy color, polycythemia
Clubbing of fingers or toes
Murmurs
Congestive heart failure
Distention of neck veins
Enlarged liver
Ascites
Weakness
Dizziness, syncope, coma

---

faintness, dizziness, syncope, and coma. In most cases they are caused by anoxia or thrombosis (complication of polycythemia).

Weakness is a symptom that may be secondary to the other causes of dyspnea or may be present secondary to myocardial failure (Table 4-2).

Patients with congenital heart disease may appear ruddy in color if significant polycythemia is present. Those with long-standing right-to-left shunting of blood may reveal clubbing of the fingers or toes (Fig. 4-8). Patients with high-velocity shunts will demonstrate murmurs and often associated thrills. Those who have developed myocardial failure may show distention of the neck veins, enlarged and tender liver, ascites, or other signs.

Defects that result in significant shunting will produce murmurs that can be detected by auscultation. Cardiac catheterization is done to reveal the pressure and oxygen content of the various heart chambers and great vessels. Under normal conditions little difference is noted between oxygen content of the vena cava, right atrium, right ventricle, and pulmonary artery. With a defect in the atrial septum, the oxygen content in the right atrium is higher than in the vena cava. Angiocardiography provides visualization of the chambers of the heart, aorta, and pulmonary artery so that abnormal flow patterns can be identified. Electrocardiography has limited value and is primarily used to demonstrate ventricular hypertrophy.

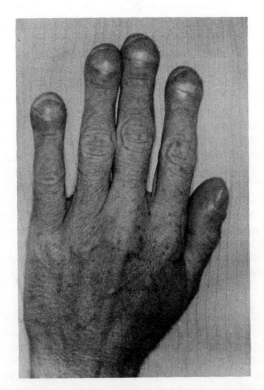

FIG. 4-8. Clubbing of fingers secondary to congenital heart disease.

MEDICAL MANAGEMENT

Successful treatment by surgical means is now available for patent ductus arteriosus, pulmonary valvular stenosis, coarctation of the aorta, atrial septal defect, ventricular septal defect, transposition of the great vessels, and valvular anomalies involving the tricuspid, mitral, and aortic valves.[4] The frequency of operative complications increases in the order in which the preceding conditions are listed. The surgical mortality for closure of patent ductus arteriosus is about 2%.[4]

Generally patients with physical signs of congenital heart disease who do not have symptoms should not undergo corrective surgery. Exceptions are patent ductus arteriosus, ventricular septal defects, and coarctation of the aorta because of the high risk of infective endocarditis or endarteritis if the defect is not corrected.

Digitalis is the keystone to therapy for patients with right or left ventricular failure. Patients with polycythemia are protected against thrombosis by anticoagulation therapy or venesection and by prevention of dehydration. (For more details concerning the management of congestive heart failure and endocarditis and endarteritis, see Chapter 2.)

The surgical correction of the adult type of coarctation of the aorta occasionally can be complicated by gangrene of the small intestines as a result of the pressure caused by rapid filling and distention of the branches of the abdominal aorta, with resulting necrosis of the tissues supplied by these vessels.[4]

Patients with tetralogy of Fallot may be helped by the Blalock-Taussig operation, which makes an artificial ductus arteriosus that bypasses the pulmonary stenosis. However, the preferred treatment is to correct the ventricular septal defect and pulmonary stenosis surgically if the clinical situation allows.

Medical management includes dealing with the complications of congenital heart disease, such as brain abscesses, infective endocarditis or endarteritis, cerebrovascular problems, congestive heart failure, acute pulmonary edema, bleeding problems, and associated emotional problems.

DENTAL MANAGEMENT
Medical considerations

The prime concern with the asymptomatic patient with congenital heart disease is the prevention of infective endocarditis or endarteritis following dental procedures that produce transient bacteremias. Patients with patent ductus arteriosus, ventricular septal defect, coarctation of the aorta, and valvular anomalies are most prone to these infections, and patients who have had surgery to correct congenital lesions also are susceptible during the healing phase. It would appear that most patients who have had surgery to correct a congenital heart lesion would not be susceptible to endocarditis if at least 3 months had elapsed since the surgery. However, before performing any dental treatment for these patients their physician (surgeon) should be consulted regarding the patient's status and need for prophylactic antibiotic coverage to prevent endocarditis.

TABLE 4-3. Dental management of patient with congenital heart disease

Medical consultation

Drugs—confirmation

Current status

Presence of congestive failure

Prevention of infective endocarditis (or endarteritis)

Prevention of excessive blood loss if surgery performed
    Anticoagulation medication
    Depletion of fibrinogen
    Thrombocytopenia

The prophylactic antibiotic coverage to prevent infective endocarditis in the patient with congenital heart disease is the same as for patients with rheumatic heart disease. Patients who have just had a congenital heart lesion corrected by surgery should receive the coverage regimen used for patients with an artificial heart valve (Chapter 2).

No routine dental procedures should be done for patients with symptomatic congenital heart disease without complete consultation with the patient's physician. Patients with polycythemia may have clinical bleeding tendencies, and this should be evaluated before any surgical procedure is attempted. Patients who have bleeding problems should not be operated on until the proper steps have been taken to avoid this complication. This will involve working with the patient's physician or a hematologist. Patients receiving anticoagulants should be managed as described in Chapter 20.

The patient with congestive heart failure secondary to congenital heart disease should not receive any routine dental care until the heart failure has been dealt with and then only after consultation with the patient's physician (Table 4-3).

Treatment planning considerations

The patient with congenital heart disease who is asymptomatic can receive any indicated dental treatment as long as antibiotics are used to prevent infective endocarditis. The patient with symptoms secondary to the congenital heart disease may have

to have an altered plan of treatment depending on the complication and its severity. Some patients may be able to receive only urgent dental care and then with some risk.

Oral complications

There are usually no oral complications directly related to congenital heart disease. The facial skin and oral mucosa may appear bluish in color in patients with the central type of cyanosis. Patients who have significant polycythemia may have a ruddy color to the face and oral mucosa. If thrombocytopenia is present, the patient may show evidence of small hemorrhages secondary to minor trauma in the oral mucosa. If significant leukopenia is present the patient may develop oral infection out of proportion to the etiologic factor(s) involved.

Emergency dental treatment

Asymptomatic patients with congenital heart disease can receive any indicated dental treatment for emergency problems as long as they are protected with antibiotics from infective endocarditis or endarteritis. Patients who are symptomatic should not be treated until consultation with a physician. Even then the treatment selected should be as conservative as possible—analgesics for pain and antibiotics for infections. Dehydration must be avoided in patients with acute oral infection since the complications related to polycythemia will be increased in frequency and severity (infarction of organs and depletion of coagulation factors).

REFERENCES

1. Fortuin, N.J., et al.: Cardia murmurs and other manifestations of valvular and acyanotic congenital heart disease. In Harvey, A., editor: Osler's the principles and practice of medicine, ed. 19, New York, 1976, Appleton-Century-Crofts, pp. 272-297.
2. Friedman, W.F., and Braunwald, E.: Congenital heart disease. In Thorn, G.W., et al., editors: Harrison's principles of internal medicine, ed. 8, New York, 1977, McGraw-Hill Book Co., pp. 300-350.
3. Hurst, J.W.: The heart, arteries and veins, ed. 4, New York, 1978, McGraw-Hill Book Co., pp. 750-901.
4. Julian, O.C.: Cardiovascular surgery, ed. 2, Chicago, 1970, Year Book Medical Publishers, Inc.
5. Silber, E.N., and Katz, L.N.: Heart disease, New York, 1975, Macmillan Publishing Co., Inc., pp. 565-697.

5

ISCHEMIC HEART DISEASE

Coronary atherosclerotic heart disease may be asymptomatic or symptomatic. When it is symptomatic it is referred to as ischemic heart disease. The symptoms result because of oxygen deprivation consequent to reduced perfusion to a portion of the myocardium of the heart. Other conditions, such as embolism, coronary ostial stenosis, coronary artery spasm, and congenital abnormalities, may also cause ischemic heart disease. In this chapter coronary atherosclerosis and its myocardial complications will be considered.

GENERAL DESCRIPTION
Incidence

It is estimated that about 40 million Americans (20% of the population) have one or more cardiovascular diseases; 34 million have hypertension, 4.2 million have coronary heart disease, 1.85 million have rheumatic heart disease, and 1.82 million have stroke.[8] The mortality per year caused by cardiovascular disease has been declining each year since 1950. Over 40% of this decline occurred during the last 5 years. In 1979 cardiovascular disease accounted for more than 50% of the deaths in the United States. Even now, 1 out of every 3 men and 1 out of every 10 women will develop significant cardiovascular disease before the age of 60. Coronary heart disease is still the leading cause of death after the age of 40 years in men and 50 years in women. Over 500,000 Americans die of heart attacks per year. Myocardial infarction and heart-related sudden death account for about 33% of deaths of those over 35 years of age. Although the incidence of coronary atherosclerotic heart disease had been increasing during the past 30 years, there is now some evidence that it has peaked and is on a decline.[8] The incidence and severity of the disease increase with age.

The process starts as coronary atherosclerosis with the appearance of fatty streaks in the walls of the coronary vessels.[7] Essentially all Americans over the age of 25 years have fatty streaks in their coronary vessels. A raised fibrous plaque may be found in as many as 80% of American men and 65% of American women over the age of 40.[6,11,13]

Autopsies on American military personnel killed during the Korean War showed that 15% had significant coronary artery disease. The mean age for this study was 22.1 years. During the Vietnam War, autopsies on military personnel killed in battle showed 45% to have significant coronary artery disease. Again the mean age of the study was 22.1 years. It is clear from these two studies that an increase in the incidence of asymptomatic coronary artery disease had occurred in young American adults during approximately a 20-year period.[13]

Studies on autopsied patients in the United States showed that between the ages of 30 and 39 years just less than 20% of the patients had more than 50% occlusion of one or more coronary arteries. Between the ages of 40 and 49 years this increased to over 40% of the patients.[5,6,11,13] The Framingham study[5] revealed that 8% of men between the ages of 30 and 44 years and 18% between the ages of 55 and 62 years had coronary atherosclerotic heart disease. These data show the incidence of coronary artery disease and prevalence of coronary atherosclerotic heart disease in American men and, to some extent, women.

Etiology

The cause of coronary atherosclerosis is not known at present. It appears to be related to some major risk factors, minor risk factors, and possible risk factors.[6]

The major risk factors most often mentioned are age, sex, familial history, serum lipid level, diet, hypertension, cigarette smoking, and abnormal glucose tolerance.

The incidence of coronary atherosclerosis increases with age. However, this may reflect the effects of other risk factors acting for a longer time rather than a direct effect of aging.

Men are much more prone to clinical manifestations of coronary atherosclerosis than are women of childbearing age. Between the ages of 35 and 44 years the risk is 5.2 times higher for men.[14] Infarction and sudden death are rare in premenopausal women.[8] After menopause there is a rapid reduction in this sex difference; between the ages of 65 and 74 years the risk falls to 2.3 times higher for men.[14] The sex difference in incidence of coronary atherosclerotic heart disease is more marked in whites than blacks.

Recent studies have confirmed that individuals who have either parents or siblings affected by coronary atherosclerotic heart disease before the age of 50 years have a greater risk of developing the disease at a younger age than those who do not have such a history. This risk factor may be as high as 5:1.[6]

Elevation of serum lipid levels has been demonstrated to be a risk factor. Individuals with cholesterol levels greater than 300 mg/100 ml had a four times greater risk of developing coronary atherosclerotic heart disease than those with cholesterol levels below 200 mg/100 ml. Individuals with elevated triglyceride or beta-lipoprotein levels also have shown an increased risk for the disease.[2,6,7]

A diet rich in one or more of the following increases the risk: total calories, saturated fats, cholesterol, sugars, and salts.

Increased blood pressure appears to be one of the most influential risk factors in coronary atherosclerotic heart disease. The Framingham study[5] showed that angina, myocardial infarction, and nonsudden death were all significantly correlated with elevated blood pressure (greater than 140/90 mm Hg). Sudden death in men was related only to elevation of systolic blood pressure, and no correlation of sudden death in women was found with increased blood pressure. The evidence suggests that hypertension has its impact primarily on the rate of development of coronary atherosclerosis rather than as a primary cause in its development.

The risk of developing coronary atherosclerotic heart disease or risk of death from the disease is from two to six times higher in cigarette smokers than in nonsmokers. The increased risk appears to be proportional to the number of cigarettes smoked per day. Pipe and cigar smoking carry little risk of developing the disease.[2,3,6]

Patients with diabetes mellitus have been found to have a greater incidence of coronary atherosclerotic heart disease, to have more extensive lesions, and to develop the condition at an earlier age than persons who do not have diabetes.

Minor risk factors include obesity, sedentary living pattern, personality type, and psychosocial tensions.

It would appear that no single factor per se is responsible for the development of coronary atherosclerosis but that a multiplicity of factors contributes to its development.

The evidence suggests that modification of risk factors that can be controlled, such as smoking, hypertension, blood cholesterol level, and diabetes, will reduce or modify the clinical effects of the disease.

Pathophysiology and complications

Coronary atherosclerosis appears to begin with the accumulation of lipid-laden macrophages in the intima of the blood vessel. A fibrous reaction to the presence of fatty material then occurs, causing the intima to increase in thickness. The lipid-laden macrophages then rupture, releasing additional lipid material into the extracellular areas of the intima. This material then undergoes crystallization and calcification, and an additional fibrous tissue response follows in an attempt to encapsulate the lipid mass. As the thickness of the intima increases, the size of the lumen of the vessel may be reduced and atrophy of the medial portion of the vessel may occur (Figs. 5-1 and 5-2).

There is a tendency for the greatest changes to occur at areas of arterial bifurcation, which sug-

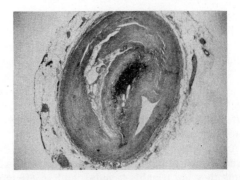

FIG. 5-2. Photomicrograph of cross-section of coronary artery partially occluded as a result of coronary atherosclerotic heart disease. (Courtesy W. O'Conner, M.D., Lexington, Ky.)

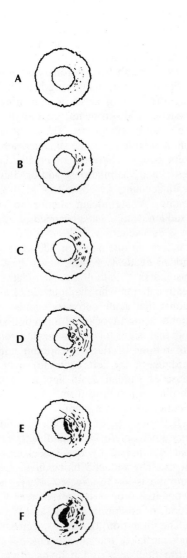

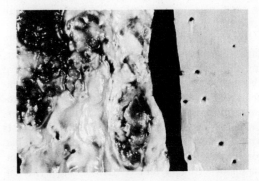

FIG. 5-3. Postmortem specimen demonstrating atherosclerotic changes in wall of aorta on the left. The specimen on the right is a normal aorta. (Courtesy W. O'Conner, M.D., Lexington, Ky.)

FIG. 5-1. Pathologic sequence in coronary atherosclerotic heart disease. **A,** Lipid-laden macrophages in intima; **B,** fibrous tissue reaction in intima; **C,** macrophages rupture, releasing additional lipids into vessel wall; **D,** increased fibrous connective tissue response to lipid material decreasing lumen size; **E,** calcification of plaque in vessel wall; **F,** endothelial cells become damaged and thrombosis occurs that may obstruct coronary blood flow.

gests that mechanical factors may stimulate the atherosclerotic process.

The lumen of the artery may be narrowed circumferentially or eccentrically, depending on the location and extent of the lesion. Microthrombi may develop on the endothelial surface overlying the developing lesion, which may lead to thrombosis and total occlusion of the vessel or to embolism.

The intraarterial complications of coronary atherosclerosis are luminal narrowing, intramural hemorrhage, thrombosis, embolism, and aneurysm (Fig. 5-3). Intramural hemorrhage occurs because of the weakening of the intimal tissues and may lead to thrombosis. It also may serve as an irritant and cause a reflex reaction that results in spasm of collateral vessels.

Coronary thrombosis is usually found in the segment of the artery that contains an advanced atherosclerotic lesion. Once thrombosis has occurred, it may become encapsulated and undergo fibrous organization and recanalization.

Aneurysms do not develop very often in diseased coronary arteries; however, when they are found they are usually saccular, and an effective lumen for blood flow remains.

Narrowing of the lumen of a coronary artery may lead to decreased blood flow to a portion of the heart muscle, resulting in myocardial ischemia. Myocardial ischemia may be manifested clinically as brief pain (angina pectoris), prolonged pain (myocardial infarction), or sudden death.

Patients with brief pain (angina pectoris) usually have coronary atherosclerotic disease. However, angina may occur in patients with hypertensive disease, valvular heart disease, and anemia. Patients who have coronary atherosclerosis will demonstrate brief episodes of pain more often if hypertension also is present. In one study of 177 patients with a history of brief chest pain, only 16% had coronary atherosclerosis only. Most had a combination of coronary atherosclerosis and hypertension and/or valvular heart disease.

The normal heart extracts about 65% to 75% of the oxygen that reaches it through the coronary vessels. During increased function, coronary vasodilation can increase the blood flow four to five times. The heart obtains additional oxygen for increased function by increasing the flow rather than by increasing the amount of oxygen it extracts from the blood that passes through the coronary vessels.

Myocardial ischemia accelerates anaerobic metabolism; thus a glucose molecule that would yield 32 high-energy phosphate bonds by aerobic process will give only 2 high-energy phosphate bonds. The results of this shift in metabolic process are that less energy is produced, creatine phosphate is depleted, adenosine triphosphate is depleted, lactate and pyruvate accumulate, and potassium and phosphate concentrations increase. These effects then may lead to a rapid failure of the myocardial

cell sodium pump with resulting decrease in the calcium-sodium intracellular ratio. This reduced ratio leads to decreased actin-myosin contractile sites to develop force or tension within the muscle.

Sudden death in the absence of demonstrable acute myocardial infarction is the largest single cause of death from coronary atherosclerosis.

Some type of underlying heart disease is found in about 90% of cases of sudden death. This approaches 100% if death occurs within 1 hour after the onset of symptoms. The prodromal symptoms that most often precede sudden death include chest pain, cough, shortness of breath, fainting, dizziness, and palpitations and/or fatigue. Sudden death accounts for about 15% to 30% of all natural deaths. A significant number of patients with "sudden death" have been saved by cardiopulmonary resuscitation (CPR) administered by bystanders. In one study of 400 patients saved from sudden death 35% were saved by CPR given by bystanders.[14] Pathologic examinations of sudden-death patients who died outside of a hospital have shown that acute coronary occlusion and demonstrable acute myocardial infarction are uncommon and that signs of old subendocardial infarctions (infarctions of the myocardium under the endocardium of the left ventricle) are common. The cause of sudden death appears to be ventricular fibrillation resulting from interruption of the electrical conduction system.

If the degree of ischemia resulting from coronary atherosclerosis is significant, the myocardium that is supplied by that vessel may undergo necrosis. The reduced blood flow may result from thrombosis in the affected artery, the effects of a hypotensive episode, an increased demand for blood, or emotional stress.

The infarction, or area of necrosis, may be subendocardial or transmural (Fig. 5-4), in which the entire thickness of the myocardium is involved. The cellular sequence that takes place is as follows (Fig. 5-5): (1) during the first several hours no histologic changes can be seen; (2) about 12 hours after the infarction the muscle fibers appear eosinophilic on histologic examination; (3) after about 18 hours the cytoplasm begins to clump, the capillaries are dilated, and neutrophils begin to infiltrate the dying muscle tissue; (4) by 24 hours the leuko-

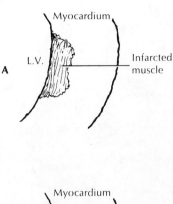

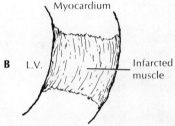

FIG. 5-4. Myocardial infarction. A, Subendocardial infarction; B, transmural infarction.

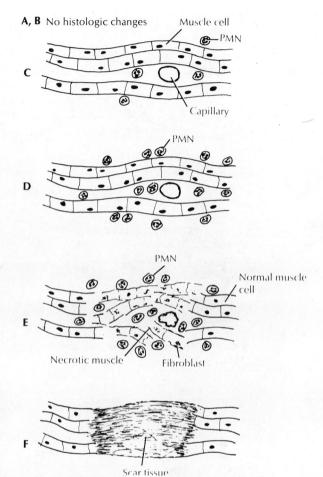

FIG. 5-5. Cellular sequence occurring in myocardial infarction (time approximate). A, One to 11 hours—no histologic changes; B, 12 hours—eosinophilic appearance of muscle fibers; C, 18 hours—clumping of cytoplasm, dilatation of capillaries, and infiltration of polymorphonuclear leukocytes (PMNs); D, 24 hours—marked infiltration of polymorphonuclear leukocytes; E, 72 hours—removal of necrotic tissue and formation of scar; F, 3 weeks—scar tissue formed.

cytic infiltration is marked (Fig. 5-6); (5) after 48 to 72 hours the nuclei of the myocardial fibers become indistinct and the cross-striations become altered but not lost; (6) after 72 hours the process of removal of affected muscle fibers begins at the area between nonaffected muscle and infarcted muscle; (7) by the third week replacement of necrotic muscle by scar tissue becomes apparent; and (8) by the end of the fourth week the necrotic muscle fibers have been removed and replaced by scar tissue (Fig. 5-7).

The causes of death in patients who have had acute myocardial infarctions include ventricular fibrillation, cardiac standstill, congestive heart failure, and rupture of the heart wall (Fig. 5-8). Rupture of the heart secondary to infarction most often occurs during the third or fourth day after infarction. The rupture usually occurs at the periphery of the infarction, at the junction of necrotic and healthy muscle. Rupture of the heart wall occurs only in transmural infarctions. Depending on the location of the infarction, the ventricular septum may rupture or papillary muscles may tear.

Death also may be caused by thromboembolic complications. The embolism may originate from the left ventricle or systemic veins. In the case of embolism from a mural thrombus in the left ventricle, the site of damage may be the brain, coronary arteries, or mesenteric arteries.

Transmural infarctions may cause a pericarditis

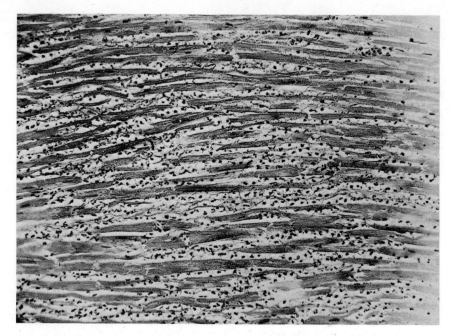

FIG. 5-6. Photomicrograph of myocardial infarction (24 to 48 hours). (Courtesy Jesse E. Edwards, M.D., St. Paul, Minn.)

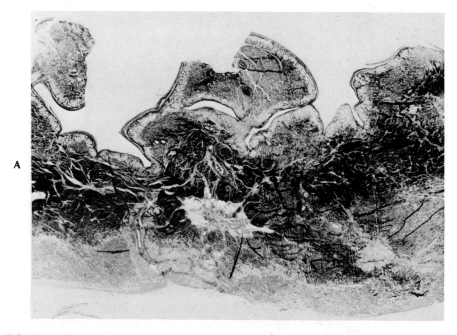

FIG. 5-7. A, Gross appearance of healed myocardial infarction. (Courtesy Jesse E. Edwards, M.D., St. Paul, Minn.)

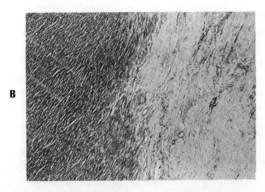

B

FIG. 5-7, cont'd. B, Photomicrograph of healed myocardial infarction (1 month). Courtesy W. O'Conner, M.D., Lexington, Ky.)

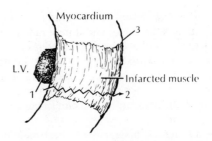

FIG. 5-8. Complications of transmural infarction. *1,* Mural thrombosis may give rise to embolism to brain, coronary arteries, or mesenteric arteries; *2,* myocardial wall may rupture; *3,* pericarditis may lead to tamponade.

that usually is of only passing interest. However, if a hemorrhagic effusion occurs during an episode of a fibrinous pericarditis secondary to a transmural infarction, cardiac tamponade and death may result.

The prognosis for patients who have healed myocardial infarctions varies. In one study of 329 patients with healed infarction at autopsy, about one third were found to have died from noncardiac causes; the other patients died of cardiovascular causes.[6] Of the patients who died of cardiac causes, 38% had sudden deaths without recurrent acute myocardial infarction, 27% died of congestive heart failure, and 34% died as a result of complications of an acute myocardial infarction.

CLINICAL PRESENTATION
Symptoms

A most important symptom of coronary atherosclerotic heart disease is pain. The pain may be brief, as in angina pectoris resulting from temporary ischemia of the myocardium, or it may be prolonged, as in myocardial infarction. Ischemic myocardial pain results when there is an imbalance between the oxygen supply to the muscle and the oxygen demand of the muscle. Atherosclerotic narrowing of the coronary arteries is an important cause of this imbalance. If the imbalance is severe enough, necrosis of the involved portion of the heart muscle may result. The exact mechanism or agents involved in producing the cardiac pain are not known.

Ischemic myocardial pain of the brief nature is usually described as an aching, heavy, squeezing pressure or tightness in the midchest region. The area of discomfort is about the size of the fist. The pain may radiate down the left or right arm, to the neck, to the lower jaw, to the palate, or to the tongue. In rare cases it may be present only in one of these distant sites, and the patient will be free of central chest pain. The pain is usually brief in duration, lasting only 1 to 3 minutes if the provoking stimulus is reduced or stopped.

Patients with initial angina, progressive angina, or angina at rest are described as having an unstable form of angina. Patients with angina that has not changed in frequency or severity over a period of time are said to have stable angina.

Patients with brief pain caused by myocardial ischemia who have a stable pattern of attacks have a relatively good prognosis. Patients with unstable angina have a poor prognosis and often develop myocardial infarction within a short time.

A form of angina, Prinzmetal's variant angina, occurs at rest and is related to spasm of a coronary artery, usually with varying amounts of atherosclerosis. The prognosis depends on the degree of arterial disease.[14] Angina has been reported in individuals with normal coronary vessels.[14]

Patients with coronary atherosclerosis who develop prolonged pain resulting from myocardial ischemia usually are having an infarction of the myocardium. There may or may not be objective clinical evidence of infarction. The pain resulting from infarction is usually more severe and lasts longer—½ to 1 hour or more—but has the same character as that described previously for angina. The location is the same, and it may radiate in the same pattern as the brief pain that results from temporary myocardial ischemia. With infarction there is no relief of pain with vasodilators or cessation of activity. Neither brief nor prolonged pain resulting from myocardial ischemia is aggravated by deep breathing.

The differential diagnosis of chest pain should include acute dissection of the aorta, acute pericarditis, pulmonary embolism, and anxiety. Acute dissection of the aorta produces severe pain in the anterior chest that lasts for hours and often has its maximum intensity at the onset. It may radiate to the back and is not aggravated by deep breathing.

Acute pericarditis produces a sharp pain usually located in the pericardial region that is aggravated by deep breathing. Its onset and severity are not related to effort.

Small pulmonary emboli usually do not cause pain. The pain produced by larger emboli may be very similar to that which results from myocardial infarction. The presence of acute, distressing dyspnea may be the only clue to pulmonary embolism as the cause of the pain.

Anxiety is the most common cause of chest pain. The pain may consist of a short series of "sticks" or "stabs" or of a prolonged, dull ache. The pain rarely radiates, is not initiated by effort, is not aggravated by breathing, and is usually associated with other signs of anxiety, such as deep sighing, fatigue, or hyperventilation.

Palpitation of the heart may be present in patients who have coronary atherosclerotic heart disease. The rhythm may be normal or abnormal. The complaint (disagreeable awareness of the heartbeat) is not directly related to the seriousness of the underlying cardiac problem.

Syncope, a transient loss of consciousness resulting from an inadequate cerebral blood flow, may occur in patients who have coronary atherosclerotic heart disease.

If congestive heart failure develops as a complication of coronary atherosclerotic heart disease, dyspnea, orthopnea, paroxysmal nocturnal dyspnea, edema, hemoptysis, fatigue, weakness, and cyanosis may be present. Fatigue and weakness may be present early in the course of the disease, before the onset of congestive heart failure (see Chapter 8).

Signs

The clinical signs of early coronary atherosclerotic heart disease are few and may reflect the anxiety felt by the patient concerning the episodes of brief cardiac pain rather than being directly related to the underlying disease process. The skin may be moist and ashen. The patient may be losing weight, and some irregularity in the rhythm of the pulse may be detected.

Signs associated with advanced coronary atherosclerotic heart disease usually reflect the presence of congestive heart failure. Distention of neck veins, peripheral edema, cyanosis, ascites, and enlarged liver may be present.

Laboratory findings

Coronary atherosclerosis may be detected by coronary arteriograms before the development of coronary atherosclerotic heart disease. Also, an abnormal electrocardiogram may be detected before the development of symptomatic coronary atherosclerotic heart disease. An exercise electrocardiogram is being used with increased frequency to detect patients with coronary atherosclerotic heart disease. It is about 60% to 70% accurate in detecting patients with significant disease. However, about a 10% rate of false-positive results occurs, primarily in young people.[14]

Several new techniques to evaluate patients for evidence of coronary atherosclerotic heart disease are now being used. These include echocardiography (ultrasound), thallium-201 myocardial perfusion, technetium-99m stannous pyrophosphate, indium–111 labeled platelet imaging, and measurement of prostaglandins such as thromboxane A_2 and prosstacyline[4,12,15] (Table 5-1). The electrocardiogram is used to aid in the diagnosis of acute myocardial infarction. It is of most diagnostic value when the infarction is large, transmural, and located in the anteroseptal position and when intraventricular conduction is normal. The electrocardiographic diagnosis of acute myocardial infarction is most difficult when the infarction is small, subendocardial, and located on the lateral wall of the left ventricle and when the left bundle branch conduction system is blocked. The electrocardiogram may also be used to determine the presence of old infarctions.

Serum enzyme determinations are often very helpful in establishing the presence of an acute myocardial infarction and the extent of infarction. This method is not specific for myocardial infarction, however, because any injured or necrotic tissue will release many of the enzymes that are released following infarction of heart muscle. Thus serum enzyme results must be evaluated in light of the patient's clinical picture to be meaningful from a diagnostic standpoint.

The principal enzymes that are measured are serum glutamic-oxaloacetic transaminase (SGOT), creatine phosphokinase (CPK), and lactate dehydrogenase (LDH).[6,11] The SGOT level will increase above normal 6 to 12 hours after the infarction. It reaches a peak value approximately 24 to

48 hours after the infarction and returns to normal in about 4 to 7 days. The SGOT increase is in direct relation to the size of the myocardial infarction. The CPK level increases above normal about 6 to 8 hours after the infarction. It reaches a peak value in approximately 24 hours and returns to normal in 3 to 4 days. The LDH level increases above normal approximately 24 to 48 hours after the infarction, peaks at 3 to 6 days, and then returns to normal by 8 to 14 days. The LDH level is not as reliable diagnostically as the SGOT level (Table 5-2).

MEDICAL MANAGEMENT

The patient who has coronary atherosclerotic heart disease with a history of brief pain (angina pectoris) is medically managed by a combination of approaches. The patient may be aided in adjusting to the emotional impact of the presence of the disease. The management program may include general measures such as an exercise program; weight control; diet alteration with restriction in sodium chloride intake, cholesterol, and saturated fatty acids; cessation of smoking; and control of exacerbating conditions such as anemia, hypertension, and hyperthyroidism. Drug therapy includes nitroglycerin or a long-acting nitrate such as Nitro-Bid or Nitroglyn for pain control. Beta-adrenergic blockers, such as propranolol and nadolol, have been found to be useful in decreasing myocardial oxygen consumption. Cardiac glycosides and diuretics are often prescribed. The new calcium channel blockers, such as nifedipine and verapamil, have been found to be useful in treating angina caused by coronary artery spasm. Percu-

TABLE 5-1. Laboratory tests for coronary heart disease

Angina
   Electrocardiogram
   Exercise electrocardiogram
   Thallium-201 imaging
   Echocardiography
   Arteriography

Myocardial infarction
   Electrocardiogram
   Serum enzyme levels
   Technetium-99m stannous pyrophosphate
   Echocardiography

Experimental procedures
   Indium–111 labeled platelet imaging
   Measurement of prostaglandins
   Radiolabeled myosin–specific antibody
   Position imaging

TABLE 5-2. Laboratory tests to measure serum enzyme levels for evaluation of myocardial tissue injury or death*

Enzyme	Level increases above normal	Peak value	Level returns to normal
Serum glutamic-oxaloacetic transaminase (SGOT)	6 to 12 hours†	24 to 48 hours	4 to 7 days
Creatine phosphokinase (CPK)	6 to 8 hours	24 hours	3 to 4 days
Lactate dehydrogenase (LDH)‡	24 to 48 hours	3 to 6 days	8 to 14 days

*Enzyme results must be looked at in light of the clinical picture. Results are not specific for myocardial infarction.
†Increase is in direct relation to the size of the myocardial infarction.
‡Not as reliable as SGOT.

taneous transluminal angioplasty or coronary dilation with a small balloon is being used for the nonoperative dilation of stenotic coronary arteries.[1,14]

A patient with significant obstruction of the proximal portions of two or more of the major coronary arteries or obstruction of the left proximal anterior descending coronary artery is a candidate for a coronary bypass operation. The surgical mortality for the procedure is 2% to 3%. About 60% of patients who undergo this procedure will obtain complete relief of symptoms, and 20% to 30% will have major or partial relief. Bypass of left main coronary disease has been shown to prolong life. It is not clear if the other bypass procedures prolong survival.[1,14] Patients with unstable angina who are treated by medical or surgical means show no difference in mortality or myocardial infarction rate at the end of 3 years. However, pain relief is more complete in the patients treated by surgery.[14]

Rest is an important part of the therapeutic approach. If activity brings on chest pain, the patient is instructed to stop and rest for several minutes or longer until the pain goes away. Nitroglycerin tablets also may be taken. Bed rest (10 to 14 days) usually is recommended only when the angina syndrome first appears. A period of bed rest also is suggested for patients who have the stable type of angina that for no reason begins to occur more frequently and severely.

Patients who have significant angina are encouraged to avoid long hours of work, to take rest periods during the working day, to obtain adequate rest at night, to use mild sedatives, to take frequent vacations, and in some cases to change their occupation or retire.

Patients who have coronary atherosclerotic heart disease should avoid any of the precipitating factors that may bring on cardiac pain, such as cold weather, hot humid weather, big meals, emotional upsets, cigarette smoking, and drugs such as amphetamines, caffeine, ephedrine, cyclamates, and alcohol.

The treatment of the patient who has an acute myocardial infarction is far from ideal at present. Since about two thirds of deaths from acute myocardial infarction occur outside the hospital (50% of these are sudden deaths),[6] it is clear that there is now no effective system of therapy to deal with this problem. Several strategies have been proposed by which a potential victim might be identified and a fatal myocardial infarction possibly prevented. These include the following:

1. Identification and control of risk factors
2. Periodic monitoring by electrocardiogram of high-risk patients using an isometric stress test; monitoring and control of patients with cardiac arrhythmias
3. Long-term use of antiarrhythmic drugs for individuals with frequent ventricular premature beats, etc.; however, the drugs available at present have side effects that discourage this approach
4. Mass educational programs to reduce time between the recognition of early symptoms and the seeking of medical care
5. Establishment of fixed and mobile life-support stations

Patients with acute myocardial infarction are hospitalized as soon as possible. As a general rule, a patient with an uncomplicated myocardial infarction is kept in the coronary intensive care unit for 4 to 5 days. If the infarction is complicated by serious dysrhythmia, pump failure, or shock the stay in the coronary unit is extended.

In the past about 30% of hospital "coronary" deaths occurred just after the patients were transferred from the coronary unit to standard care facilities. This has led some hospitals to develop halfway or intermediate coronary care units. Current studies[14] show a significant reduction in hospital "coronary" deaths after transfer from the coronary intensive care unit. The length of stay in the intermediate coronary care unit is 7 to 12 days.

The present trend is for early ambulation of the patient who has had a myocardial infarction in the hospital. In some uncomplicated cases this occurs at about the eighth day of hospitalization. For most patients ambulation is started the twelfth to fifteenth day.

Pain relief is an important part of the early medical management of the patient with an acute myocardial infarction. Morphine sulfate is the drug of choice for acute pain relief. Sedatives and hypnotic medications also are used to calm the patient and ensure adequate periods of rest.

Oxygen is used during the acute period to increase the degree of oxygen saturation of the blood and keep the work load of the heart at a minimum. However, 100% oxygen should be avoided because it may cause hyperoxia, which can reduce coronary blood flow. Oxygen usually is best administered by nasal cannula.

During the first 24 hours the diet usually is liquid in nature. If no cardiac complications develop, the diet for the next few days consists of soft foods. After that a regular diet can be taken, but it should be low in saturated fats, total calories, and salt.

Straining during bowel movements can be dangerous during the first several days following an infarction. Wetting agents such as docusate sodium are given to the patient to soften the stool and avoid straining.

Most studies of patients with myocardial infarction have shown a significant reduction in mortality and thromboembolic complications by the use of anticoagulants. Patients may be given anticoagulants during the acute phase of infarction and for as long as 2 years thereafter.

The hemodynamic benefit of digitalis during the early postinfarction period in patients who have no evidence of congestive heart failure remains unproved.

Some physicians give a polarizing solution of potassium, glucose, and insulin IV during the early postinfarction period. There appears to be some question of whether this therapy is beneficial. Atropine may be used in patients who have severe bradycardia and profound hypotension.

The development of dysrhythmias in patients who have had an acute myocardial infarction constitutes an emergency problem that must be treated aggressively.

The prime purpose of the rehabilitation program for patients who have had myocardial infarction is to return them to as normal a life as possible. The patient is encouraged to return to his previous life-style. If this is not possible because of medical restrictions, an attempt is made to alter the patient's life-style in a way that is consistent with his cardiac reserve but still allows him to use his full physical and emotional capacities.

Two prime concerns of many patients that must be dealt with effectively during rehabilitation are the possibilities of returning to their occupation and of resuming an active sex life. The physical status of the individual patient and his emotional reaction to the events must be considered in developing the rehabilitation program. Patients with uncomplicated first myocardial infarctions usually can return to an active life-style in about 6 to 8 weeks.[6]

There is no conclusive evidence that physical conditioning during the postinfarction period exerts a beneficial effect on the course of the disease.[6] Physical conditioning does not appear to alter the collateral development or electric stability of the heart to reduce the rate of subsequent myocardial infarctions or increase the patient's life expectancy. However, a reduction in symptoms does occur, and many patients have an improved sense of well-being and improved function. These positive factors warrant an active conditioning program for the patient who has had an infarction.

Strenuous physical exertion is contraindicated during the first 6 months after a myocardial infarction. During the first 3 months, as soon as the patient is physically and emotionally ready, walking is the best physical activity. Most patients should not drive cars during the first 3 months. After this time, swimming, golf, and bowling are good activities. Playing competitive games, shoveling snow, chopping trees, pushing stalled cars, lifting weights, etc. should be avoided.

Some physicians do not recommend jogging because of the variable environmental conditions that are experienced, but they often suggest the use of a stationary bicycle.[6]

Retirement is not indicated for most patients. However, a reduction in total number of work hours, longer lunch hours, and more rest periods and vacations usually are indicated.

DENTAL MANAGEMENT
Medical considerations

Patients who have the stable form of angina without a history of infarction generally have a much lower risk of complications occurring in the dental office than patients who have unstable angina or a history of a recent myocardial infarction.

Patients who have had a recent myocardial infarction should not receive any routine dental care until 6 months after the infarction (possible complications decrease with time).[10] Even after this time the dentist should consult with the patient's

TABLE 5-3. Dental management of patient with angina pectoris

Morning appointments

Short appointments

Reduction of stress and anxiety:
  Patient should be able to express fears
  Premedication—diazepam, 5 to 10 mg
  Nitrous oxide—hypoxia must be avoided

Nitroglycerin tablets available; may use prophylactic

Local anesthesia with epinephrine 1:100,000—aspirate, inject slowly; no more than three cartridges

Avoidance of use of vasopressors to control local bleeding

Avoidance of use of vasopressors in gingival packing material

If patient becomes fatigued or develops significant changes in pulse rate or rhythm during appointment, termination of appointment

TABLE 5-4. Dental management of patient with history of myocardial infarction

Consultation with patient's physician concerning management

No routine dental care until at least 6 months after infarction

Patients on anticoagulant therapy who need deep scaling or surgical procedures:
  Check prothrombin time
  Have physician reduce prothrombin time to 1.5 to 2 times normal
  Give antibiotics

Morning appointments

Short appointments

Reduction of stress and anxiety—premedication with diazepam

Local anesthesia with epinephrine 1:100,000—aspirate, inject slowly; no more than three cartridges

Avoidance of use of vasopressors to control local bleeding

Avoidance of use of vasopressors in gingival packing material

If patient becomes fatigued or develops significant changes in pulse rate or rhythm during appointment, termination of appointment

physician before beginning dental treatment. The physician should be informed of the basic nature of the dental care to be rendered and the dental management plan based on what has been learned about the patient from the medical history and physical examination. Important medical points and medications should be confirmed, and information concerning the presence of other medical problems the patient may have and the patient's present status should be sought.

The dental management plan that is developed for the patient with a history of myocardial infarction should include the following considerations. First, what is the patient's current status in regard to presence of congestive heart failure, hypertension, and angina? Second, what medications is the patient taking?

Patients with a history of coronary atherosclerotic heart disease should be given short morning appointments, and may be premedicated with 5 to 10 mg of diazepam (Valium) before the appointment in an attempt to reduce anxiety. The approach of the office staff and dentist should be one of openness so that feelings of fear can be expressed by the patient and dealt with in a constructive way to reduce the patient's anxiety toward the

dental personnel and process. Effective local anesthesia is a must for these patients. Nitrous oxide analgesia can be used as long as hypoxia is avoided. Epinephrine in the concentration of 1:100,000 can be used safely, even if the patient has hypertensive disease. Usually no more than three cartridges of anesthetic should be given during any single appointment. This concentration of epinephrine can be tolerated very well and should lead to no complications unless injected intravascularly; therefore aspiration for blood should be done before the anesthetic solution is slowly deposited. Vasopressors must not be used to control local bleeding or used in gingival packing materials. The patient with an old infarction may still be receiving anticoagulant medication. If surgical procedures or extensive scaling procedures are planned, the dosage of anticoagulant should be reduced by the patient's physician. A prothrombin

TABLE 5-5. Dental management of patient with history of stable angina who develops chest pain during dental appointment

I. Stop dental procedure

II. Give patient nitroglycerin tablet(s) (from patient's own medication, if possible) under tongue
  A. If pain is relieved within 15 minutes:
    1. Let patient rest and continue with procedure
    or
    2. Terminate appointment and reschedule for another day
    3. If possible inform patient's physician of what happened
  B. If pain is not relieved within 15 minutes:
    1. Take patient's blood pressure and pulse
    2. If patient's condition is stable, call physician and arrange for patient to be seen; if patient must be transported, attend him until patient is in hands of his physician or is being managed by hospital emergency room personnel

TABLE 5-6. Dental management of patient with history of unstable angina or myocardial infarction who develops chest pain during dental appointment

I. Stop dental procedure

II. Give patient nitroglycerin tablet(s) from patient's own medication, if possible) under tongue and measure blood pressure and pulse
  A. If pain is relieved within 15 minutes and patient's condition is stable, terminate appointment and inform patient's physician of what happened
  B. If pain is not relieved within 15 minutes:
    1. If patient's condition is stable call physician and attend patient when transported for emergency hospital care
    2. If patient's condition is unstable provide immediate emergency care, call physician, and attend patient when transported for emergency hospital care

time that is 1.5 to 2 times normal should be obtained on the day of the dental procedure (Tables 5-3 and 5-4).[10]

Patients who are receiving antihypertensive agents or digitalis may be prone to nausea and vomiting; thus excessive stimulation of the gag reflex should be avoided. Antisialogogues should not be used in patients who have coronary atherosclerotic heart disease unless the patient's physician has been consulted, because these drugs tend to cause tachycardia. Antiarrhythmic agents such as quinidine and procainamide may cause nausea and vomiting, hypotension, and, on occasion, agranulocytosis. Any medication the patient is taking must be identified, and the *Physicians' Desk Reference* must be checked for side effects and drug interactions.

If at any time during the dental appointment a patient with coronary atherosclerotic heart disease becomes fatigued or develops a significant change in pulse rate or rhythm, the appointment should be terminated. Thus it is important for the dentist to tell the patient to inform him or her if at any time during the appointment he becomes fatigued, notes a change in heart rate, etc.

Patients who have angina pectoris should bring their nitroglycerin medication with them to every dental appointment. Prophylactic nitroglycerin

may be considered for patients who have frequent attacks. If pain develops during the dental appointment all work should be stopped, and the patient should take a nitroglycerin tablet and be allowed to relax. Up to three tablets can be given during a 15-minute period. If after 15 minutes the patient is free of pain, the dentist can consider completing the work planned for the appointment. Patients who have the stable form of angina pectoris with no history of myocardial infarction can usually tolerate continuation of the dental appointment once they are free of pain and relaxed. Usually the appointment should be discontinued for patients who have a history of myocardial infarction or unstable angina. These patients should be observed for 10 to 15 minutes after the pain has been relieved by nitroglycerin. Their physician should be called and informed of what happened. If the physician wants to see the patient, then the patient should be so informed. Otherwise the patient should be told to go home and relax for the remainder of the day if possible (Table 5-5).

If the pain is not relieved within 15 minutes after nitroglycerin is taken, the possibility of a myocardial infarction must be considered and emergency steps taken. If the patient's pulse and blood pressure are stable, the patient's physician should be called and immediate arrangements made for the patient to be seen. Appropriate transportation should be arranged for the transfer. Patients who do not have a physician or whose physician cannot be reached should be taken to the nearest emergency facility or physician's office, depending on the local circumstances.

If the patient's status becomes unstable before the transfer, appropriate emergency lifesaving procedures should be started. Regardless of whether the patient's condition is stable or not, the dentist must accompany him during the transfer (Table 5-6).[10]

Treatment planning modifications

Patients who have had a myocardial infarction within the last 6 months should not receive any routine dental treatment. In general it also is best that patients who have unstable angina receive no routine dental treatment, since they are at high risk for myocardial infarction. The stress of the dental appointment could be a precipitating factor for the infarction.

Patients who have the stable form of angina or who had a myocardial infarction at least 6 months ago can receive any indicated dental treatment. Before dental treatment is begun the patient's physician should be contacted whenever possible to confirm the dental management plan.

Oral complications

There are no oral lesions associated directly with coronary atherosclerotic heart disease. Drugs used in the treatment of this disease and its complications may result in oral changes. Some of these drugs may cause allergic or toxic reactions that can result in oral ulceration and infection. Patients who are receiving dicumarol may have significant bleeding problems following trauma or surgical procedures.

Patients who have coronary atherosclerotic heart disease with brief pain may rarely have the pain referred to the lower jaw. The pattern of onset of pain caused by physical activity and its disappearance with rest will usually serve as clues to its cardiac origin.

Emergency dental treatment

In general, patients who have stable angina or a history of an infarction that occurred at least 6

TABLE 5-7. Emergency dental care for patient with history of recent* myocardial infarction

Consultation with physician
Strong analgesic agents for pain control
Antibiotics for control of infection
Sedative pulpal medication in place of extraction or endodontic procedures
Formocresol pulpotomy to avoid extraction

*Within 6 months.

months ago can receive any indicated dental emergency treatment.

Patients who have unstable angina must be judged on an individual basis, including consultation with the patient's physician regarding the type of emergency dental care provided.

Patients who have emergency dental problems during the 6-month period after an infarction should be treated in as conservative a manner as possible, with pain relief as the primary objective. The patient's physician must be consulted and the planned dental approach discussed in detail before any treatment is rendered. Strong analgesic agents should be used for pain control and antibiotics for infection. Sedative pulpal medications should be considered in place of extraction or endodontic procedures. Pulpotomy with formocresol may have to be performed in certain instances to avoid extraction. The endodontic procedure or extraction can be performed at a later date. This approach also may have to be used for patients who have unstable angina (Table 5-7).

REFERENCES

1. Braunwald, E., and Cohn, P.F.: Ischemic heart disease. In Peterdorf, R.G., et al., editors: Harrison's principles of internal medicine, ed. 10, New York, 1983, McGraw-Hill Book Co., pp. 1423-1442.
2. Chung, E.K., editor: Controversy in cardiology: the practical clinical approach, New York, 1976, Springer-Verlag New York, Inc.
3. Dawber, R.T., and Kammel, W.B.: Susceptibility to coronary heart disease, Mod. Concepts Cardiovasc. Dis. **30:** 671-676, 1961.
4. Felner, J.M.: Techniques of echocardiology. In Hurst, J.W., editor: The heart, ed. 5, New York, 1983, McGraw-Hill Book Co., pp. 1773-98.
5. Gordon, T., and Kammel, W.B.: Premature mortality from

coronary heart disease: the Framingham study, J.A.M.A. **215:**1617-1625, 1971.

6. Hurst, J.W.: The heart arteries and veins, ed. 4, New York, 1978, McGraw-Hill Book Co., pp. 1094-1362.

7. Hurst, J.W., et al.: Atherosclerotic coronary heart disease: angina pectoris, myocardial infarction, and other manifestations of myocardial ischemia. In Hurst, J.W., editor: The heart, ed. 5, New York, 1983, McGraw-Hill Book Co., pp. 1009-1149.

8. Kammel, W.B.: Incidence, prevalence, and mortality of cardiovascular disease. In Hurst, J.W., editor: The heart, ed. 5, New York, 1983, McGraw-Hill Book Co., pp. 621-629.

9. Kammel, W.B., et al.: Serum cholesterol, lipoprotein and risk of coronary heart disease: the Framingham study, Ann. Intern. Med. **74:**1, 1971.

10. McCarthy, F.M.: Emergencies in dental practice, Philadelphia, 1968, W.B. Saunders Co.

11. Pitt, B., et al.: Myocardial infarction. In Harvey, A., editor: Osler's the principles and practice of medicine, ed. 19, New York, 1976, Appleton-Century-Crofts, pp. 341-363.

12. Ross, R.: Coronary heart disease: factors influencing atherogenesis. In Hurst, J.W., editor, The heart, ed. 5, New York, 1983, McGraw-Hill Book Co., pp. 935-949.

13. Silber, E.M., and Katz, L.M.: Heart disease, New York, 1975, Macmillan Publishing Co., Inc., pp. 760-820.

14. Young, J.B., and Luchi, R.J.: Coronary heart disease. In Rose, L.F., and Kaye, D., editors: Internal medicine for dentistry. St. Louis, 1983, The C.V. Mosby Co., pp. 524-540.

15. Zaret, B.L., and Berger, J.J.: Techniques of nuclear cardiology. In Hurst, J.W., editor: The heart, ed. 5, New York, 1983, McGraw-Hill Book Co., pp. 1803-1843.

6

DENTAL MANAGEMENT OF PATIENTS WITH SURGICALLY CORRECTED CARDIAC AND VASCULAR DISEASE

There is general agreement among physicians and dentists that patients who have congenital heart disease and rheumatic heart disease are more susceptible than the general population to infective endocarditis or infective endarteritis. These infections can develop following dental procedures that cause transient bacteremias. It is current practice to protect a susceptible patient with prophylactic antibiotics just before and after all dental procedures to minimize the chance of endocarditis or endarteritis.

The risk of these diseases occurring following dental treatment in a patient who has a surgically corrected cardiovascular lesion is less clearly defined, and the guidelines for prevention are more vague.

The purpose of this chapter is to consider the risk of endocarditis or endarteritis in a patient who has undergone corrective surgery for any type of cardiac or vascular disorder and to suggest guidelines for the dental management of such patients with respect to the need for protection against these serious complications. The following surgical procedures will be considered: (1) closure of an atrial or ventricular septal defect, (2) ligation or resection of ductus arteriosus, (3) commissurotomy for diseased cardiac valve(s), (4) prosthetic replace-

ment of diseased cardiac valve(s), (5) coronary artery bypass graft, (6) arterial graft, (7) implantation of a transvenous pacemaker, and (8) heart transplantation.

GENERAL DESCRIPTION, CLINICAL PRESENTATION, AND SURGICAL MANAGEMENT
SURGICALLY CLOSED SEPTAL DEFECT

Three anatomic types of defects are found that involve the atrial septum. These are, in order of frequency, (1) ostium secundum, (2) sinus venosus, and (3) ostium primum.

For an ostium secundum defect in an asymptomatic infant with a left-to-right shunt greater than 2:1, surgical closure usually is postponed until the child is about 6 years of age. The operation is recommended even in older individuals who have pulmonary hypertension, as long as the left-to-right shunting of blood exists. Systemic pulmonary hypertension with a balanced shunt or right-to-left shunting is a contraindication for surgery. Usually, a patient with an ostium secundum defect is treated if the heart is enlarged, heart failure is present, arrhythmia is present, or the shunt is large. The patient is not treated if the shunt is small or if the patient is asymptomatic, has normal heart

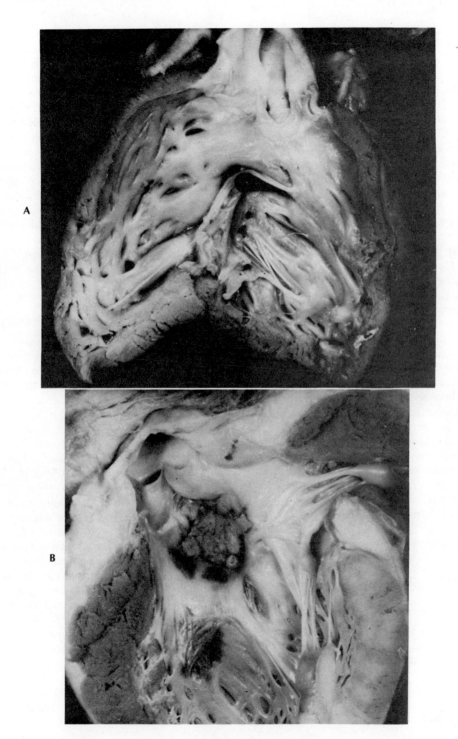

FIG. 6-1. A, Ventricular septal defect. **B,** Ventricular septal defect closed by use of Dacron patch. (Courtesy Jesse E. Edwards, M.D., St. Paul, Minn.)

size, or has developed pulmonary hypertension with reversal of shunt. The defect is closed with sutures.[8,15,16]

A sinus venosus defect is located high in the septum near the opening of the superior vena cava. The indications for surgical repair are the same as for ostium secundum defect. The defect is often larger than the ostium secundum type and requires a patch graft of pericardium or Dacron.[8,15]

The ostium primum defect is a more serious lesion than ostium secundum or sinus venosus defect. Most patients who have ostium primum defect will not survive into adulthood without surgical repair of the defect. Ostium primum is a round defect located low in the septum and often is associated with malformations of atrioventricular valves. One complication of surgery is injury to the conduction system, which can result in a heart block. This can necessitate a pacemaker on a permanent basis. The defect is closed with a patch graft of pericardium or Dacron[8,15,16] (Fig. 6-1). A small ventricular septal defect is compatible with a relatively normal life expectancy and may close spontaneously, particularly during infancy and childhood. Large defects eventually lead to increased pulmonary vascular resistance and right-to-left shunting. Once the shunt has changed from left to right to right to left, the lesion may be inoperable.[4,17] A child who has a small defect and normal pulmonary artery pressure does not require an operation unless there is a history of endocarditis.[8,15]

Most patients who have large defects are operated on before they reach adulthood. Small lesions are treated by primary closure, and larger lesions are closed by a Dacron or pericardial patch.[8,15,16]

LIGATED OR RESECTED DUCTUS ARTERIOSUS

Endarteritis and pulmonary hypertension are two complications found in untreated patients who have patent ductus arteriosus (Fig. 6-2). A 17-year-old patient who has a patent ductus arteriosus has about one half the life expectancy of a comparable normal individual. The operative risks are small for patients who have patent ductus arteriosus without cardiac failure; the mortality under these circumstances is less than 0.5%. If patients with cardiac failure are included, however, the operative mortality increases to about 2% to 3%. When the complications of patent ductus arteriosus and the shortened life expectancy and the low operative risk of patients with the condition are considered, corrective surgery is indicated in asymptomatic children or young adults. A patient over the age of 30 years with patent ductus arteriosus who is asymptomatic and has a normal-sized heart is commonly not treated. Repair is complicated in adults because of enlargement of adjacent vessels and presence of atherosclerotic lesions. The operative risk rises greatly in a patient with right-to-left shunting and/or pulmonary hypertension, to the point where surgery is contraindicated.[8,15,18]

Repair is performed by cutting the ductus and suturing the cut ends closed or by suturing the ductus closed without resection.[8,15,18]

COMMISSUROTOMY FOR DISEASED CARDIAC VALVE(S)

Mitral valve surgery usually consists of either a closed or open mitral commissurotomy (release of adhesions or valve leaflets) or the prosthetic replacement of the valve. The presence of a murmur, even with an enlarged left atrium and right ventricle, is not an indication for mitral valve surgery. Surgery is indicated for a patient who has progressive symptoms of congestive heart failure or who has developed systemic emboli from the left atrium.[1,2]

Closed mitral commissurotomy may be the treatment of choice for a patient who has isolated noncalcific mitral stenosis without regurgitation. The appendage of the left atrium is opened and a finger inserted into the atrium, and then an attempt is made to separate the valve leaflets. If this fails, a small hole is made in the left ventricle and a transventricular dilator is inserted and guided to the mitral valve, separating the valve.[1,3]

Open mitral commissurotomy is selected when the patient has had a previous closed commissurotomy, atrial clots are suspected, or valvular replacement is a strong possibility. Access is gained through the wall of the left atrium so that the top of the valve can be viewed. The valve leaflets are then incised.[1,2,4]

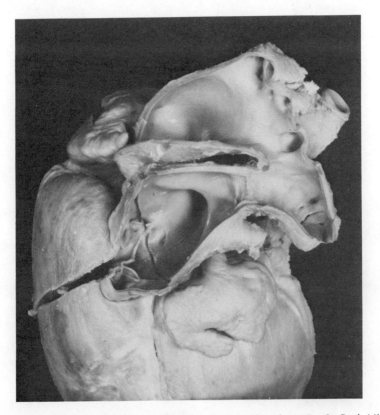

FIG. 6-2. Patent ductus arteriosus. (Courtesy Jesse E. Edwards, M.D., St. Paul, Minn.)

PROSTHETIC REPLACEMENT OF DISEASED CARDIAC VALVE(S)

A patient who has significant functional alteration of one or more cardiac valves is a candidate for the surgical placement of a prosthetic valve(s). Prosthetic valve replacement is indicated in a patient with a defective valve who has developed: (1) progressive congestive heart failure, (2) systemic emboli from the left atrium, and/or (3) endocarditis.[1,2]

A number of prosthetic valves have been designed and tested in laboratory animals and humans.[11] Two general types of valves are now being used, mechanical valves and tissue valves (Table 6-1). In both types there are a number of variations in design and materials used in construction (Figs. 6-3 to 6-5). During open heart surgery the prosthet-

TABLE 6-1. Types of prosthetic valves now in use

Mechanical valves
Caged ball
Cloth-covered
Non-cloth-covered
Central disc and conical occluder
Tilting disc
Tissue valves
Aortic valve homograft
Porcine aortic valve xenograft
Bovine pericardial xenograft
Dura mater homograft

From Lefrak, E.A., and Starr, A.: Cardiac valve prostheses, New York, 1979, Appleton-Century-Crofts.

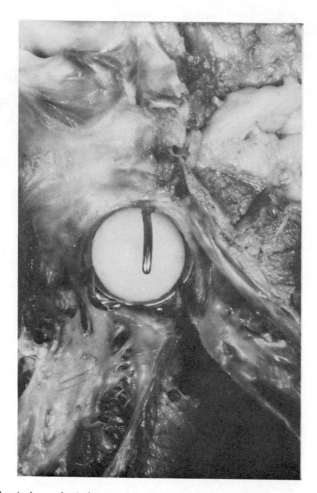

FIG. 6-3. Mechanical prosthetic heart valve. (Courtesy Jesse E. Edwards, M.D., St. Paul, Minn.)

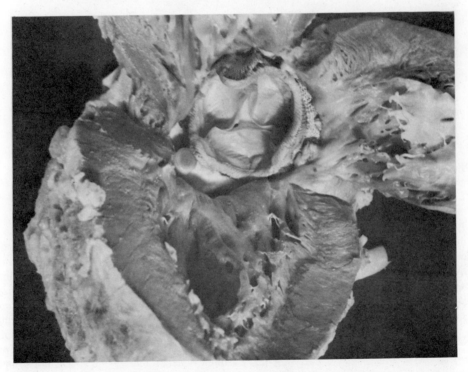

FIG. 6-4. Tissue prosthetic heart valve. (Courtesy Jesse E. Edwards, M.D., St. Paul, Minn.)

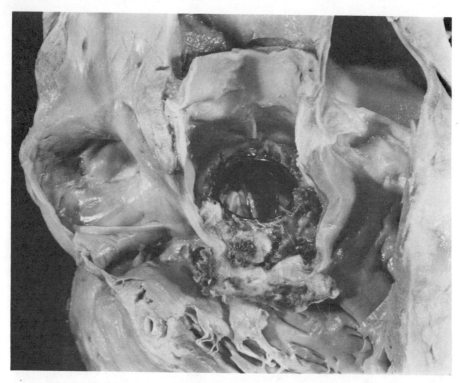

FIG. 6-5. Mechanical prosthetic heart valve with prosthetic heart endocarditis. (Courtesy Jesse E. Edwards, M.D., St. Paul, Minn.)

ic valve is sutured to the surrounding tissues, replacing the diseased valve, which is removed. Prosthetic valve failure involves: (1) excessive thrombosis on and around the valve, leading to systemic emboli, (2) infection at the site of attachment to cardiac tissues, and (3) mechanical failure of valve components.

CORONARY ARTERY BYPASS GRAFT

Before a coronary artery bypass graft (CABG) procedure is selected for a patient who has significant coronary artery disease, the natural history of the disease must be considered (Fig. 6-6). The available reports have shown that symptoms do not always correlate with risk of death or myocardial infarction. A person may develop myocardial infarction or sudden death without a history of pain. Thus angiography may be indicated by reasonable suspicion for the presence of coronary disease in the absence of clinical symptoms.[6]

In a study of 112 patients who were advised to have a CABG and refused, the following observations were reported[6]: (1) data available at the time of catheterization correlated poorly with subsequent death or survival, (2) 55% of the patients were dead within 2 years, (3) symptom complex or crescendo of pain was associated with increased mortality, (4) major stenosis of the proximal left coronary artery was the most significant predictor of early death, and (5) the absence of symptoms or number of infarcts did not correlate with either survival or death.

Indications for CABG surgery are (1) tight stenosis of the proximal left coronary system, (2) severe vessel disease, and (3) crescendo-type anginal pain. As the number of coronary vessels involved by atherosclerotic narrowing increases, the death rate increases, and surgery becomes more advisable.[6]

Single, nondominant coronary disease is not as-

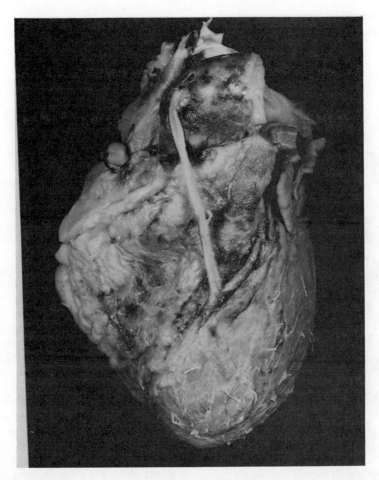

FIG. 6-6. Coronary artery bypass graft. (Courtesy Jesse E. Edwards, M.D., St. Paul, Minn.)

sociated with early death and often is successfully treated by medical means.[6] A patient with poor ventricular function is a candidate for coronary artery surgery only when severe, life-threatening coronary atherosclerosis is present. Smoking is an important factor in the patient who develops pulmonary complications during the postoperative period. Some physicians will not perform elective surgery for the patient who continues to smoke.

Most grafts are performed by taking a section of saphenous vein from the leg and connecting it to the aorta and then to the involved coronary vessel distal to the stenotic lesion. Closure of the graft after surgery is one of the major concerns with coronary artery bypass surgery. The skill of the surgical team and the graft flow rate at the time of surgery are two important factors in determining the long-term patency of the graft. A flow rate below 20 ml/mm is associated with a high rate of graft closure.[6]

ARTERIAL GRAFT

Arterial grafts are used to replace segments of large arteries such as the aorta that have developed an aneurysm secondary to severe atherosclerotic disease (Fig. 6-7). The material most commonly used for the graft is Dacron. Autogenous tissues also may be used for replacement of segments of large or small arteries.

Infections of arterial grafts are not common;

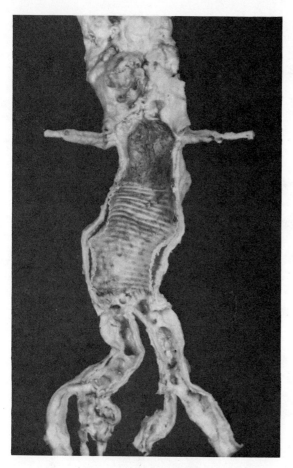

FIG. 6-7. Dacron arterial graft sutured into place. (Courtesy Jesse E. Edwards, M.D., St. Paul, Minn.)

however, one major cause of infection appears to be wound contamination from the skin or from infected lymph nodes. Hematogenous implantation of bacteria on the uncovered surface of the graft following transient bacteremias also may occur after surgical manipulation of the genitourinary tract or oral cavity.[12,14,19]

IMPLANTATION OF TRANSVENOUS PACEMAKER

When significant blockage has occurred in the conduction system of the heart, a pacemaker may have to be used to maintain a relatively normal cardiac rhythm. Temporary and permanent pacemakers are used (see Chapter 5).

Three types of temporary pacemakers are used. *External pacemakers* are the simplest and are used in emergency situations. Electrodes are placed at the scapula and right sternal border on the skin. Care must be taken to avoid pain, severe muscle spasms, and burns. Placement of a *percutaneous pacemaker* consists of passing a wire through the skin into the left ventricle and then attaching the wire to the skin by the suture. *Transvenous pacemakers* consist of a bipolar catheter that is inserted, under fluoroscopic observation, through the external jugular vein into the right ventricle and a battery-operated pacemaker that is attached to the catheter. If a "soft" catheter is used, the fluoroscope is not needed for insertion.[5] A patient with a fixed complete heart block usually has a transvenous pacemaker inserted. This is then replaced by a permanent pacemaker implant.[7]

Several types of permanent pacemakers are available. A transvenous pacemaker that is wired to a generator buried in the subcutaneous tissues is the most commonly used type (Fig. 6-8). Others consist of electrode implants on the epicardium or left atrium and ventricle. Some pacemakers may have a receiving coil that is implanted in the subcutaneous tissues and an impulse generator that transmits radio signals to the implanted coil located externally.

Chung[4] reports that only about 5% to 6% of the patients who have transvenous pacemakers develop a problem with infection. The mortality is low, about 2%. Endocarditis is uncommon but can occur. Most of the infections with pacemakers, however, involve the local area around the generator, which is remote from the heart. Infections involving the electrode catheter may lead to endocarditis.

TRANSPLANTATION OF HEART

A patient with end-stage heart disease for whom no other treatment is available is a candidate for cardiac transplantation. The procedure is complex and carries many operative and postoperative risks. Tissue matching of donor and recipient is most important. The recipient's immune response is then suppressed by chemotherapeutic agents, and the operation is performed with the timing

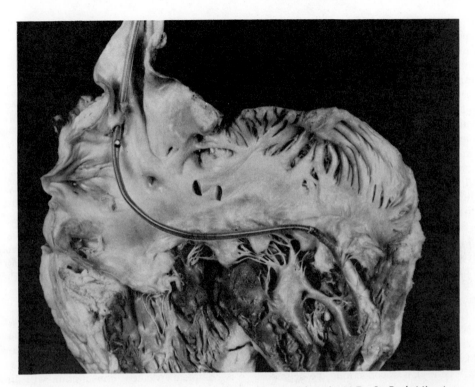

FIG. 6-8. Transvenous pacemaker. (Courtesy Jesse E. Edwards, M.D., St. Paul, Minn.)

based on the death of the donor. Usually two operating teams are needed, one to remove the heart from the donor and the other to transplant the donor's heart into the recipient.

There have been over 325 recipients of human heart transplants in the world. The University Medical Center of Stanford has performed over 137 heart transplants. The current survival figures from Stanford show that about 68% of the patients survive for 1 year, and that 56% are alive at the end of 5 years. These results are equal to the success rates for cadaver renal allografts.[1,17]

The Stanford program incorporates several major advancements in the management of the heart transplant patient. Careful tissue typing is most important in the selection of a donor heart. By the use of antithymocyte globulin and serial measurements of T-lymphocytes, the immunologic rejection reaction can be monitored and combated and reduced levels of corticosteroids and azathioprine (an antimetabolic agent) can be used. This re-

duces the frequency and severity of infections and toxic side effects caused by these agents. The problem of accelerated graft atherosclerosis of the coronary arteries is dealt with by the use of oral anticoagulants (warfarin sodium), a platelet antagonist (dipyridamole), and the control of serum lipid levels.[1,17]

Although the number of transplant patients is small at present, these patients may require dental care. In addition, if the current trend continues, medical centers across the country may soon begin to provide heart transplantation as a treatment alternative for selected patients. When this occurs, the number of heart transplant patients will increase, and there will be a greater number of transplant patients seeking dental care.

DENTAL MANAGEMENT
Medical considerations

Patients who have had surgical procedures to correct cardiac or vascular defects have varying degrees of susceptibility to endocarditis and endarteritis, depending on the location of the surgery, the material used for the correction or replacement, and in some cases the length of time since surgery.

For example, experimental work with dogs has shown that cardiac and arterial grafts made of Dacron may become completely covered by repair tissue (endocardium or endothelium) and are not susceptible to endocarditis or endarteritis once this has occurred. However, a significant number of Dacron grafts never become completely covered, and small defects remain that are susceptible to endocarditis or endarteritis.[13] In contrast, procedures that use autogenous tissues to close or replace the defect remain susceptible to endocarditis only until healing has occurred at the surgical site.

Prosthetic valve replacements are susceptible to infective endocarditis or prosthetic valve endocarditis (PVE), because these valves are attached to surrounding cardiac tissues by numerous nonabsorbable sutures. Thus the site of attachment remains susceptible to infection from transient bacteremias.

Each of the surgical procedures discussed in this chapter will be reviewed concerning the degree of susceptibility to infection from transient dental bacteremias and the type of antibiotic coverage that would best protect the patient from developing endocarditis or endarteritis.

SURGICALLY CLOSED SEPTAL DEFECT

The type of septal defect and the material used to close it must be determined by medical consultation. Small septal defects closed by absorbable sutures are susceptible to endocarditis only during the immediate postoperative period. Once healing has occurred, a patient who had a septal defect closed by absorbable sutures is no longer susceptible to endocarditis and does not require antibiotic coverage for dental treatment. A patient with septal defects that have been repaired by a patch of pericardial tissue also is susceptible to endocarditis only during the immediate postoperative period. Once healing has occurred, this patient is no longer considered susceptible to the disease.

Although healing usually would be complete in 1 to 3 weeks, the patient is usually given antibiotic prophylaxis for any dental treatment received during the first 6 months after surgery. This

TABLE 6-2. Regimen B—prophylactic antibiotic coverage to prevent infective endocarditis in high-risk adult dental patients

A. Patients not allergic to penicillin
   1 million units of aqueous crystalline penicillin G mixed with 600,000 units of procaine penicillin G, IM, administered at least 30 minutes before dental procedure and 1 g streptomycin, IM, followed by 500 mg penicillin V, orally, every 6 hours for eight doses.

B. Patients allergic to penicillin
   1 g of vancomycin, IV, 30 minutes to 1 hour before dental procedure followed by 500 mg erythromycin, orally, every 6 hours for eight doses.

Recommended by the American Heart Association for control of subacute bacterial endocarditis following dental procedures. From Kaplan, E.L.: Prevention of bacterial endocarditis, Circulation **56:**139A-143A, 1977. By permission of the American Heart Association, Inc.

practice is recommended by the American Heart Association.[9] Regimen B is usually recommended (Table 6-2) during the healing stages and then regimen A (Table 6-3) or no coverage once healing is complete. Medical consultation will direct the choice.

A patient who had septal defect closed with a Dacron patch is considered to be susceptible to endocarditis during the immediate postoperative period and to remain less susceptible thereafter because of incomplete coverage of the Dacron patch by endocardial tissues. Regimen B is usually recommended during the first 6 months after surgery. Regimen A (see Table 6-3) may be used thereafter based on the results of medical consultation.

LIGATED OR RESECTED DUCTUS ARTERIOSUS

A patient with a surgically corrected ductus arteriosus remains susceptible to endarteritis during the immediate postoperative period, that is for the first 6 months after surgery. This patient is given antibiotic coverage, using regimen B, during any dental treatment. After the 6-month postoperative period, a patient with a ductus arteriosus corrected by resection is no longer considered to be susceptible to endarteritis and is not given antibiotic prophylaxis when receiving dental treatment.

A patient whose patent ductus arteriosus was closed by sutures would be given regimen B for the

TABLE 6-3. Regimen A—prophylactic antibiotic coverage to prevent infective endocarditis in adult dental patients

I. Patients not allergic to penicillin
  A. 1 million units of aqueous crystalline penicillin G mixed with 600,000 units of procaine penicillin G, IM, administered at least 30 minutes before dental procedure followed by 500 mg Penicillin V, orally, every 6 hours for eight doses *or*
  B. 2 g of penicillin V, orally, at least 30 minutes before dental procedure followed by 500 mg Penicillin V, orally, every 6 hours for eight doses.

II. Patients allergic to penicillin or who are receiving low penicillin dosage to prevent recurrent attacks of rheumatic fever
  1 g of erythromycin, orally, at least 1½ to 2 hours before dental procedure followed by 500 mg erythromycin, orally every 6 hours for eight doses.

Recommended by the American Heart Association for control of subacute bacterial endocarditis following dental procedures. From Kaplan, E.L.: Prevention of bacterial endocarditis, Circulation 56:139A-143A, 1977. By permission of the American Heart Association, Inc.

6 months after surgery when receiving any dental treatment. After that time, no coverage is indicated. In rare cases, the ductus may become patent again because of defective sutures, etc. If this occurs, the patient would become susceptible to endarteritis once again. Thus it is important to determine by medical consultation the method used to correct the ductus arteriosus, the patient's current status, and the need for antibiotic prophylaxis.

COMMISSUROTOMY FOR DISEASED CARDIAC VALVE(S)

A patient who has had either an open or closed commissurotomy to improve cardiac valvular function remains susceptible to endocarditis and must be given regimen B before and after all dental procedures. The dentist should consult with the patient's physician whenever possible before rendering any dental care.

PROSTHETIC REPLACEMENT OF DISEASED CARDIAC VALVE(S)

In a recent report[20] involving 4,586 patients in whom 4,706 prosthetic valves had been placed, 45 cases of PVE occurred. This represented an in-cidence of 0.98%. PVE was described as either early or late. The early cases occurred within 2 months of the surgical implantation of the prosthetic valve and had an 88% mortality (14 of 16 patients). Early PVE is thought to be caused by contamination at the time of surgery. Late PVE occurred 2 months or longer after surgery and had a mortality of 38% (11 of 29 patients). Late cases of PVE were thought to be caused by transient bacteremias. One late case of PVE followed dental manipulation; others followed urinary tract infections, wound infections, surgical procedures, trauma, etc. In 22 cases no apparent portal of entry for the infecting agent was identified. The overall mortality of this group of patients (early and late PVE) was 56% (25 of 45 patients).

Karchmen et al.[10] reported on 43 cases of late PVE in which the mortality was 53% (23 of 43 patients). Nine patients reported that dental procedures were performed before the onset of symptoms of PVE. In addition, two patients were reported to have severe periodontal disease. Thus a total of 11 patients may have had a dental cause for their PVE. The authors reported that three of the nine patients who had received dental treatment before the onset of PVE had been given prophylactic antibiotics but did not describe the drug used or the dosage.

Dismukes[5] reported on 38 cases of PVE, 19 early and 19 late, with an overall mortality of 50%. Four patients with late PVE appeared to have an associated dental cause, and one of these patients had received prophylactic antibiotics.

These reports show that PVE is associated with a significant mortality and that dental procedures may serve as a source of infection. A patient with a prosthetic heart valve(s) must be given antibiotic coverage before and after all dental procedures. The coverage recommended by the American Heart Association[9] is regimen B (see Table 6-2). These coverages are different from those for the patient with rheumatic or congenital heart disease and reflect the greater risk involved in terms of mortality and morbidity. Ideally, a patient who is going to receive a prosthetic heart valve should have all indicated dental treatment performed before the valve is placed. Whenever posible, the patient's physician should be consulted before any dental treatment is performed.

CORONARY ARTERY BYPASS GRAFT

Except for the immediate postoperative period, CABG patients do not appear to be susceptible to endarteritis[13] and therefore require no prophylactic antibiotic coverage for dental procedures. Regimen B is recommended when indicated during the immediate postoperative period. The patient's current cardiac status and the need for prophylactic antibiotics should be established through consultation with the patient's physician before any dental treatment is performed.

ARTERIAL GRAFT

From 1963 to 1974, 859 vascular grafts were placed in patients at the Virginia Medical Center.[12] There were 22 cases of graft infection (2.5%). A review of the literature by Liekweg et al.[12] showed 153 cases of graft infection, which represented an incidence of infection ranging from 0.25% to 6.0%. There were 52 deaths, which represented a 34% mortality. The longest interval from implantation to symptoms of infection was 87 months with a mean of 27 weeks. Synthetic grafts appear to be much more susceptible to infection than autogenous grafts.

The following recommendations are made for a patient with an arterial graft who is going to receive dental treatment: (1) consult with the patient's physician; (2) give prophylactic antibiotic coverage, using regimen B, for all dental procedures for any patient who has an arterial graft that has been in place less than 6 months; (3) no coverage appears to be indicated for autogenous grafts that have been in place more than 6 months; and (4) because small areas of incomplete pseudointimal lining may be present in an older synthetic graft, which would render the graft susceptible to bacterial infection, it may be best to give the patient antibiotic coverage before and after all dental procedures. The final decision to give coverage or not should be made in consultation with the patient's physician. Because of the decreased risk of infection it would appear that regimen A would be adequate.

IMPLANTATION OF TRANSVENOUS PACEMAKER

Bryan et al.[3] in a recent report on endocarditis related to transvenous pacemakers concluded that the problem is rare and does not support the use of prophylactic antibiotic therapy during procedures that are likely to cause transient bacteremias. The 1977 report by the American Heart Association Committee on Rheumatic Fever and Endocarditis[9] stated that indwelling transvenous cardiac pacemakers appear to present a low risk of endocarditis; however, the report left it open to the dentist and physician to choose whether to employ prophylactic antibiotics during dental and surgical procedures in patients with pacemakers. If it is decided to give coverage it would appear that regimen A (Table 6-3) would be adequate. Electrical equipment, such as Cavitron, electric vitalometer, and electric cautery equipment, should not be used on a patient who has a cardiac pacemaker because of possible interference with the function of the pacemaker.

TRANSPLANTATION OF HEART

Under no circumstances should dental care be provided to a heart transplant patient before consultation with the patient's physician has occurred. Endocarditis does not appear to be a problem in these patients once healing has occurred. However, infection is an ever-present danger for the heart transplant patient because of the suppression of the patient's immune system. Therefore prophylactic antibiotic therapy is recommended for all dental procedures. The dosage should be established by consultation with the patient's physician. The patient is usually taking oral anticoagulants and therefore potentially has a bleeding problem. The level of anticoagulation may have to be reduced by the patient's physician before any surgical procedures are begun (the prothrombin time should be two times normal or less), and the dentist must be prepared to deal with excessive bleeding by the use of splints, thrombin, pressure, etc. (Chapter 20).

The heart transplant patient who is receiving steroids may not be able to adjust to the stress of various dental procedures and may require additional steroids before and after these dental procedures to protect against an acute adrenal crisis (see Chapter 16).

Treatment planning modification

A patient being prepared for surgery to correct a cardiac or vascular defect should be referred for an evaluation of dental status. A patient found to have active dental disease should receive dental care before surgery to correct the cardiovascular defect. This is most important for a patient who is going to receive a prosthetic heart valve. The patient will require prophylactic antibiotic coverage, using regimen B, for any dental treatment that is needed after the cardiovascular surgery. This involves the injection of penicillin and streptomycin followed by oral penicillin or, if the patient is allergic to penicillin, an IV drip of vancomycin followed by oral erythromycin. Most dentists are not prepared to give parenteral antibiotics, so a special visit to the physician would be required before each dental appointment. The patient allergic to penicillin would most likely have to be hospitalized for each dental appointment so that the IV drip of vancomycin could be given.

The basic problem faced when dental treatment is planned for a patient who is about to have or has already undergone cardiovascular surgery (especially placement of a prosthetic heart valve) relates to the retention of teeth in cases where the level of dental repair is moderate to poor. A patient who has advanced periodontal disease may be best advised to have his teeth extracted and dentures constructed. This would be most advisable for the patient with a prosthetic heart valve who is allergic to penicillin. The same consideration would be involved for a patient who has extensive caries and has shown little interest in improving his level of oral hygiene or diet.

Patients who have a very high level of dental health should be encouraged to keep their teeth, but they must be advised of the problems involved when dental care is provided after cardiovascular surgery.

Recommendations concerning retention of teeth for a patient who has a dental status that falls between the extremes of poor and very good are more difficult to make. The risks involved regarding endocarditis or endarteritis, the steps needed to prevent these complications, and the costs involved must be discussed with the patient and his cardiovascular surgeon. Then the patient can make an informed decision based on the value he places on retention of his natural teeth. A patient with poor oral hygiene who has failed to become motivated to improve his level of home care should be encouraged more strongly to become edentulous and have dentures constructed.

A patient who is considered susceptible to endocarditis or endarteritis must be given the appropriate antibiotic coverage regimen at the time the new dentures are inserted. The patient should be examined the next day, and if sore spots have developed the dentures must be adjusted.

Once an antibiotic coverage period is started, as much dental treatment as possible should be performed during this coverage period. Under very special circumstances, the coverage period may be extended to 5 to 7 days. At least 1 week should elapse after completion of a coverage period before another is started (Chapter 2).

Emergency dental care

A patient with a surgically corrected cardiac or vascular defect who remains susceptible to endocarditis or endarteritis must be given the appropriate antibiotic coverage regimen when receiving emergency dental care. Once antibiotic coverage has been started, any emergency dental procedure can be performed unless the patient is taking an anticoagulant, has congestive heart failure, etc. (see Chapters 5 and 8).

Medical consultation should be obtained, particularly if the patient is still in the immediate postoperative phase (the first 6 months) or has a transplanted heart, before any dental care, even emergency care, is initiated.

REFERENCES

1. Austen, W.G.: Heart transplantation after ten years, N. Engl. J. Med. **298:**682-683, 1978.
2. Boake, W.C., and Kroncke, G.M.: Pacemaker complications. In Varriale, P., and Naclerio, E.A., editors: Cardiac pacing: a concise guide to clinical practice, Philadelphia, 1979, W.B. Saunders Co., pp. 229-238.
3. Bryan, C.S., et al.: Endocarditis related to transvenous pacemakers: syndromes and surgical implications, J. Thorac. Cardiovasc. Surg. **75:**758-762, 1978.
4. Chung, E.K.: Complications and malfunctions of artificial cardiac pacing. In Chung, E.K., editor: Artificial cardiac pacing: a practical approach, Baltimore, 1978, The Williams & Wilkins Co., pp. 327-346.
5. Dismukes, W.E.: Prosthetic valve endocarditis, Circulation **48:**365-377, 1973.
6. Eleland, W.P.: Closed mitral valvotomy. In Longmore, D.B., editor: Modern cardiac surgery, Baltimore, 1978, University Park Press, pp. 45-47.
7. Feola, M.: Techniques of permanent pacing. In Chung, E.K., editor: Artificial cardiac pacing: practical approach,

Baltimore, 1978, The Williams & Wilkins Co., pp. 223-239.

8. Friedberg, C.K.: Diseases of the heart, vol. II, ed. 3, Philadelphia, 1976, W.B. Saunders Co., pp. 1187-1299.

9. Kaplan, E.L.: Prevention of bacterial endocarditis, Circulation **56:**139A-143A, 1977.

10. Karchmen, A.W., et al.: Late prosthetic valve endocarditis, Am. J. Med. **64:**199-206, 1977.

11. Lefrak, E.A., and Starr, A.: Cardiac valve prostheses, New York, 1979, Appleton-Century-Crofts, pp. 41-67.

12. Liekweg, W.G., et al.: Infections of vascular grafts: incidence, anatomic location, etiologic agents, morbidity and mortality. In Duma, R.J., editor: Infections of prosthetic heart valves and vascular grafts: prevention, diagnosis and treatment, Baltimore, 1977, University Park Press, pp. 239-252.

13. Moore, W.S.: Experimental studies relating to sepsis in prosthetic vascular grafting. In Duma, R.J., editor: Infections of prosthetic heart valves and vascular grafts: prevention, diagnosis and treatment, Baltimore, 1977, University Park Press, pp. 267-287.

14. Moore, W.S.: Infection in prosthetic vascular grafts. In Rutherford, R.B., et al., editors: Vascular surgery, Philadelphia, 1977, W.B. Saunders Co., pp. 385-397.

15. Perloff, J.K.: Congenital heart disease. In Beeson, P.B., et al., editors: Cecil textbook of medicine, ed. 15, Philadelphia, 1979, W.B. Saunders Co., pp. 1149-1172.

16. Rosenthal, A.: When to operate on congenital heart disease. In Chung, E.K., editor: Controversy in cardiology: the practical clinical approach, New York, 1976, Springer-Verlag, New York, Inc., pp. 136-152.

17. Stinson, E.B., and Shumway, N.E.: The national heart hospital lecture: transplantation of the heart. In Longmore, D.B., editor: Modern cardiac surgery, Baltimore, 1978, University Park Press, pp. 3-19.

18. Szarnicki, R.J.: Results of patent ductus arteriosus ligation in infants and children. In Longmore, D.B., editor: Modern cardiac surgery, Baltimore, 1978, University Park Press, pp. 163-167.

19. Szilagyi, D.E.: Antibiotic prophylaxis in vascular grafting. In Duma, R.J., editor: Infections of prosthetic heart valves and vascular grafts: prevention, diagnosis, and treatment, Baltimore, 1977, University Park Press, pp. 323-342.

20. Wilson, W.R.: Prosthetic valve endocarditis: incidence, anatomic location, cause, morbidity and mortality. In Duma, R.J., editor: Infections of prosthetic heart valves and vascular grafts: prevention, diagnosis and treatment, Baltimore, 1977, University Park Press, pp. 3-17.

7

HYPERTENSIVE DISEASE

Hypertensive disease has been defined as a sustained elevation of the diastolic blood pressure that results from increased peripheral arteriolar resistance and leads to cardiac, renal, retinal, and cerebrovascular complications. The first indication of the disease most often is an increase in blood pressure. Increased blood pressure may be the only finding for a variable period of time. The term *hypertension* or *high blood pressure* is used to describe the patient who has an elevation in blood pressure greater than 140/90 mm Hg.[11,13,14,16]

Patients who have a blood pressure between 140/90 and 160/95 mm Hg are described as being borderline hypertensives. Definite hypertension is present when the blood pressure is found to be greater than 160/95 mm Hg. Most authors define the severity of definite hypertension based on the level of the diastolic pressure: mild hypertension between 95 and 104 mm Hg, moderate between 105 and 114 mm Hg, and severe 115 mm Hg or greater.[3,9]

The diagnosis of hypertensive disease should be made only by the physician. In the early stages of the condition it may be impossible even for the physician to make the diagnosis. This is because the patient may be hypertensive yet show no evidence of retinal, cerebral, renal, or cardiac involvement. The changes, as they develop, will allow the diagnosis to be established.[10,13,14,16] However, patients who have sustained moderate to severe elevation in blood pressure are treated as if they have hypertensive disease even if they do not show retinal, cerebral, renal, or cardiac involvement.

The dentist can play a very important role in the life of the individual who has hypertensive disease. If patients are unaware of their condition, the dentist, as a member of the health team, may be the first to detect the elevation of blood pressure or symptoms of hypertensive disease or both. Patients with hypertensive disease may be in danger in the dental office, since any procedure or drug that causes an elevation of blood pressure may precipitate a myocardial infarction or cerebrovascular accident. By obtaining an adequate health history and measuring the blood pressure of all patients, the dentist will be able to detect these individuals before starting any dental treatment. By prompt referral of the hypertensive patient, a medical diagnosis can be established and early treatment begun, which may prolong the life of the patient.

Once under medical care, the hypertensive patient may return for dental treatment. The dentist must be careful to avoid dangerous drug interactions between certain agents used in dentistry and medications used to treat hypertension. In addition, every effort must be made by the dentist to reduce as much as possible the stress and anxiety often associated with dental treatment, which can cause an increase in blood pressure.

GENERAL DESCRIPTION
Incidence

Just a few years ago only about one half of the individuals who had hypertension were aware of the problem.[9,11] Now this has increased to about 70%. The increased detection of hypertension appears to be the result of the numerous screening programs across the country.[14,16] It has been estimated that about 35 million Americans have definite hypertension and about 25 million have borderline hypertension. In a Caucasian, suburban population (Framingham, Massachusetts) 20% of the adults were found to have a blood pressure above 160/95 mm Hg and 45% to have a blood pressure above 140/90 mm Hg.[16] Screening of 160,000 people took place as part of the Hypertension Detection and Follow-up Program, and 10,940 were found to be hypertensive (7%). Mild hypertension (diastolic pressure less than 105) was found in 71% of these and moderate to severe hypertension in 28.5%.[3,7,8]

About 10% of the individuals with hypertension have an associated underlying condition that explains the presence of the hypertension. This form of hypertension is called secondary hypertension. The other 90% of the people with hypertension have essential hypertension, which has no known cause.[4]

Hypertension occurs early in a higher percentage of blacks than whites. The incidence of hypertension in American blacks may be as high as 17% to 25%.[11] Women develop hypertension slightly more commonly than men but appear to tolerate it better.

A hypertension detection project undertaken by dentists in Bergen County, New Jersey, demonstrates how common this disease is and the impact of a screening program by dentists.[1,2] During the project 1071 adult dental patients were screened for hypertension. Of these, 126 (12%) were found to have sustained hypertension; 68 of these patients knew of their condition, and 58 were unaware of the problem. Of the 58 patients who had possible hypertensive disease, seven were lost to follow-up. Of the remaining 51 patients, 44 had hypertensive disease and were placed under medical treatment.

Thus in the Bergen County project 44 patients with undetected hypertensive disease were found, representing an incidence of 4.1% in the adult population studied. Seven patients were referred who did not have hypertensive disease for a 13.6% rate (7 of 51) of false-positive identifications. The preceding data demonstrate the impact the dental profession could have in the detection of hypertensive disease if blood pressure recordings were performed on all patients.

Etiology

As stated earlier, the majority of patients with hypertension have no cause established for their disease. The remainder of patients have underlying systemic disease that produces hypertension as a complication.

A few systemic conditions will cause hypertension that results only in the increase of systolic blood pressure. These conditions are thyrotoxicosis, anemia, arteriovenous fistula, and psychogenic disorders.[4] The majority of conditions that cause hypertension lead to an elevation of both diastolic and systolic blood pressure. These conditions include renal disease, endocrine problems, neurogenic problems, and conditions of unknown cause. The endocrine problems include acromegaly, adrenocortical hyperfunction, and pheochromocytoma. The neurogenic problems include brain tumors, cerebrovascular accidents, poliomyelitis, and psychogenic disorders.[3,11,13,16]

Patients who have hypertension resulting from unilateral renal disease such as renal artery obstruction or pyelonephritis can, once detected, be cured of the hypertension by surgical correction of the defect or removal of the diseased kidney. About 1% of all patients with hypertensive disease will have correctable renovascular disease.[3,16]

In a few patients with secondary hypertension, a tumor of the adrenal medulla, pheochromocytoma, will be responsible for their hypertension. This lesion is surgically treatable.

Hyperfunction of the adrenal gland caused by a tumor of the adrenal cortex or by cortical hyperplasia may cause secondary hypertension in a few cases. These conditions also are surgically treatable.

Weight gain has been demonstrated to cause an increase in blood pressure.[16] The most common cause of endocrine hypertension is oral contraceptives. About 5% of women taking "the pill" will have a blood pressure greater than 140/90.[16]

Hypertension develops earlier and with greater severity in successive generations with hypertensive predecessors.

Pathophysiology and complications

The blood pressure is measured by the use of an instrument that records the diastolic and systolic

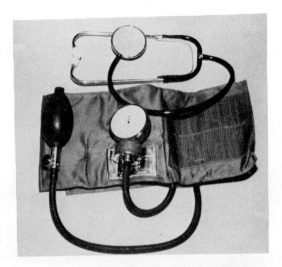

FIG. 7-1. Standard blood pressure cuff and stethoscope.

levels (Fig. 7-1). The diastolic pressure represents the total resting resistance in the arterial system following passage of the pulsating force produced by contraction of the left ventricle. The pulsating force is modified by the degree of elasticity of the walls of larger arteries and the resistance of the arteriolar bed. The pressure at the peak of ventricular contraction is the systolic blood pressure. The difference between the diastolic and systolic pressures is termed *pulse pressure*.

Many factors may alter the blood pressure. Increased viscosity of the blood may cause an elevation of blood pressure as a result of an increase in the peripheral resistance to flow. A decrease in blood volume or tissue fluid volume will reduce blood pressure, and an increase in blood volume or tissue fluid volume will increase blood pressure. A decrease in elasticity of the larger arteries will increase blood pressure, because the arteries will fail to distend with the systolic thrust. Increased cardiac output associated with exercise, fever, and thyrotoxicosis will increase the blood pressure. One of the most important clinical causes of increased blood pressure is an increase in peripheral arteriolar resistance.[11,13,16]

Blood pressure is modified by reflex arcs of the autonomic nervous system. Changes in arteriolar tone, lumen size, and cardiac output can be initiated through the autonomic nervous system.

Hormones can increase the smooth muscle tone of arterioles, which results in increased peripheral resistance and increased blood pressure. Epinephrine and norepinephrine, which are produced by the adrenal medulla, may increase smooth muscle tone. Renin, a hormone produced by the kidney, can also increase smooth muscle tone.

Renin levels have been found to be high in about 20% of hypertensive patients, normal in about 60%, and low in 20%.[14] Renin can cause an increase in blood pressure through angiotensin II. Renin activates the formation of angiotensin I, which activates formation of angiotensin II. Angiotensin II causes the increase in blood pressure by stimulating the release of aldosterone from the adrenal cortex. Aldosterone increases sodium retention and increases extravascular fluid levels. Angiotensin II also increases blood pressure by causing vasoconstriction of small blood vessels.[14]

The normal blood pressure increases from infancy (70/45 mm Hg), early childhood (80/55 mm Hg), and adolescence (100/75 mm Hg) to adulthood. The upper normal level for adults is 140/90 mm Hg. In about one third of the population, a transient period of increased blood pressure may occur in early adulthood and is the usual finding beyond the age of 60 years. On an individual basis such increases may be of little significance, but data based on large numbers of people indicate that occasional rises in the resting blood pressure are associated with shortening of the life span. Untreated sustained elevations in blood pressure carry an even greater risk in terms of shortening the life span. This is true for systolic as well as diastolic pressures.[10,11,13]

It has been estimated that untreated hypertension reduces the life span by 10 to 20 years. Even mild hypertension that has not been treated for 7 to 10 years increases the risks of complications such as stroke, and heart attack.[16]

Complications of essential hypertension include renal failure, cerebrovascular accident, coronary insufficiency, myocardial infarction, congestive heart failure, and blindness. The hypertension precedes the onset of vascular changes in the kidney, heart, brain, and retina that may lead to these clinical complications.

CLINICAL PRESENTATION
Signs and symptoms

Most cases of essential hypertension follow a chronic course. Sustained hypertension may be the only sign present for a number of years. The patient is usually asymptomatic at first and is unaware of the problem. The "early" symptoms of hypertension are occipital headache, vision changes, ringing ears, dizziness, and weakness and tingling of the hands and feet. If there is significant kidney, brain, heart, or eye involvement, there will be other signs and symptoms related to these organ systems (Table 7-1).

Funduscopic examination of the eyes may show early changes of hypertension consisting of hemorrhages, narrowed arterioles, exudate, and, in more advanced cases, papilledema. In more advanced cases the left ventricle may be enlarged, and a tapping left ventricular apical beat can often be observed in the thin individual. Renal involvement can result in hematuria, proteinuria, and renal failure.[3,11,13,16] Hypertensive persons may complain of fatigue and coldness of the legs as a result of peripheral artery changes that occur in advanced hypertension.

These findings may be seen in patients who have essential hypertension. They also may be present in patients who have secondary hypertension. However, additional signs or symptoms may be present that are associated with the underlying disease. Hypertension that is severe and has an abrupt onset before the age of 35 has about a 50% probability of having a secondary cause.[14]

Children who have acute glomerulonephritis may complain of malaise, fever, anorexia, vomiting, and generalized edema. Adults who have acute glomerulonephritis may complain of malaise and at times a dull headache. Patients with pyelonephritis usually have weight loss, fatigue, dysuria, and lumbar pain.

Patients who have pheochromocytoma may complain of anxiety, profuse perspiration, headaches, pallor, palpitations, and vomiting. These symptoms are caused by the release of norepinephrine by the tumor cells. The attacks may last minutes or hours, and frank angina pectoris may occur.

Patients who have primary aldosteronism experience episodes of generalized muscular weakness, paralysis, paresthesia, polyuria, polydipsia, and cardiac irregularity as a result of the associated hypokalemia.

Pure diastolic hypertension is very rare, and when it occurs it is found in children or young adults. Pure systolic hypertension may be found in older patients.[3]

Laboratory findings

A 1980 report of the Joint National Committee on Detection, Evaluation and Treatment of High Blood Pressure recommended that patients who have sustained hypertension be screened using hematocrit, urinalysis (protein, blood, glucose), and blood chemistry (potassium, creatinine, cholesterol, blood glucose, uric acid) laboratory tests.[9] An electrocardiogram and chest x-ray film also were suggested. These tests serve as the baseline laboratory values that should be obtained before initiating therapy. If clinical and laboratory findings suggest the presence of an underlying cause for the hypertension, then additional tests should be ordered.[6,16]

TABLE 7-1. Signs and symptoms of hypertensive disease

Signs
  Early
    Increased blood pressure
    Narrowing of retinal arterioles
    Retinal hemorrhages
  Advanced
    Papilledema
    Cardiac enlargement—left ventricle
    Hematuria
    Proteinuria
Symptoms
  Occipital headache
  Failing vision
  Ringing ears
  Dizziness
  Weakness
  Tingling of hands and feet
  Congestive heart failure
  Angina pectoris
  Renal failure

MEDICAL MANAGEMENT

There is not complete agreement among physicians on when and how to treat varying degrees of hypertension. Factors that have been given in favor of medical treatment of patients with essential hypertension include the following: a minimal elevation of either systolic or diastolic blood pressure increases morbidity and mortality; labile hypertension is associated with an increase in morbidity and mortality; and effective drugs with minimal side effects are now available to treat hypertension. Also, some available data suggest that treatment decreases the incidence of vascular complications and increases longevity. Adequate therapy also may reverse cardiac and retinal changes. The incidence of death from heart failure secondary to hypertension has been reported to be greatly decreased since the advent of drug therapy for hypertension.[3,6,11,13]

Factors contraindicating treatment of patients with essential hypertension include the following: drugs are expensive and produce a financial burden on the patient; some of the drugs are toxic and have significant side effects; when severe renal damage is present, therapy is difficult and less effective and may be dangerous; and if significant cerebral or coronary artery disease is present, therapy may be dangerous, because a decrease in perfusion pressure and a reduction in arterial flow may result.[3,6,11,13]

It appears that most physicians believe that essential moderate to severe hypertension should be treated to prevent complications and halt the progression of complications that are already present. On the other hand, some workers in the field believe that the clinical course of mild essential hypertension is so benign and prolonged that treatment is not justified unless multiple risk factors for coronary atherosclerotic heart disease are present.[5] All observers appear to agree, however, that malignant essential hypertension must be treated.

The following are factors that lead most physicians to prescribe more vigorous therapy for patients who have essential hypertension. The prognosis of hypertension in men is worse than in women. The prognosis is worse in blacks than in whites. The higher the diastolic pressure, the worse the prognosis. If there is a family history of hypertension, the prognosis is worse. In the presence of changes in optic fundi, cerebrovascular disease, and congestive heart failure, the prognosis is worse.[3,6,11,13]

There are factors that may allow the physician to recommend less vigorous therapy. Patients who are obese may be able to reduce their blood pressure by weight reduction and restriction of sodium intake. If patients are older at the time of onset, they may be allowed to maintain the higher pressure because of the shorter life expectancy and poor tolerance to antihypertensive drugs of older people. Women may tolerate moderate elevation of blood pressure for many years without serious consequences. Systolic hypertension secondary to arteriosclerosis of the aorta and great vessels may not have to be treated.

Several general measures are suggested in the treatment of hypertension. These include relief of stress, dietary control, regular exercises, and elimination of cigarette smoking.[4,6] Although the long-term effectiveness of techniques used in stress reduction (yoga, biofeedback, meditation) has not been demonstrated, they do aid the patient's sense of well-being and may help in changing life-style. Dietary control consists of restriction of sodium chloride intake, calories, cholesterol, and saturated fatty acids. Drug therapy is indicated for most hypertensive patients.[4,16]

Treatment of patients who have uncomplicated essential hypertension usually consists of starting with the drugs least likely to produce side effects. More vigorous treatment is reserved for patients with serious hypertension in whom milder forms of therapy have failed. In young patients with severe hypertension and in any patient with malignant hypertension, the side effects of the stronger antihypertensive agents must be accepted. Once treatment of essential hypertension has been started, it must be continued with good medical supervision.

The Joint National Committee on Detection, Evaluation and Treatment of High Blood Pressure recently made the following general recommendations[9]:

1. Any group measuring blood pressure should have resources available for referral, confirmation, and follow-up of the patient.
2. Virtually all patients with diastolic pressure of two

or more readings of 105 mm Hg or greater should be treated with antihypertensive drug therapy.

3. For persons with diastolic pressures of 90 to 104 mm Hg, treatment should be based on individual circumstances concerning presence of risk factors such as family history, sex, etc.
4. Evaluation of patients with high blood pressure can be limited to a few baseline laboratory tests in most cases.
5. A step approach should be used in treatment.
6. Treatment of patients with high blood pressure includes plans for facilitating long-term maintenance of blood pressure control.

The Committee recommended the following courses of action for patients, depending on what the initial blood pressure measurement was. All adults found to have a diastolic blood pressure of 115 mm Hg or greater should be referred for medical evaluation and treatment. All adults found to have a diastolic blood pressure of 95 to 114 mm Hg should have their blood pressure measurement repeated within a month. Individuals with an initial diastolic blood pressure recording of 90 to 95 mm Hg should have their blood pressure rechecked within 3 months.

Recommended action by the Committee for persons with these blood pressure measurements is as follows. Patients with diastolic pressure of 115 mm Hg or greater should receive immediate medical evaluation and treatment. Treatment also is suggested for patients with a diastolic pressure of 105 to 114 mm Hg. Patients with a diastolic pressure of 90 to 104 mm Hg should be evaluated on an individual basis for presence of risk factors to decide the need for treatment. Persons under 35 years of age with an initial systolic blood pressure recording of 150 mm Hg or greater should be referred. For individuals over 35 an initial systolic pressure of 160 mm Hg or greater should lead to referral. Patients with a repeated diastolic pressure of less than 90 mm Hg should have their blood pressure measured every year.

The purpose of rechecking the blood pressure is to identify individuals whose diastolic pressure has returned to normal and to identify persons with sustained elevation of diastolic pressure. At each visit the blood pressure should be checked twice with the patient in a seated position, and the two measurements should be averaged.

The medical evaluation of the patient with elevated diastolic blood pressure should include a determination of the severity of blood pressure increase and a search for any complications by means of history, physical examination, and the recommended baseline laboratory tests.[9] More complex diagnostic procedures designed to discover specific causes of secondary hypertension, such as primary aldosteronism, renovascular disease, and pheochromocytoma, should be reserved for the following:

1. Individuals who have a history and examination findings that suggest the presence of secondary hypertension
2. Individuals who are under the age of 30 years, since this age group contains the greatest prevalence of correctable causes of secondary hypertension
3. Individuals in whom drug therapy has proved to be inadequate or unsatisfactory
4. Individuals with accelerated or malignant hypertension

Four progressive steps are used to treat patients with hypertension as defined earlier[3] (Table 7-2).

1. The first step involves initial treatment with a drug that decreases intravascular fluid volume. The primary drug used for this purpose is a thiazide diuretic. Many patients with mild to moderate hypertension can be managed very well with this drug along with modification of controllable risk factors such as smoking and salt intake.
2. If thiazide diuretics fail to control the disease, the second step in treatment is to add a drug that blocks adrenergic neurons. Reserpine, clonidine, prazosin, or methyldopa may be used.
3. The patient who does not respond well to the second step of management will move to the third step in treatment, which is the addition of a stronger drug that inhibits vascular reactivity—hydralazine.
4. Patients with severe hypertension who are not responsive to the third step of management are treated with a stronger drug that blocks adrenergic neurons—guanethidine.

The principal side effects of the thiazides are decreased blood volume, hypokalemia, hyperglycemia, gastrointestinal irritation, weakness, photo-

TABLE 7-2. Side effects of and precautions with commonly used antihypertensive drugs

Drug	Common side effects	Special considerations
Diuretics		
Thiazide and thiazide-derived diuretics	Hypokalemia, hyperuricemia	Digitalis and hypokalemia, gout, renal insufficiency, pancreatitis
Loop diuretics	Hypokalemia, hyperuricemia	Excessive diuresis, hyponatremia, ototoxicity (IV), gout, digitalis and hypokalemia
Potassium-sparing agents		
Spironolactone	Hyperkalemia, lethargy, gynecomastia, mastodynia, gastrointestinal symptoms, menstrual irregularities	Hyperkalemia, renal failure
Triamterene	Hyperkalemia, nausea, weakness, leg cramps	Hyperkalemia, renal failure
Adrenergic-inhibiting agents		
Clonidine	Drowsiness, fatigue, dry mouth, constipation, dizziness	Rebound hypertension, concomitant use of other central nervous system depressants
Guanethidine	Postural hypotension, diarrhea, weakness, nasal stuffiness, retrograde ejaculation, bradycardia	Heart failure, renal failure, severe bradycardia
Methyldopa	Drowsiness, fatigue, dizziness, dry mouth	Hepatic disease, hyperpyrexia, hemolytic anemia (Coombs positive)
Metoprolol	Bradycardia, anorexia, nausea, lightheadedness, insomnia, fatigue	Heart failure, asthma, diabetes, peripheral vascular disease
Nadolol	See metoprolol	See metoprolol
Prazosin	Postural dizziness, palpitations, headache, drowsiness, weakness, nausea	Postural syncope (first dose)
Propranolol	See metoprolol	See metoprolol
Rauwolfia alkaloids	Nasal congestion, depression, lethargy	Mental depression, peptic ulcer disease
Vasodilators		
Hydralazine	Headache, tachycardia, palpitations, nausea	Coronary artery disease, lupuslike syndrome (rare at recommended doses)
Minoxidil	Tachycardia, palpitations, edema, hypertrichosis, mastodynia	Coronary artery disease, fluid retention, congestive heart failure

From Joint National Committee on Detection, Evaluation and Treatment of High Blood Pressure, U.S. Department of Health and Human Services, Public Health Service: 1980 report, National Institutes of Health, NIH Publication No. 81-1088, December 1980. Permission of National High Blood Pressure Education Program.

sensitivity, impotency, and, in rare cases, blood dyscrasias. Side effects of rauwolfia drugs include drowsiness, nasal congestion, bradycardia, mental depression, nightmares, and impairment of sympathetic cardiovascular reflex while under general anesthesia. Methyldopa may cause orthostatic hypotension, drowsiness, depression, dry mouth, impotency, fluid retention, and liver disease. Hydralazine may cause headache, tachycardia, palpitations, exacerbation of angina or congestive heart failure, and a lupuslike mesenchymal reaction. Guanethidine may cause orthostatic hypotension, weakness on exertion, bradycardia, diarrhea, and symptomatic cardiovascular disease[9] (see Table 7-2).

DENTAL MANAGEMENT
Medical considerations

It is important to identify the patient with severe, undiagnosed hypertensive disease before starting dental treatment, because the stress and anxiety associated with dental procedures may raise the patient's blood pressure to dangerous levels. In a patient with diseased vessels and an already high blood pressure, the additional increase in blood pressure may result in a cerebrovascular accident or a myocardial infarction. In addition, the dentist may use an excessive amount of local anesthetic containing a strong vasopressor, which can cause a significant increase in blood pressure. The dentist also may use a strong vasopressor to control local bleeding or to retract gingival tissues in preparation for taking impressions of teeth cut for gold castings. All of these procedures can result in significant elevation of the blood pressure, which in the normal patient would not be dangerous but in the undetected hypertensive patient could be life threatening.

It is important for the dentist to know which patients are receiving medical treatment for hypertensive disease. Many are treated with strong antihypertensive drugs that have significant side effects and possibly may interact with agents used in dentistry.

Many known hypertensive patients may be receiving medical treatment for complications of hypertensive disease such as cardiac failure or myocardial infarction. The drugs used to manage these problems must be identified, since they will necessitate modification of the dental management plan.

TABLE 7-3. Dental management of hypertensive patient: detection

History
  Signs
  Symptoms
Blood pressure
  Baseline for emergency management
  Screen for hypertensive disease
History of past illness
Medications patient may be taking
  Physicians' Desk Reference
  Drug information center
  Physician

The first task of the dentist is to identify by blood pressure measurement and history those patients who may have significant hypertension (Table 7-3). Two blood pressure recordings should be taken on all new patients during the first dental appointment, and the results should be averaged. This average figure represents the blood pressure for that day. The blood pressure is recorded for two reasons. First, it serves as a baseline from which to make decisions for the emergency management of the patient should an untoward systemic reaction occur later during dental treatment. Second, it is used to screen patients (along with a medical history) to identify those who have or may have hypertensive disease.

A complete medical history should be obtained from each patient (see Chapter 1). Included in the history are questions concerning the presence of symptoms associated with hypertensive disease. The patient should be asked if he is taking any medications. If the patient does not know the name of the drug, the *Physicians' Desk Reference (PDR)* can be used to identify it. The patient's pill, tablet, or capsule is matched with pictures of various manufacturers' medications. Once the medication has been identified, the section of the *PDR* that describes the drug should be consulted. Here the drug action, side reactions, and drug interactions can be obtained.

Based on information (average of two blood pressure recordings and history) obtained from a patient during the first dental examination appoint-

TABLE 7-4. Dental management of hypertensive patient: patient grouping based on clinical and history findings

Group	Patient
I	Normal
II	Initial average blood pressure greater than 140/90 mm Hg with no symptoms of hypertensive disease
III	Under treatment of physician at present
IV	Has been treated but discontinued treatment program or is not following it—"out of control"
V	Symptoms of hypertensive disease and blood pressure greater than 140/90 mm Hg

TABLE 7-5. Dental management of group II hypertensive patient

Patient with diastolic blood pressure of 115 mm Hg or greater—refer for medical evaluation and treatment

Repeat blood pressure recording at next appointment or within 1 month for all other patients in this group

  If repeat blood pressure recording is normal, continue with dental care

  If repeat blood pressure recording is also elevated, refer patient for medical evaluation; after medical evaluation and treatment, have patient return for management as in group III

ment, five separate groups of patients can be identified (Table 7-4).

Group I Patients who have no history of hypertensive disease, have no symptoms of hypertension, and have normal blood pressure

Group II Patients who have no history of hypertensive disease, have no symptoms of hypertension, but have initial average blood pressure reading greater than 140/90 mm Hg

Group III Patients who are being treated by physician for hypertension at present

Group IV Patients who have been treated for hypertension but who discontinued their treatment program or who are not following it as they should and are "out of control"

Group V Patients who have blood pressure greater than 140/90 mm Hg and reveal symptoms of hypertensive disease but who have never been to physician for diagnosis or treatment

GROUP I

For the patient in group I, the dentist may continue with all dental work. The patient should be recalled at least once a year for remeasurement of blood pressure.

GROUP II

The patient in group II gives no symptoms of hypertensive disease. If the diastolic pressure is 115 mm Hg or greater (average of two recordings taken during first dental appointment), the appointment should be concluded and the patient referred to a physician for evaluation and treatment. Patients under 35 years of age who have a systolic average of 150 mm Hg or greater should also be referred. Patients over 35 years of age who have a systolic average of 160 mm Hg or greater should be referred. Once the patient is under medical treatment, he should return for dental care and be managed as described for patients in group III.

If the diastolic recording is less than 115 mm Hg and greater than 90 mm Hg, the first dental appointment can be continued. It is best that this be an examination-type appointment and that no dental treatment be rendered. A second appointment should be made for these patients, and at that time two blood pressure recordings should be made and the results averaged. If the average diastolic recording is greater than 90 mm Hg, the patient should be referred for medical evaluation and treatment.

Patients who have repeated blood pressure recordings below 140/90 mm Hg can have their dental treatment continued and should be recalled at least once a year for dental evaluation and remeasurement of the blood pressure (Table 7-5).

Patients who had a moderate elevation of blood pressure at the first appointment but had a normal blood pressure at the second appointment should be treated as normotensive patients. Anxiety about the first dental appointment would be the most likely reason for the moderate elevation of blood pressure.

TABLE 7-6. Dental management of group III hypertensive patient

Consult with patient's physician
Identify patient
Identify medical problem
Establish current status (presence of other disease)
Confirm medications
Identify general dental needs
Explain dental management plan
Ask for comments and suggestions
After physician's response, finalize dental management plan

TABLE 7-7. Dental management of group IV hypertensive patient

Refer to physician for treatment
Have patient return after control has been regained
Manage as in group III

GROUP III

The patient in group III has hypertensive disease that is under good medical control. After all examination procedures have been completed and dental diagnoses established and a tentative treatment plan has been developed, the dentist should discuss the following points with the patient's physician:

1. Identify the patient and his dental problem. Ask what the patient's current medical status is and confirm the medications with which the patient is being treated.
2. Describe in general terms the type of dental treatment you are planning.
3. Describe your management plan for the patient in light of his medical status.
4. Ask the physician for suggestions regarding the management plan.

When you have received the physician's replies to these points, the final dental management plan can be established (Table 7-6).

GROUP IV

The patient in group IV has hypertensive disease that is not under good medical control. Patients who, for whatever reason, have failed to follow their medical treatment program and are "out of control" should be referred back to their physician. When their disease is under control these patients can return for completion of the examination and receive dental treatment. They would then be managed the same as patients in Group III (Table 7-7).

GROUP V

The patient in group V has overt signs and symptoms of hypertensive disease and is not under a physician's care. This patient would be referred to a physician. After a medical diagnosis has been established and the patient's disease is under control, the patient can return for dental care. This patient too would then be managed the same as a group III patient (Table 7-8).

• • •

An attempt should be made by the dentist to develop an approach to the management of all patients that will reduce the stress and anxiety associated with dental treatment as much as possible. This is of particular importance in dealing with the hypertensive patient. A critical factor in providing an "anxiety-free" situation is the relationship established among the dentist, office staff, and patient. An attempt should be made to establish an atmosphere in which patients are encouraged to express their fears and concerns about dental treatment (Table 7-9).

Anxiety can be reduced for many patients by premedication with diazepam (Valium) the night before and the day of the dental appointment. Barbiturates can be used, but they present more problems because of drug interactions, which will be discussed later.

Hypertensive patients should be scheduled for treatment in the morning rather than in the afternoon, when they may be stressed from the day's activities. Long appointments should be avoided. If the patient becomes overstressed during the appointment, it should be terminated and the patient scheduled for another day.

Since many of the antihypertensive agents have as a side effect the tendency to produce acute episodes of postural hypotension, sudden changes in

TABLE 7-8. Dental management of group V hypertensive patient

Refer to physician for treatment
Have patient return and manage as in group III

TABLE 7-9. Dental management of hypertensive patient: reduction of stress and anxiety

Atmosphere of openness and support
Explanation of treatment plan—honesty
Dealing with fears and concerns
Premedication—diazepam, sedatives (reduced dosage)
Nitrous oxide (avoid hypoxia)
Morning appointments
Avoidance of long appointments
Dismissal of patient if appears to be overstressed

the patient's position during dental treatment should be avoided. In addition, when the patient is dismissed the dental chair should be returned to an upright position slowly and the patient supported as he gets out of the chair, until it is clear that he has obtained good balance.

General anesthesia in the dental office is not indicated for patients who are taking antihypertensive drugs, because the anesthetic can precipitate serious episodes of hypertension. Nitrous oxide analgesia can be used with the hypertensive patient, provided the equipment is functioning well and hypoxia is avoided. Hypoxia can cause a rapid increase in blood pressure, which could be dangerous in a patient with hypertensive disease.

Some of the stronger antihypertensive drugs cause as a side reaction a rather severe mental depression in some patients. Although there is little the dentist can do to control or alter the depression, an awareness of this complication may explain various mood changes observed in patients. If severe depression is observed in a patient who is taking antihypertensive drugs, the dentist should talk with the patient about the possibility that the depression is related to the medication. The dentist should recommend that this patient see his physician.

A local anesthetic with epinephrine in a concentration of 1:100,000 or less (remember that a *lower* concentration is indicated by a *higher* figure in the ratio, for example, 1:200,000) is recommended for use in patients who are receiving antihypertensive drug therapy, particularly for procedures that will last longer than 30 minutes. It is important that good anesthesia be obtained, and this would be difficult without the very small amount of vasopressor. The basis for giving a vasopressor to a hypertensive patient is to ensure adequate anesthesia to eliminate any pain, which in turn would produce the release of larger amounts of endog-

enous catecholamines. However, as a rule of thumb, no more than three cartridges of anesthetic solution should be given for any dental appointment. For very short procedures it may be desirable to give a local anesthetic without a vasopressor, if an adequate level of anesthesia can be obtained. It is most important to aspirate before injecting the local anesthetic, because even a small amount of vasopressor accidentally injected into the vascular system could increase blood pressure. The anesthetic should be injected slowly. Epinephrine should not be used as a vasopressor in the anesthetic for a patient who is being treated with monoamine oxidase (MAO) inhibitors, such as pargyline (Eutonyl), because these drugs will greatly potentiate the actions of the vasopressor. Patients being treated with MAO inhibitors should be given a local anesthetic containing a very small concentration of a vasopressor other than epinephrine; phenylephrine (Neo-Synephrine) or nordefrin (Cobefrin) may be used. For short procedures, a local anesthetic without a vasopressor may be considered for patients who are taking MAO inhibitors.

Vasopressors should not be used to control local bleeding problems in the hypertensive patient. When doing crown and bridge procedures for hypertensive patients, gingival packing material that contains a vasopressor must not be used (Table 7-10).

Central nervous system depressants (barbiturates, narcotics, antianxiety drugs) should not be given to patients who are taking MAO inhibitors. The MAO inhibitors prolong and intensify the actions of depressant drugs. If it has been at least 2

TABLE 7-10. Dental management of hypertensive patient: drug considerations

Antihypertensive drugs

Side effect of nausea and vomiting

Side effect of postural hypotension
  Sudden change in position
  Supporting patient when getting out of chair

Avoidance of general anesthetics, since severe hypotension may result

Potentiation of effects of barbiturates—if used, dosage of sedative should be reduced

Central nervous system depressants should not be used in patients taking MAO inhibitors

Side effect of severe depression

Nitrous oxide

Avoidance of hypoxia since marked elevation of blood pressure can occur

Epinephrine

Use of weak concentration (1:100,000) in local anesthetic

No more than three cartridges of local anesthetic should be used

Aspiration before injection; slow injection

Gingival packing material that contains a vasopressor should not be used

Vasopressor should not be used to control local bleeding

Epinephrine should not be used in patients taking MAO inhibitors, such as pargyline

weeks since a patient has taken a MAO inhibitor, the central nervous system depressants can be used.

Many of the other antihypertensive agents also will potentiate the actions of barbiturates. Barbiturates can still be used in patients who are receiving these medications; however, the usual dosage must be reduced. Before using a barbiturate in a patient who is receiving antihypertensive medication, the dentist should consult the patient's physician concerning the dosage. In addition, sedative medications may cause hypotensive episodes in patients who are taking certain antihypertensive agents and must be used with care. Once again the specific antihypertensive drug(s) a patient is being treated with should be looked up in the *PDR*, significant side effects and drug interactions noted, and the appropriate action taken.

Many of the antihypertensive agents cause a tendency for nausea and vomiting. Excessive stimulation of the gag reflex during dental treatment in patients taking these drugs may bring on nausea and vomiting and should be avoided.

Treatment planning modifications

No routine dental procedures should be performed for the patient who has hypertension and is not receiving medical management. Patients who are receiving good medical management and have no complications such as renal failure or congestive heart failure can receive any indicated dental treatment. If complications are present, the treatment plan may have to be modified.

Oral complications

There are not many oral complications associated with hypertensive disease itself. Patients who have malignant hypertension have been reported to develop facial palsy on occasion.[15] Patients who have severe hypertension have been reported to bleed excessively following surgical procedures or trauma. However, excessive bleeding in hypertensive patients is not common, and when observed it is usually found in patients who have coarctation of the aorta.[12] Patients who are receiving antihypertensive agents may complain of dry mouth. The mecurial diuretics may cause oral lesions on an allergic or toxic basis. Facial and oral paresthesias have been reported in patients who take acetazolamide. Lichenoid reactions have been reported with methyldopa, propranolol, and labetalol.[15]

Emergency dental care

To identify the hypertensive patient, all patients being seen for emergency dental treatment should have a health history and a blood pressure recording taken. Patients under good medical management can receive any needed emergency dental treatment. Patients who have severe hypertension (diastolic pressure greater than 115 mm Hg) should receive only conservative dental treatment for their emergency problem. This would include antibiotics for infection and analgesics for pain. Surgical procedures should be avoided in these patients.

Hypertensive patients who are receiving emergency dental care should not be given a local anesthetic that contains more than a 1:100,000 concentration of epinephrine, and local bleeding must not be controlled with a vasopressor.

REFERENCES

1. Berman, C.L.: Screening dental patients for hypertension, D. Survey, p. 46, November 1974.
2. Berman, C.L., Guarino, M.A., and Giovannoli, S.M.: High blood pressure detection by dentists, J. Am. Dent. Assoc. **87**:359-363, 1973.
3. Dustan, H.P.: Pathophysiology of hypertension. In Hurst, J.W., editor: The heart, ed. 5, New York, 1983, McGraw-Hill Book Co., pp. 1171-1181.
4. Gunnells, J.C., Jr.: Treatment of systemic hypertension. In Hurst, J.W., editor: The heart, ed. 5, New York, 1983, McGraw-Hill Book Co., pp. 1196-1212.
5. Freis, E.D.: Should mild hypertension be treated? N. Engl. J. Med. **307**:306-309, 1982.
6. Hall, W.D., Wollam, G.L., and Tuttle, E.P., Jr.: The diagnostic approach to the patient with hypertension. In Hurst, J.W., editor: The heart, ed. 5, New York, 1983, McGraw-Hill Book Co., pp. 1196-1212.
7. Hypertension Detection and Follow-up Program Cooperative Group: Five-year findings of the Hypertension Detection and Follow-up Program. I. Reduction in mortality of persons with high blood pressure, including mild hypertension, JAMA **242**:2562-2571, 1979.
8. Hypertension Detection and Follow-up Program Cooperative Group: Five-year findings of the Hypertension Detection and Follow-up Program. II. Mortality by race, sex, and age, JAMA **242**:2572-2577, 1979.
9. Joint National Committee on Detection, Evaluation and Treatment of High Blood Pressure, U.S. Department of Health and Human Services, Public Health Service: 1980 report, National Institutes of Health, NIH Publication No. 81-1088, December 1980.
10. Moser, M., et al.: Report of the Joint National Committee on Detection, Evaluation and Treatment of High Blood Pressure: a cooperative study, JAMA **237**:255-261, 1977.
11. Peart, W.S.: Arterial hypertension. In Beeson, P.B., and McDermott, W., editors: Textbook of medicine, ed. 14, Philadelphia, 1975, W.B. Saunders Co., pp. 981-992.
12. Rose, L.F., Godfrey, P., and Steinberg, B.J.: Dental correlations. In Rose, L.F., and Kaye, D., editors: Internal medicine for dentistry, St. Louis, 1983, The C.V. Mosby Co., pp. 572-575.
13. Russell, R.P.: Systemic hypertension. In Harvey, A., editor: Osler's the principles and practice of medicine, ed. 19, New York, 1976, Appleton-Century-Crofts, pp. 370-392.
14. Singh, S.: Systemic hypertension. In Rose, L.F., and Kaye, D., editors: Internal medicine for dentistry, St. Louis, 1983, The C.V. Mosby Co., pp. 465-475.
15. Scully, C., and Clawson, R.A.: Cardiovascular disease. In Medical problems in dentistry, London, 1982, Wright PSG, pp. 29-33.
16. Williams, G.H., and Branonwald, E.: Hypertensive vascular disease. In Petersdorf, R.C., et al., editors: Harrison's principles of internal medicine, ed. 10, New York, 1983, McGraw-Hill Book Co., pp. 1475-1488.

8

CONGESTIVE HEART FAILURE

One of the most common causes of death in the United States is congestive heart failure.[3] Patients who have untreated or poorly managed heart failure are high-risk patients, because serious medical complications such as infection, cardiac arrest, excessive bleeding, cerebrovascular accident, and myocardial infarction can occur in the dental office as complications secondary to receiving dental treatment. The purpose of this chapter is to present the basic pathophysiology, clinical findings, medical management, and dental management for the patient with congestive heart failure. The emphasis is directed toward the role of the dentist in detecting these patients based on history and clinical findings, referring the patient for medical diagnosis and management, and then with close consultation with the physician developing a dental management plan so that effective and safe dental care can be rendered for the patient.

At times the patient who has untreated or poorly managed heart failure will be seen in need of emergency dental care. The management of these problems also will be considered in this chapter. In general under these conditions no dental care should be rendered other than analgesics for pain control and antibiotics for infection until consultation with a physician.

Under no circumstances should elective, routine dental care be rendered to a patient who has signs and symptoms of congestive heart failure. Once the patient is under good medical control and an effective dental management plan has been established with input from the patient's physician, routine dental care may be delivered.

GENERAL DESCRIPTION
Incidence and etiology

Congestive heart failure is much like anemia in that it represents a symptom complex that can be caused by any number of specific disease processes. The three most common causes of congestive heart failure are cardiac valvular disease, coronary atherosclerotic heart disease and its complications, and hypertensive disease. Other causes include thyrotoxicosis, rheumatic fever, congenital heart disease, severe anemia, chronic obstructive lung disease, and pulmonary hypertension. With the recent increases in the frequency of coronary atherosclerotic heart disease and hypertensive disease alone, the number of individuals susceptible to congestive heart failure in the United States is increasing greatly, and the dentist must be prepared to recognize patients who have congestive heart failure and be able to manage them properly.

Congestive heart failure may involve the failure of the left ventricle, right ventricle, or both ventricles. Most of the acquired disorders that may lead to congestive heart failure result usually in failure of the left ventricle. This often is followed by failure of the right ventricle. Initial failure of the right side of the heart is much less common and is associated with certain of the congenital heart defects or with emphysema. By the time most patients are seen for medical treatment, failure of both sides of the heart has usually occurred.

Pathophysiology and complications

Congestive heart failure is the end stage of a disproportion between the hemodynamic load and

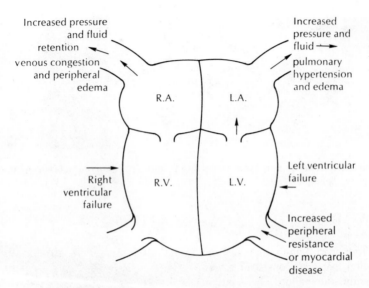

Increased pressure
and fluid
retention

venous congestion
and peripheral
edema

Increased
pressure and
fluid

pulmonary
hypertension
and edema

R.A.   L.A.

Right
ventricular
failure

R.V.   L.V.

Left ventricular
failure

Increased
peripheral
resistance
or myocardial
disease

FIG. 8-1. Effects of right and left side heart failure.

the capacity of the heart to handle the load. This imbalance can occur with chronic increase in the load or damage to the myocardium. In most cases a combination of these two factors is involved. Chronic congestive heart failure usually evokes compensatory adjustments consisting of increased peripheral resistance, redistribution of the blood flow to heart and brain, and increased erythropoietic activity to increase the oxygen-carrying capacity of the blood.

Failure of the heart most often begins with left ventricular failure brought about by either increased work load or disease of the heart muscle. The increased work load may result from aortic valve disease, anemia, arterial hypertension, etc. Direct effects on the myocardium may be the result of infections, rheumatic fever, or infarction. The outstanding symptom of left ventricular failure is dyspnea, which results from blood accumulation in the pulmonary vessels. Acute pulmonary edema is often associated with left ventricular failure. Left-side heart failure leads to pulmonary hypertension, which increases the work of the right ventricle pumping against the increased pressure and often leads to right-side heart failure as well. In fact the most common cause of right-side heart failure is preceding failure of the left ventricle. An

important feature of left ventricular failure is the retention of sodium and water and the insufficient emptying of the left ventricle during systole.[3]

Failure of the right side of the heart alone is uncommon. The most common cause of pure right-side heart failure is emphysema. Systemic venous congestion and peripheral edema are the major results of failure of the right side of the heart (Fig. 8-1).

Ventricular failure will lead to dilation and hypertrophy of the ventricle in an attempt to compensate for its inability to keep up with the work load.

The increased erythropoietic activity of the bone marrow in response for the need to increase the oxygen-carrying capacity of the blood can lead to polycythemia, thrombocytopenia, and leukopenia. The clinical results of these changes are the same as those described in Chapter 4 that occur following the right-to-left shunting of blood that results from congenital heart lesions. These include susceptibility to infection as a result of the decrease in circulating white blood cells and excessive bleeding following trauma or surgical procedures brought about by the reduction in circulating platelets and coagulation factors (depleted as a result of thrombosis in small vessels).

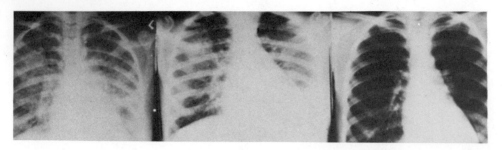

FIG. 8-2. Chest x-ray films demonstrating resolving pulmonary edema from left to right. (Courtesy J. Noonan, M.D., Lexington, Ky.)

CLINICAL PRESENTATION
Signs

Patients with overt heart failure may demonstrate a gallop rhythm that may consist of a ventricular, atrial, or summation gallop. The ventricular gallop occurs in the dilated heart during left ventricular filling. The atrial gallop results from the forceful presystolic distention of the ventricle by atrial contraction. The summation gallop consists of a triple rhythm that occurs during tachycardia because of coincidence of atrial and ventricular gallops.[3]

A pulsus alternans—a regular alternation of one strong beat with one weak beat—may be present.

The circulation time is usually prolonged. Decholin time, the measurement of arm-to-tongue circulation time, is prolonged beyond the normal 10 to 15 seconds.

Radiographs of the chest may show enlargement of one or more of the heart chambers and the presence of pulmonary venous congestion and edema (Fig. 8-2).

Evidence of systemic venous congestion may be detected by the presence of distended neck veins, large tender liver, peripheral edema (Fig. 8-3), ascites (Fig. 8-4), and cyanosis. In addition, the patient may appear ruddy in color because of polycythemia and may show clubbing of the fingers (Fig. 8-5, Table 8-1).

Symptoms

Exertional dyspnea and fatigue in a patient suggest the possibility of beginning left-side heart failure. Indications of overt heart failure include

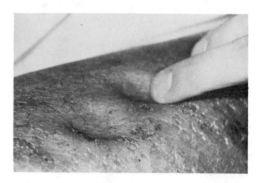

FIG. 8-3. Pitting pretibial edema in patient with congestive heart failure. (Courtesy N. Wood, D.D.S., M.S., Ph.D., Chicago, Ill.)

the following: orthopnea, paroxysmal nocturnal dyspnea (patient wakes gasping for breath), periodic breathing consisting of alternate periods of hyperventilation and apnea, and weakness. The patient may have a low-grade fever (Table 8-2).

Laboratory findings

The laboratory findings of greatest importance to the dentist relate to the status of the red blood cells, white blood cells, platelets, and coagulation mechanism. Many patients who have congestive heart failure will demonstrate polycythemia, thrombocytopenia, and leukopenia. In addition, the amounts of circulating coagulation factors may be depleted, possibly resulting in prolongation of the prothrombin time and partial thromboplastin time.

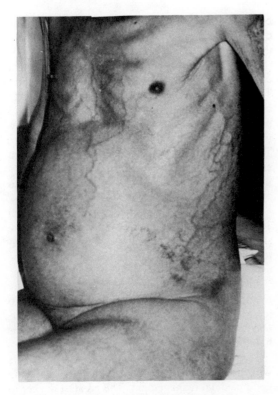

FIG. 8-4. Ascites. (Courtesy P. Akers, D.D.S., Evanston, Ill.)

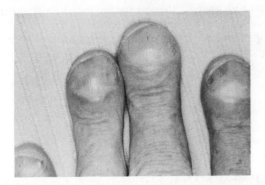

FIG. 8-5. Clubbing of fingers in patient with congestive heart failure.

TABLE 8-1. Signs and symptoms of congestive heart failure

Signs	Symptoms
Gallop rhythm	Fatigue and weakness
Pulsus alternans	Dyspnea on exertion
Prolonged circulation time	Orthopnea
Cardiac enlargement shown on chest radiographs	Paroxysmal nocturnal dyspnea
Distended neck veins	Periods of hyperventilation
Large, tender liver	
Peripheral edema	Low-grade fever
Ascites	
Cyanosis	

TABLE 8-2. Dental management of patient with congestive heart failure

I. Consultation with patient's physician
   A. Medications—confirmation
   B. Present status—routine dental care for patients under good medical management and control
   C. Nature of underlying problem
      1. Valvular disease
      2. Hypertensive disease
      3. Myocardial infarction
      4. Hyperthyroidism
      5. Emphysema

II. Patients receiving digitalis
   A. Prone to nausea and vomiting
   B. Avoidance of stimulating gagging

III. Patients receiving dicumarol
   A. Patient may have bleeding problem
   B. Prothrombin time should be brought to 1½ to 2 times normal if any invasive procedures are planned
   C. Adjustment of medication by physician

IV. Polycythemia
   A. Thrombocytopenia and decreased fibrinogen levels may be present
   B. Patient may have bleeding problem
   C. Avoidance of dehydration
   D. If white count is depressed, antibiotics are administered to avoid postoperative infection

V. Patient is placed in upright position in dental chair

MEDICAL MANAGEMENT

Several factors relating to the prognosis for the patient who has congestive heart failure are important. The initial response to medical treatment is critical. A lack of response after several days of vigorous medical treatment usually indicates a poor prognosis for the patient.[3] The type of underlying cardiac disease also is important; for example, the patient with mitral stenosis has a much better prognosis than a patient with disease of the myocardium resulting from coronary atherosclerotic heart disease. The reason is that the diseased valve can be surgically opened or replaced, whereas there is no way to replace the necrotic muscle that results from myocardial infarction. The presence of significant ventricular dilation is generally a poor sign.

The medical treatment of the patient who has congestive heart failure usually starts with rest to keep the demands on the heart at a minimum. A semirecumbent position in bed is best to reduce the effects of pulmonary congestion and edema. The patient may be allowed to have bathroom privileges. Minimal exercise that produces no symptoms is allowed for some patients.[3]

The diet is adjusted so that it is low in sodium. At first sodium-free milk (Lanalac), fruit juices, and bananas are given. The water should have a low sodium content. Once improvements are observed, the sodium content in the diet can be increased to about 1 g per day. Obese individuals are usually put on a weight-reduction program.

Digitalis is indicated for most patients with cardiac failure. Once the patient has started taking digitalis it will usually be needed the rest of his life. The drug is not used in most cases of cardiac enlargement or murmur unless dyspnea or edema is present.

Digitalis increases the force of contraction of the cardiac muscle fiber and thus helps overcome the effects of myocardial failure. In addition, the drug is helpful in patients who have a slow rate of ventricular contraction or have atrial fibrillation. In patients with atrial fibrillation, enough of the drug is administered so that the heart rate remains within normal range after mild exercise.

Unless the patient has a preexisting conduction impairment, digitalis rarely causes heart block with bradycardia. The drug may cause a disturbance in the cardiac rhythm consisting of premature beats or atrial tachycardia. The use of a thiazide diuretic without potassium replacement increases the likelihood of these effects.[3]

Diuretic agents are important in the management of the patient who has congestive heart failure. They are used whenever there is increasing edema or dyspnea or when a weight gain of more than 3 pounds occurs during a 7-day period. The commonly used diuretics are mercurials and thiazides. The untoward effects include electrolyte depletion and dehydration. Potassium supplement is usually indicated for patients who are receiving diuretics to avoid cardiac dysrhythmias.[3]

Patients who have severe dyspnea may be given 10 to 20 mg of morphine for 1 or 2 days to promote sleep and reduce the strenuous work of the respiratory muscles.[3] Barbiturates or tranquilizers may be used for the same purpose.

Patients who have acute pulmonary edema may require either an actual or bloodless phlebotomy to reduce the blood volume returning to the heart. Oxygen may be used, and at times thoracentesis may be indicated.

Pregnancy may be tolerated in some patients with congestive heart failure who are receiving good medical management. The greatest danger to the woman with congestive heart failure occurs at the seventh to eighth month of pregnancy, at which time previously undetected heart disease may manifest itself.[3]

The patient with congestive heart failure needs to be evaluated carefully to find the underlying cause of the problem. Once this has been accomplished, specific therapy for the initiating problem should be rendered when appropriate.

In summary, the medical management of the patient with congestive heart disease consists of the following:

1. Increasing cardiac output
2. Decreasing the work load of the heart
3. Improving myocardial contractility
4. Mobilizing excess tissue fluid
5. Detecting and treating the underlying cause when possible

DENTAL MANAGEMENT
Medical considerations

No patient with untreated congestive heart failure should be treated for for routine dental needs until he has been referred for medical management.[1,2] Once the congestive heart failure is under good medical management and the underlying cause has been identified, the patient should be encouraged to return for dental care. The dental management plan then must deal with the problems related to the congestive heart failure and the underlying medical problem. The patient who has congestive heart failure resulting from rheumatic heart disease can serve to demonstrate the problems involved and how they can be managed.

Following detection, referral, and medical treatment, the patient may return for routine dental care. Consultation with the patient's physician confirms that the patient is under good medical control and is being treated with digitalis, a thiazide diuretic, dicumarol, potassium supplementation, and 250 mg per day of oral penicillin to prevent recurrent attacks of rheumatic fever. The patient still has a significant degree of polycythemia; however, the platelet count and white blood cell count are within normal ranges. The prothrombin time is being maintained at about three times the normal value.

The following problems relate directly to the congestive heart failure and its medical management. Patients taking digitalis are more prone to develop nausea and vomiting during dental treatment. Procedures that may cause gagging should be done with extra care in these patients, since gagging may trigger nausea and vomiting. If surgical procedures are planned or if the patient develops oral infection, dehydration must be prevented, since thrombosis may occur that could result in infarction of various organs. Patients under good control may still have some degree of pulmonary edema. Thus if any evidence of pulmonary congestion develops with the patient in the supine chair position, the patient should be placed in an upright position for the remaining dental treatment. In this patient the white blood cell count and platelet count are normal, and no special attention would have to be paid to prevent postoperative infection or bleeding relating directly to these elements. If the patient complains of weakness or fatigue developing during the dental appointment, the appointment should be terminated and the patient given an appointment on another day. In general, morning appointments are best for these patients (see Table 8-2).

The problems that must be considered that relate to the underlying cause of the heart failure, rheumatic heart disease, including the following. The patient must be protected by prophylactic antibiotic coverage during and following all dental procedures in order to prevent infective endocarditis. Because the patient is taking a low daily dosage of oral penicillin, the oral flora may contain penicillin-resistant bacteria; thus erythromycin should be selected for the antibiotic coverage. The physician should be consulted as to whether or not the patient should continue taking the oral penicillin during the periods of erythromycin coverage. (See Chapter 2 for dosage, etc.) If scaling or surgical procedures are planned, the physician should be asked to reduce the dicumarol dosage, and the patient should be managed as described in Chapter 20.

The dentist must be prepared to recognize and deal with any of the serious medical emergencies that may arise at any time during the dental visit in patients with a history of congestive heart failure.

Treatment planning modifications

In general the patient with congestive heart failure who is under good medical management can receive any indicated dental treatment as long as the dental management plans deal effectively with the problems presented by the heart failure and its underlying cause.

Oral complications

There are usually no oral complications directly related to congestive heart failure other than infection, spontaneous gingival bleeding, ecchymoses, and petechiae, which may result from the effects of the polycythemia (thrombocytopenia, leukopenia, and thrombosis).[2]

Emergency dental care

Dental emergencies in the patient who has untreated congestive heart failure should be dealt with in as conservative manner as possible. Good analgesic agents for pain control and antibiotics for control of infections should be given after consultation with a physician. All other dental procedures should be avoided if at all possible until the patient is under good medical control.

REFERENCES

1. Accepted dental therapeutics, ed. 39, Chicago, 1982, American Dental Association, pp. 3-25.
2. Lynch, M.A.: Diseases of the cardiovascular system. In Lynch, M.A., editor: Burket's oral medicine, diagnosis and treatment, ed. 7, Philadelphia, 1977, J.B. Lippincott Co., pp. 375-395.
3. Ross, R.S., et al.: Management of the patient with congestive heart failure. In Harvey A., editor: Osler's the principles and practice of medicine, ed. 19, New York, 1976, Appleton-Century-Crofts, pp. 255-272.

9

PULMONARY DISEASE

Many types of pulmonary disorders may compromise routine dental care and require special management of the patient. Two of the more commonly encountered pulmonary diseases, bronchial asthma and tuberculosis, will be discussed in this chapter.

Bronchial asthma

GENERAL DESCRIPTION
Incidence and etiology

Bronchial asthma is a syndrome consisting of dyspnea, cough, and wheezing caused by bronchospasm, which results from a hyperirritability of the tracheobronchial tree.[5] It is a worldwide problem, but the exact incidence is unclear. It is estimated, however, that 6 to 8 million Americans suffer from bronchial asthma.[4] Of interest is the fact that asthma is uncommon among certain populations, such as West Africans and Eskimos.[5] This observation has not been explained. It is primarily a disease of children and young adults, with males affected more often than females, especially during childhood.

Asthma is a multifactorial disease for which the exact cause is not well defined. Two types of asthma are classically described, allergic (extrinsic) asthma and idiosyncratic (intrinsic) asthma, although these classifications frequently overlap.[5]

Epidemiology

Allergic, or extrinsic, asthma is the most common form of asthma and is usually seen in children and young adults. There is generally an associated family history of allergic diseases in addition to positive skin testing to various allergens. There are elevated serum levels of immunoglobulin E (IgE) in affected individuals. Allergic asthma is often seasonal and may be associated with various grasses or pollen.[5] Approximately 50% of asthmatic children become asymptomatic by adulthood.[4]

The idiosyncratic or intrinsic type of asthma is, in contrast, usually not associated with a family history of allergy. Patients are usually nonresponsive to skin testing to allergens and demonstrate normal IgE levels. This form of asthma is generally seen in middle-aged adults, and its onset is frequently associated with an upper respiratory infection.[5,13] Of interest is the fact that 10% of patients who have intrinsic asthma demonstrate salicylate intolerance.[13]

Asthma may be precipitated by a number of substances or events. Some of the more common include airborne substances (pollen, dust), aspirin and nonsteroidal antiinflammatory drugs (especially in adults who have the triad of asthma, nasal polyps, and sinusitis), environmental pollutants (smoke, chemicals), respiratory infections (viruses), exercise (especially in cold, dry weather), and emotional stress (implicated in at least 50% of asthmatics).[5,6,13]

Pathophysiology

The most striking macroscopic finding in the asthmatic lung is the occlusion of bronchi and bronchioles by thick, tenacious mucous plugs (Fig. 9-1). The characteristic histologic findings in

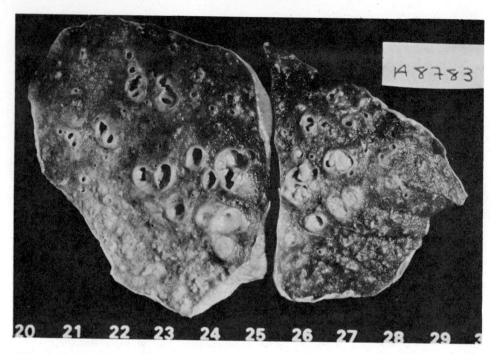

FIG. 9-1. Section of lung with bronchioles occluded by mucous plugs. (Courtesy A. Golden, M.D., Lexington, Ky.)

asthma include (1) thickened basement membrane of the bronchial epithelium, (2) edema, (3) hypertrophy of the mucous glands, and (4) hypertrophy of the bronchial wall muscle.[7] All of these changes result in decreased diameter of the airway.

Sequelae and complications

In terms of serious complications, asthma is relatively benign. It is estimated that between 50% and 80% of patients can expect a relatively good prognosis, especially those whose disease develops during childhood.[5] However, a small percentage of patients can be expected to develop status asthmaticus, the most serious manifestation of asthma. Status asthmaticus is a particularly severe asthmatic attack that is refractory to usual therapy and can lead to death in a matter of minutes. It is often associated with a respiratory infection.[11] Although death directly attributable to asthma is relatively uncommon, the disease is estimated to cause 6000 deaths per year in the United States.[4]

CLINICAL PRESENTATION
Signs and symptoms

The typical symptoms of asthma consist of paroxysms of dyspnea, cough, and wheezing. The onset is usually sudden, with a tightness in the chest and commonly a cough. Respirations become difficult and are accompanied by wheezing. Tachypnea and prolonged expiration are characteristic. The termination of an attack is commonly accompanied by a productive cough. Episodes usually are self-limiting.[4]

Laboratory findings

Laboratory tests for asthma are nonspecific, and any one test alone is not diagnostic. Commonly ordered tests include the following: chest x-ray (for hyperinflation), skin testing (for specific allergens), sputum smears (for eosinophilia), arterial blood gases, and spirometry (to assess pulmonary function).

TABLE 9-1. Common medications used to treat asthma

Methylxanthines
Theophylline (Elixophyllin, Tedral)
Aminophylline

Beta-adrenergic stimulators
Epinephrine (Adrenalin)
Isoproterenol (Isuprel)
Isoetharine (Bronkosol)
Ephedrine (Bronkolixir)
Terbutaline (Brethine)

Chromones
Cromolyn sodium (Intal)

Corticosteroids
Beclomethasone (Vanceril)
Dexamethasone (Decadron)
Prednisolone (Delta-Cortef)
Prednisone (Deltasone)

TABLE 9-2. Dental management of asthmatic patients

I. Identification and assessment by history
  A. Type of asthma (allergic vs. idiosyncratic)
  B. Precipitating factors
  C. Age at onset
  D. Frequency and severity of attacks
  E. How usually managed
  F. Medications being taken
  G. Necessity of emergency care

II. Avoidance of known precipitating factors

III. Medical consultation for severe, active asthmatic

IV. Drug considerations
  A. For recent corticosteroid use, consideration of need for supplementation (see Chapter 16)
  B. If patient uses metered-dose inhaler, instruction to bring it to each appointment and keep it readily available
  C. Consideration of premedication if needed for anxiety—nitrous oxide or diazepam
  D. Avoidance of, if possible:
    1. Antihistamines
    2. Anticholinegics
    3. Narcotics
    4. Aspirin
    5. Nonsteroidal antiinflammatory drugs
    6. Penicillin

V. Provision of stress-free environment

MEDICAL MANAGEMENT

Avoidance or elimination of any known precipitating factor is the first step in preventing asthmatic attacks. For persons who have known allergies, desensitization injections may also be of some help.

The mainstay of asthma treatment is drug therapy. Drugs commonly used to treat asthma generally fall into four categories, which are the methylxanthines, beta-adrenergic stimulators, chromones, and corticosteroids. A common approach is for the asthmatic to use a metered dose spray or inhaler of a beta-adrenergic stimulator for immediate relief. The corticosteroids are used in acute episodes and also in chronic asthma in which the nonsteroidal medications have proved ineffective. Table 9-1 is a list of common preparations used to treat asthma.

DENTAL MANAGEMENT
Prevention of potential problems (Table 9-2)

The goal of management for asthmatic dental patients must be to prevent an acute asthmatic attack. The first step to achieve this goal is to iden-tify asthmatics by history and learn as much as possible about their problem.

Through a good history, the dentist should be able to ascertain the type of asthma (allergic vs. nonallergic), precipitating factors, age at onset, frequency and severity of attacks, how attacks are usually managed, and whether it has been necessary to go to an emergency room for treatment for an acute attack. All known precipitating factors should be avoided. For a severe asthmatic, consultation with the physician would be advised.

The history should also reveal what medications the patient is taking and whether or not corticosteroids have ever been necessary. If so, adrenal suppression may be a concern and require steroid supplementation (see Chapter 16). It is also helpful to determine the compliance of the patient in taking medications and to determine how well controlled the asthma is. Other than the corticosteroids, the drugs used to treat chronic asthma pose no particular management problems. Patients should bring their aerosol inhalers to each appointment.

Since emotional upset is implicated commonly in asthmatic attacks, the dentist should strive for a stress-free environment and the use of sedative premedication when appropriate. Good pain control is essential. Drugs to be avoided if possible include antihistamines and narcotics, because they cause histamine release and respiratory depression. Anticholinergics such as scopolamine should also be avoided. Nitrous oxide and diazepam are both acceptable.

Finally, aspirin, nonsteroidal antiinflammatory drugs, and penicillin should be avoided because of their potential for allergenicity.[4]

Treatment planning modifications

No specific treatment planning modifications are required.

Oral complications

There are no specific oral complications.

Emergency dental care

The same precautions also apply to the provision of emergency dental care.

Tuberculosis

Tuberculosis is a disease that is of concern to the dentist from at least three standpoints. First, it is an infectious disease and as such, is communicable in its active state. The dentist is in a high-risk population for the disease and may contract it from a patient, or patients may contract the disease from a dentist who has an active case.

Second, on rare occasions tuberculosis may be manifested in the oral cavity, thus the dentist must be alert to include tuberculosis in the differential diagnosis of oral lesions or unexplained cause.

Finally, the dentist may be the first person to discover that a patient has tuberculosis. This may be discovered as a result of history, review of systems, and physical evaluation. An immediate referral to a physician may save the patient's life or at least decrease the morbidity of the disease.

GENERAL DESCRIPTION
Incidence and epidemiology

The occurrence of tuberculosis has decreased drastically in the last century. Around the turn of the century in the United States there were approximately 500 new cases of active tuberculosis per 100,000 population identified every year. In 1969 this rate had fallen to less than 20 cases per 100,000 population.[2] By 1982 the case rate was approximately 11 per 100,000.[12] Although the present rate for the nation as a whole is very low, certain areas such as inner-city ghettos and poor rural communities still may have occurrence rates several times that of the national average. As might be expected from these statistics, tuberculosis is prevalent in areas of dense population and poor socioeconomic conditions, and as such remains a significant health problem in many areas of the world today.

A way of determining incidence is to examine the number of persons who react to the tuberculin skin test (purified protein derivative [PPD]). In the early twentieth century, surveys in St. Louis and Philadelphia showed that over 50% of the general population reacted to the test. In contrast to this, from 1955 to 1969 only 3% of 540,000 naval recruits demonstrated definite positive reactions.[3]

It is believed that the dramatic decrease in the incidence of tuberculosis can be attributed to improvement in sanitation and hygiene measures more than any other factor.

Etiology

In most cases of human tuberculosis the causative agent is *Mycobacterium tuberculosis,* an acid-fast nonmotile rod that is an obligate aerobe. Since it is an aerobe, it exists best in an atmosphere of high oxygen tension; therefore it most commonly infects the lung. Although *M. tuberculosis* is by far the most common causative agent in human infection, other species of mycobacteria are occasionally encountered, such as *M. bovis, M. avium,* and "atypical" mycobacteria.

The typical mode of transmission of the bacteria is by way of infected, airborne droplets of mucus or saliva that have been forcefully expelled from the lungs, most commonly by coughing but also by sneezing and talking. The size of the expelled droplets appears to be important in transmission.

The smaller droplets evaporate rapidly, leaving the bacteria and other solid material as floating particles that can be easily inhaled. The larger droplets quickly settle to the ground. Transmission by way of fomites rarely, if ever, occurs.[1] Transmission by ingestion rarely occurs since the advent of pasteurized milk. A secondary mode of transmission by ingestion can occur when a patient coughs up infected sputum and then swallows it. It is through this mechanism that oral lesions of tuberculosis may be initiated, with the posterior dorsal surface of the tongue being the most common site of involvement.

Pathophysiology

Tuberculosis can affect virtually any organ of the body; however, the lung is by far the most common site of infection. A typical infection of pulmonary tuberculosis begins with the inhalation of an infected droplet into the lung. The droplet is carried into the alveoli, where the bacteria settle out and begin to multiply. The infection progresses locally and may involve local and regional lymph nodes. Distant dissemination through the bloodstream may also occur during this period; however, it is believed that the vast majority of the disseminated bacteria are destroyed by natural host defenses. Approximately 4 to 5 weeks after infection, a hypersensitivity to the bacteria develops. This is manifested by conversion of the tuberculin skin test (PPD) from negative to positive. Meanwhile, the nidus of infection has become a productive tubercle that can then demonstrate central necrosis and caseation. Cavitation can also occur, resulting in the dumping of organisms into the airway for further dissemination either into other lung tissue or to the outside by means of forceful expulsion (Fig. 9-2).

The course of the infection may be interrupted by a variety of factors, including host resistance, host immune capabilities, and degree of virulence of the mycobacterium. Once the infection is successfully interrupted, the lesion heals spontaneously and then may undergo inspissation, hardening, encapsulation, and calcification. Even though the lesion is "healed," a few bacteria will remain in a dormant state.

If the infection is not interrupted, dissemination of bacilli can occur through the lung parenchyma,

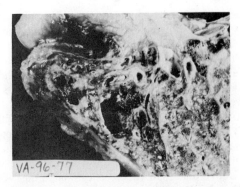

FIG. 9-2. Gross specimen of tuberculous lung demonstrating cavitation (Courtesy R. Powell, M.D., Lexington, Ky.)

resulting in extensive pulmonary lesions and lymphohematogenous spread. A widespread infection with multiple organ involvement is termed *miliary tuberculosis.*

Primary pulmonary tuberculosis is seen most commonly in infants and children; however, cavitation is rare in this age group. The majority of children produce no sputum, and, even if some bacilli are present in the bronchi, the child usually swallows the sputum on awakening in the morning.

The expression of the disease differs somewhat in teenagers and adults in that lymph node involvement and lymphohematogenous spread are not prominent features; however, cavitation commonly occurs. The most common form of the disease found in adults is termed *reinfection tuberculosis.*[10] This occurs as a result of the reactivation of persistent dormant viable bacilli and probably represents a relapse of a previous infection.

The reason for relapse is usually inadequate treatment of the primary infection in addition to influences such as illnesses, immunosuppressive agents, and age. This form of the disease is usually confined to the lungs, and cavitation is a common finding.

Sequelae and complications

The manifestations of tuberculosis are extremely varied; however, some of the more common sequelae include progressive primary tuberculosis, cavitary disease, pleuritis and pleural effusion, meningitis, and disseminated or miliary tuberculosis. Isolated organ involvement, other than lung, can also occur and commonly affects the pericardium, peritoneum, kidney, adrenal glands, and bone, especially the spine.[1] The tongue and other tissues of the oral cavity can also be involved; however, this is uncommon.[8]

Aside from the complications associated with individual organ involvement, the ultimate concern is death. The mortality from tuberculosis has paralleled the precipitous drop of its incidence in the United States. In 1830 it is estimated that 400 deaths per 100,000 population were caused by tuberculosis. In 1976 there were 1.5 deaths per 100,000 population from tuberculosis. The advent of effective chemotherapy has probably been the most significant reason for the decreased mortality of the disease.

CLINICAL PRESENTATION
Signs and symptoms

A characteristic feature of most patients who have tuberculosis is the complete lack of signs and symptoms until the lesions have become extensive. The exceptions to this are a positive skin test or radiographic findings. Once symptoms become apparent, they are usually nonspecific and could be associated with any infectious disease. They include lassitude and malaise, anorexia, weight loss, night sweats, and fever.[1,10] The character of the fever associated with tuberculosis is unusual in that the patient is usually not debilitated by a temperature that reaches 103° to 104° F (39.4° to 40° C) and may even be unaware of its presence. The temperature elevation commonly occurs in the evening or during the night and is accompanied by profuse sweating.

Specific local symptoms of the disease depend on the organ involved. Cough is associated with pulmonary tuberculosis, although it may be quite late in appearance. It is commonly seen in cavitary disease. The sputum produced is characteristically mucopurulent, and hemoptysis (blood in the sputum) is common. Dyspnea is also seen in advanced pulmonary disease. Radiographic findings in pulmonary tuberculosis differ with the age of the patient. The radiographic findings in tuberculosis are not pathognomonic, and the diagnosis is not made from radiographs alone.[10]

Manifestations of other organ involvement may include localized lymphadenopathy with development of sinus tracts, back pain over the affected spine, gastrointestinal disturbances in intestinal tuberculosis, dysuria or hematuria in renal involvement, heart failure, or neurologic deficits. Physical examination may be inconclusive.

Laboratory findings

The tuberculin skin test (Mantoux) is the most useful and reliable method of determining if a person has been infected with *M. tuberculosis*. A positive test means that a person has been infected and that there are viable organisms present. It does not mean that the person is infectious. Infectiousness is determined by other methods. Tuberculin is a standardized PPD of culture extract of *M. tuberculosis*. Specifically, PPD-S is used as the international testing standard. The test is administered by an intradermal injection of 0.001 mg of PPD-S. The test is then read 48 to 72 hours later, and evidence of induration is noted. An area of induration of less than 5 mm in diameter is considered a negative result. An area of induration between 5 and 9 mm is considered inconclusive, and the test is usually repeated. If the repeat result is 5 to 9 mm of induration, it probably indicates infection with a mycobacterium other than *M. tuberculosis*. An area of induration 10 mm or greater is considered positive.[1] A positive test necessitates a physical examination, radiographic evaluation, and, if necessary, sputum culture to rule out active disease.

The definitive diagnosis of tuberculosis must be based on the culture and identification of *M. tuberculosis* or other species from body fluids or tissues.[1] A tentative diagnosis is commonly made from detection of acid-fast bacilli in smears; however, this must be verified by culture. Multiple specimens should be obtained for culturing to ensure positive results. It commonly takes several weeks for growth to occur.

Other laboratory studies such as sedimentation rate, complete blood count, and urinalysis usually are not helpful in delineating the disease.

MEDICAL MANAGEMENT

With the initiation of chemotherapy, a cure is almost always assured provided proper selection of drugs is made and patient compliance is optimal.

TABLE 9-3. Some commonly used antituberculous drugs

Isoniazid (INH)
Rifampin
Pyrazinamide
Ethambutol
Streptomycin

Several antituberculous drugs are in use today from which the physician may select an appropriate regimen. It is common to administer a combination of drugs (usually two or three) rather than a single drug, since development of resistance is markedly decreased by combination therapy. Table 9-3 is a listing of the more common antituberculous drugs in use today. The chemotherapeutic regimen of choice today is a 9-month course of isoniazid and rifampin.[11] This is a much reduced regimen from that of only a few years ago, which called for three or four drugs to be administered for 18 to 24 months. Successful treatment depends largely on correct drug choice, adequate length of time for therapy, and good patient compliance. With proper therapy relapse after treatment (early or late) is uncommon.

Early reversal of infectiousness after the initiation of adequate chemotherapy is achieved in most cases.[1,10] Even in cases of moderately advanced disease, negative sputum cultures are achieved after 3 or 4 months of treatment. Based on this rapid reversal of infectiousness, patients are usually hospitalized only a few weeks if at all and then are allowed to go home and are rechecked for positive sputum cultures periodically. Within 3 to 4 months the large majority of patients are able to return to a normal life-style as long as they continue the chemotherapy. In some extremely ill patients corticosteroids may be used in conjunction with the antituberculous drugs. Surgery is infrequently indicated.

The patient who has had a negative skin test and then, on retesting, converts to positive has been infected with *M. tuberculosis*. Once it is established by physical examination and radiographic examination that the disease is not active, the patient may be given a course of chemotherapy to prevent active disease from developing. Most commonly chemotherapy is provided by the oral administration of isoniazid daily for approximately 12 months. Even though this usually prevents active disease from occurring, the person usually retains the hypersensitivity to tuberculin and remains positive on skin testing.

DENTAL MANAGEMENT
Medical considerations

Dental patients can be placed into four categories for the purpose of management: patients with active tuberculosis, patients with a past history of tuberculosis, patients with a positive tuberculin test, and patients with signs or symptoms suggestive of tuberculosis. Each will be discussed in detail (Table 9-4).

PATIENTS WITH ACTIVE TUBERCULOSIS

Patients with recently diagnosed active tuberculosis and positive sputum cultures should not be treated on an outpatient basis. Treatment is best rendered in a hospital setting with appropriate isolation, sterilization, mask, gloves and gown, and ventilation systems. Because of the special precautions, it is best that treatment be limited to emergency care only.

After a patient has been receiving chemotherapy and bacilli can no longer be cultured from his sputum (usually after 3 or 4 months), it is permissible to treat him on an outpatient basis in the same manner as any normal, healthy patient. The physician should be consulted to verify that the patient is no longer infectious and to determine if there are any complicating factors. If not, there need be no special precautions.

A child who has active tuberculosis and is receiving chemotherapy can usually be treated as an outpatient at any time, because bacilli are found only rarely in the sputum of a young child. Children should be considered noninfectious unless a positive sputum culture has been obtained. It is nearly impossible to define exactly what age constitutes a "child" in this instance. The two reasons that a child who had tuberculosis is considered noninfectious are the rarity of cavitary disease in children and their inability to cough up sputum effectively. As a general rule; a child under the age of 6 years can be confidently treated. In children over the age of 6 years, however, some degree of concern could exist. In this case, the physician

TABLE 9-4. Dental management of patient with history of tuberculosis

I. Patients with active tuberculosis
   A. Consult with physician before treatment
   B. Administer emergency care only (over age 6 years)
   C. Treat in hospital setting with isolation, sterilization, gloves, mask, gown, and ventilation
   D. Under age 6 years, treat as normal patient (noninfectious)
   E. When patient produces consistently negative sputum, treat as normal patient (noninfectious)

II. Patients with past history of tuberculosis
   A. Approach with caution; obtain good history of disease and treatment duration; appropriate review of systems is mandatory
   B. Should give history of periodic chest x-ray examination to rule out reactivation
   C. Consult with physician and postpose treatment if:
      1. Questionable history of adequate treatment time
      2. Lack of appropriate medical supervision since recovery
      3. Signs or symptoms of relapse
   D. If present status is "free of active disease," treat as normal patient

III. Patients with positive tuberculin test
   A. Should have been evaluated by physician to rule out active disease
   B. May receive isoniazid up to 1 year for prophylaxis
   C. Treat as normal patient

IV. Patients with signs or symptoms suggestive of tuberculosis
   A. Refer to physician and postpone treatment
   B. If treatment necessary, treat as emergency patient only

should be consulted before any treatment is begun. Of greater concern in this case are the family contacts of this patient, since the disease was more than likely contracted from an infected adult. On questioning, all family members who have had contact with the patient should give a history of skin testing and chest x-ray examination to rule out the possibility of active disease. If this history is not elicited, the physician or health department should be contacted to ensure that proper preventive action is taken.

PATIENTS WITH PAST HISTORY OF TUBERCULOSIS

Fortunately, relapse is rare in patients who receive adequate treatment for the initial infection. However, this is not the case in patients who do not receive adequate treatment. Regardless of what type of treatment he has received, it is important to approach any patient who has a past history of tuberculosis with initial caution. The dentist should be aggressive in obtaining a good past medical history that includes diagnosis, dates of treatment, and type of treatment, including drugs used. Treatment duration of less than 18 months if treated in the past or 9 months if treated recently would require consultation with the physician to determine the patient's status.

These patients should give a history of periodic physical examinations and chest x-ray films to check for evidence of reactivation of the disease since recovering from their infection. This should be current within the past 12 months. Consultation with the physician is advisable to verify the current status. If the patient's current status is verified as "free of active disease," treatment should be rendered in the normal fashion with no special precautions.

A good review of systems is mandatory for these patients, and referral to a physician is indicated if questionable signs or symptoms are present.

In summary, dental treatment should be postponed and consultation with a physician sought for patients who have the following:

1. Questionable history of proper treatment
2. Lack of appropriate medical evaluation following treatment
3. Signs or symptoms of tuberculosis suggesting a relapse

PATIENTS WITH POSITIVE TUBERCULIN TEST

A person whose skin test has recently converted to positive should be viewed as having been infected with tuberculosis. The patient should give a history of being evaluated for active disease by at least a physical examination and chest x-ray film. In the absence of active disease the patient may be given isoniazid for a period of 1 year to prevent active disease development. During this time the patient is not infectious (in the absence of active disease) and can be treated in a normal manner. No special precautions are required.

PATIENTS WITH SIGNS OR SYMPTOMS SUGGESTIVE OF TUBERCULOSIS

Any time a patient demonstrates unexplained, persistent signs or symptoms that may be suggestive of active tuberculosis, no dental care should be rendered, and the patient should be referred to a physician for evaluation.

Drug administration

There are no apparent interactions between the major antituberculous drugs and the drugs commonly used in dentistry. There are no contraindications for the use of the dental agents.

Treatment planning modifications

No treatment planning modifications are required for these patients.

Oral complications

Infrequently, tuberculosis may be manifested by oral lesions. These are most commonly seen as a painful deep ulcer on the dorsum of the tongue; however, other mucosal surfaces can be involved, including palate, lips, buccal mucosa, and gingiva.[8] Biopsy, in addition to culture, can be diagnostic if acid-fast bacilli are found. Treatment of the oral lesion is secondary to treatment of the tuberculosis. Pain can be managed symptomatically by bland mouth rinses and topical preparations such as Orabase or viscous lidocaine (Xylocaine).

The cervical and submandibular lymph nodes can become infected with tuberculosis, which is termed *scrofula*. The nodes are enlarged and painful and may form abscesses and drain (Fig. 9-3). Treatment is the usual administration of antituberculous drugs.

Emergency dental care

Dental treatment is best postponed in a patient who has active tuberculosis; however, emergency care may be required. If analgesics will not suffice,

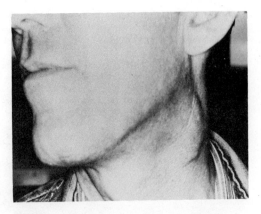

FIG. 9-3. Tuberculosis of cervical lymph node.

TABLE 9-5. Emergency dental care for patient with tuberculosis

Consultation with physician to discuss status and planned treatment
Isolation of dental operatory (special facility)
Strict aseptic procedures
Gloves, mask, gown for all personnel
Rubber dam when possible
Minimization of aerosol production by using slow-speed handpiece if possible and using air syringe judiciously
Scrubbing and sterilization of all equipment after use
Provision of only acutely necessary care

treatment should be accomplished by the procedures listed in Table 9-5.

REFERENCES

1. American Thoracic Society; Diagnostic standards and classification of tuberculosis and other mycobacterial diseases (14th edition), Am. Rev. Respir. Dis. **123**:343-358, 1981.
2. Harris, H.W., and McClement, J.H.: Tuberculosis. In Hoeprich, P.D., editor: Infectious diseases, ed. 3, Hagerstown, Md., 1972, Harper & Row, Publishers, Inc., pp. 378-404.
3. Krugman, S., and Katz, S.L.: Infectious diseases of children, ed. 7, St. Louis, 1981, The C.V. Mosby Co.
4. Malamed, S.F.: Handbook of medical emergencies in the dental office, ed. 2, St. Louis, 1982, The C.V. Mosby Co., pp. 134-143.

5. McFadden, E.R., Jr., and Austen, K.F.: Asthma. In Isselbacher, K.J., et al., editor: Harrison's principles of internal medicine, ed. 9, New York, 1980, McGraw-Hill Book Co., pp. 1203-1210.

6. McGowan, M.S.: Pulmonary disease. In Freitag, J.J., et al., editors: Manual of medical therapeutics, ed. 23, Boston, 1981, Little, Brown & Co., pp. 159-174.

7. Robbins, S.L., and Cotran, R.S.: Pathologic basis of disease, ed. 2, Philadelphia, 1979, W.B. Saunders Co., pp. 838-841.

8. Shafer, W.G., et al.: A textbook of oral pathology, ed. 4, Philadelphia, 1983, W.B. Saunders Co., pp. 341-344.

9. Stead, W.W.: Present chemotherapy for tuberculosis, J. Inf. Dis. 146:698-704, 1982.

10. Stead, W.W., and Bates, J.H.: Tuberculosis. In Isselbacher, K.J., et al., editors: Harrison's principles of internal medicine, New York, 1980, McGraw-Hill Book Co. pp. 700-711.

11. Summer, W.R., and Permutt, S.: Acute lower airway obstruction: asthma. In Shibel, E.M., and Moser, K.M.: Respiratory emergencies, St. Louis, 1977, The C.V. Mosby Co., pp. 152-169.

12. Tuberculosis—United States, 1982, Morbidity and Mortality Weekly Report 32:87, 1983.

13. Weiss, E.B.: Bronchial asthma, Clin. Symp. 27:3-72, 1975.

10

LIVER DISEASE

The dentist may encounter patients with one of many liver disorders. These patients may be of significant interest, because the liver plays such an important and vital role in metabolic functions. Impairment of liver function can lead to abnormalities of the metabolism of amino acids, ammonia, protein, carbohydrates, and lipids. In addition, many biochemical functions such as coagulation and drug metabolism may be adversely affected.

In considering the effects of liver disease on the provision of dental care, we have chosen two of the more common disorders for illustrative purposes. Therefore this chapter will deal with alcoholic liver disease and viral hepatitis.

Alcoholic liver disease

GENERAL DESCRIPTION
Etiology and incidence

It has long been recognized that a relationship exists between excessive alcohol ingestion and liver dysfunction leading to cirrhosis. However, the exact effect of alcohol on the liver was not known until it was shown that alcohol is a direct hepatotoxic drug.[16] In light of this fact, it is curious that only 10% to 20% of heavy alcohol users ever develop cirrhosis.[15] This is probably explained by other influences, such as hereditary factors and nutritional or biochemical differences between individuals.

Pathophysiology

The pathologic effects of alcohol on the liver are expressed by one of three disease entities. These conditions may exist alone or in combination. The earliest change seen in alcoholic liver disease is a fatty infiltrate. The hepatocytes become engorged with fatty lobules and distended, with enlargement of the entire liver. No other structural changes are usually noted. These changes may be seen after only moderate use of alcohol for a brief time; however, they are considered completely reversible. With abstinence, the liver will return to normal.[27]

Alcoholic hepatitis is a second and more serious form of alcoholic liver disease. It is a diffuse inflammatory condition of the liver characterized by destructive cellular changes, some of which may be irreversible. These irreversible changes can lead to necrosis. It is felt that nutritional factors may play a significant role in the progression of this disease. For the most part, alcoholic hepatitis is considered to be a reversible condition; however, it can be fatal if damage is widespread.

The third and most serious form of alcoholic liver disease is cirrhosis, which is generally considered to be an irreversible condition characterized by progressive fibrosis and abnormal regeneration of liver architecture in response to chronic injury or insult[8] (Fig. 10-1). The insult, in this case, is chronic, heavy use of ethanol.

Although cirrhosis is generally considered to be an end-stage condition, some evidence suggests that at least partial reversibility of the process is possible with complete and permanent removal of the offending agent.[8,15]

Sequelae and complications

Cirrhosis results in the progressive deterioration of the metabolic and excretory functions of the liver and ultimately leads to hepatic failure. Hepa-

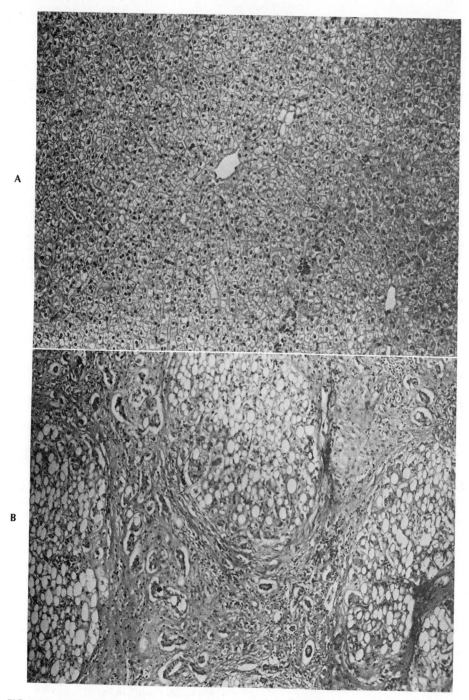

FIG. 10-1. A, Photomicrograph of normal liver architecture. **B,** Photomicrograph of liver architecture in alcoholic cirrhosis. (Courtesy A. Golden, M.D., Lexington, Ky.)

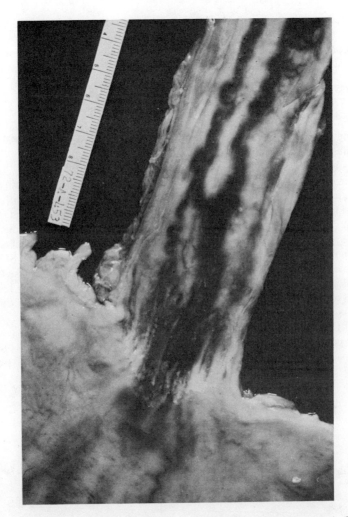

FIG. 10-2. Gross section of esophageal varices from alcoholic patient. (Courtesy A. Golden, M.D., Lexington, Ky.)

tic failure is manifested by many abnormalities. Some of the more important of these changes are generalized malnutrition, weight loss, protein deficiency (including most coagulation factors), impairment of urea synthesis and glucose metabolism, endocrine disturbances, encephalopathy, renal failure, portal hypertension, and jaundice.[8] Accompanying portal hypertension is the development of ascites and esophageal varices (Fig. 10-2).

Bleeding tendencies are a significant feature in advanced liver disease. The basis for this bleeding diathesis is in part a deficiency of coagulation factors (except factor VIII), especially the prothrombin group of factors (factors II, VII, IX, and X). This group of factors relies on vitamin K for its production. In addition to these deficiencies, thrombocytopenia may be caused by hypersplenism secondary to portal hypertension as well as an accelerated level of fibrinolysis.[13,15,20]

The combination of hemorrhagic tendencies and severe portal hypertension sets the stage for episodes of gastrointestinal bleeding, epistaxis, ecchymosis, or ruptured esophageal varices.[13] In fact, most patients with advanced cirrhosis die in hepatic coma, often precipitated by massive hemorrhage from esophageal varices or intercurrent infection.[15]

CLINICAL PRESENTATION
Signs and symptoms

With the exception of an enlarged liver, there are no clinical manifestations of a fatty liver, and the diagnosis is usually made accidentally in conjunction with another illness.

The clinical presentation of alcoholic hepatitis is often nonspecific and may include features such as nausea and vomiting, anorexia, malaise, weight loss, and fever. More specific findings may include hepatomegaly, splenomegaly, jaundice, ascites, ankle edema, and spider angiomas. With advancing disease, encephalopathy and hepatic coma may ensue, and these can terminate fatally.[15,27]

Alcoholic cirrhosis may remain asymptomatic for many years until there is finally sufficient destruction of the liver parenchyma to produce clinical evidence of hepatic failure. Ascites, spider angiomas (Fig. 10-3), ankle edema, or jaundice may be the earliest signs to develop, but, unfortunately, hemorrhage from esophageal varices is commonly seen as the presenting sign. In addition, the hemorrhagic episode may progress to hepatic encephalopathy, coma, and death. Some other, less specific signs of alcoholic liver disease include purpura, ecchymosis, gingival bleeding, and parotid gland enlargement.[6,15,18,21]

Laboratory findings

The laboratory findings in alcoholic liver disease vary from minimal abnormalities caused by a fatty liver to characteristic findings of alcoholic hepatitis and cirrhosis. These findings include elevations of bilirubin, alkaline phosphatase, serum glutamic-oxaloacetic transaminase (SGOT), and serum glutamic-pyruvic transaminase (SGPT) levels. Deficiencies of clotting factors lead to elevations in prothrombin time and partial thromboplastin time. Thrombocytopenia may be present, causing a decreased platelet count and increased bleeding time. Increased fibrinolytic activity may be evidenced by an increased bleeding time, prolonged thrombin

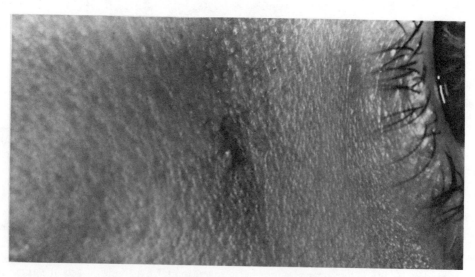

FIG. 10-3. Spider angioma. (Courtesy J. Bark, M.D., Lexington, Ky.)

time, or decreased euglobulin clot lysis time. Leukopenia or leukocytosis may be present, as may anemia.[13,15]

MEDICAL MANAGEMENT

In all forms of alcoholic liver disease, the cornerstone of treatment is withdrawal and abstinence from alcohol. In addition, strict dietary modifications are required, including a high-protein, high-calorie, and low-sodium diet. Fluid restriction as well as vitamin supplementation may be necessary. Anemia is corrected by iron replacement and folic acid supplement. Infection or sepsis is treated appropriately. Steroids may be of some benefit, although this is controversial.

Hemorrhage from esophageal varices and hepatic encephalopathy require immediate treatment. Ascites mandates measures to control fluids and electrolytes.

TABLE 10-1. Dental management of patient with alcoholic liver disease

1. Detection by
   a. History
   b. Clinical examination
   c. Repeated odor on breath
   d. Information from family members or friends

2. Referral or consultaion with a physician to
   a. Verify history
   b. Check current status
   c. Check medications
   d. Check laboratory values
   e. Obtain suggestions for management

3. Laboratory screening (if otherwise not available from physician)
   a. CBC with differential
   b. SGOT
   c. Bleeding time
   d. Thrombin time
   e. Prothrombin time

4. Minimize drugs metabolized by liver (see Table 10-3)

5. If screening tests abnormal, for surgical procedures consider using
   a. Antifibrinolytic agents (aminocaproic acid)
   b. Fresh frozen plasma
   c. Vitamin K
   d. Platelets

DENTAL MANAGEMENT
Medical considerations (see Table 10-1)

From a dental standpoint, there are two major considerations to observe with patients who have alcoholic cirrhosis. These are (1) bleeding tendencies and (2) inability to metabolize and detoxify certain drugs.

Correct dental management of patients with alcoholic liver disease first requires detection, either by history or clinical examination or both. Since alcohol abuse is commonly denied, the dentist must remain alert to the visible and obvious physical signs that suggest alcoholic liver disease. These include spider angiomas of the skin, unexplained bruising, enlargement of the parotid glands, swelling of the ankles, ascites, and jaundice, which is most evident in the scleras (Table 10-2). In addition, the patient may admit to heavy use of alcohol, or its odor may be detectable on the breath on several occasions. Family members may also volunteer this information in confidence. It should be kept in mind that alcoholism transcends the socioeconomic spectrum and is not limited to the skid-row stereotype.

If suggestive signs or symptoms are noted, the dentist should question the patient about alcohol use, including what is used, quantity on a daily or weekly basis, and for how long the use has occurred. Whether or not the patient admits to heavy use of alcohol, a high index of suspicion should be followed by a series of laboratory tests for screening purposes. A complete blood count (CBC) with differential, SGOT, bleeding time, thrombin time, and prothrombin time would be sufficient to screen for the more significant problems. Abnormal laboratory values, accompanied by abnormal clinical examination or positive history, is a basis for referral to a physician for positive diagnosis and treat-

TABLE 10-2. Signs suggestive of advanced liver disease

Spider angiomas
Jaundice (sclera)
Ankle edema
Ascites
Ecchymosis/petechiae
Parotid gland enlargement
Gingival bleeding

ment. A patient who has untreated alcoholic liver disease is not a candidate for elective, outpatient dental care and should be referred immediately to a physician. Once the patient is being managed medically, dental care may be provided after consultation with the physician regarding laboratory values and recommendations for treatment.

If a patient provides a past history of alcoholic liver disease or alcohol abuse, the physician should be consulted to verify the patient's current status, medications, laboratory status, and contraindications for medications, surgery, or other treatment.

Bleeding diatheses, as reflected in abnormal laboratory tests, should be managed in conjunction with the physician and may include fresh frozen plasma, vitamin K, platelets, and antifibrinolytic agents.

If the patient has not been seen by a physician within the past several months, it would be wise to order screening laboratory tests, including CBC with differential, SGOT, bleeding time, thrombin time, and prothrombin time.

Another significant area of concern in treating patients who have alcoholic liver disease is to eliminate or minimize the use of drugs that are metabolized principally by the liver. Table 10-3 is

a list of drugs commonly used in dentistry that are metabolized mainly by the liver. Efforts should be made to substitute other drugs, or at least decrease usual dosages, based on the severity of liver damage.

Treatment planning modifications

There are no unique treatment planning modifications required for patients who have alcoholic liver disease. However, it has been found that these patients have greater amounts of plaque, calculus, and gingival inflammation than do noncirrhotic patients.[9] This seems to be the case in any patient who is a substance abuser and to relate to oral neglect rather than any inherent property of the abused substance. Based on this observed degree of neglect and periodontal disease, the prudent practitioner would be wise not to provide extensive care until the patient demonstrates an interest in and ability to care for his dentition.

Oral complications

Neglect, as just discussed, is the most common oral complication associated with alcoholic liver disease. Spontaneous gingival bleeding is the only other significant oral complication that may be encountered, and it may in fact be the presenting complaint of the patient.[6] Ecchymosis or petechiae may also be noted intraorally.

Emergency dental care

If it becomes necessary to provide surgery for a patient who has compromised liver function, consideration should be given to using antifibrinolytic agents, such as aminocaproic acid, platelets, fresh frozen plasma, and possibly vitamin K. Therapy is best selected in consultation with the patient's physician.

TABLE 10-3. Common dental drugs metabolized primarily by liver

Local anesthetics
Lidocaine (Xylocaine)
Mepivacaine (Carbocaine)
Procaine (Novocain)*

Analgesics
Acetylsalicylic acid (aspirin)
Acetaminophen (Tylenol, Datril)
Codeine
Meperidine (Demerol)

Sedatives
Diazepam (Valium)
Barbiturates

Antibiotics
Ampicillin
Tetracycline

*Partial metabolism by liver.

Viral hepatitis

The term *hepatitis* is defined nonspecifically by *Dorland's Illustrated Medical Dictionary* as "inflammation of the liver." Hepatitis may result from a variety of causes. It may occur either as a primary disease or secondary to another disease. Examples of hepatitis occurring as a primary liver disease are viral hepatitis, drug-induced hepatitis (e.g., caused by alcohol), and toxic hepatitis (e.g., caused by halothane). Diseases in which hepatitis may occur as a secondary complication include infectious mononucleosis, secondary syphilis, and tuberculosis. The discussion here will be limited to viral hepatitis, since this disease has special implications for dentistry.

GENERAL DESCRIPTION
Etiology

Acute viral hepatitis is caused by at least three distinct viruses (types A, B, and non-A, non-B [NANB]). These viruses each have distinct antigenic properties, but the clinical expression of disease is commonly similar. Type A hepatitis was formerly called infectious hepatitis, and type B hepatitis was formerly called serum hepatitis. NANB hepatitis is a form of the disease that is essentially a diagnosis of exclusion when neither type A nor B can be identified. Table 10-4 is an explanation of the commonly used abbreviations in hepatitis terminology. Table 10-5 is a comparison of types A, B, and NANB hepatitis.

HEPATITIS A

Type A hepatitis (infectious hepatitis) is caused by the hepatitis A virus (HAV), which is an RNA-type virus. This virus was identified by electron microscopy a few years ago, and its properties are not yet completely understood. However, sensitive serologic tests for HAV and its antibody (anti-HAV) are readily available.

HEPATITIS B

Type B hepatitis (serum hepatitis) is caused by the hepatitis B virus (HBV), which is a DNA-type virus. Electron microscopy has identified at least three virus-associated particles that are related to hepatitis B infection. The intact virus (HBV), or Dane particle, is composed of an outer shell and an inner core. The outer shell is the hepatitis B surface antigen (HBsAg), and its antibody is anti-HBs. The inner core of the particle is the hepatitis B core antigen (HBcAg), and its antibody is anti-HBc. The third particle is called the hepatitis B e antigen (HBeAg), and it is an antigenic component that is believed to be related to hepatitis B infectivity. Its corresponding antibody is anti-HBe. Serologic tests are available for all these antigen-antibody systems, except for the HBcAg.

HEPATITIS NANB

Type NANB hepatitis virus is also called type C hepatitis virus. This virus is thought to be the cause of most cases of posttransfusion hepatitis. The actual virus has not been identified yet, and therefore no antigenic system or serologic tests have been developed. It is possible that several viruses may ultimately be identified in this group.

TABLE 10-4. Hepatitis terminology

Common abbreviation	Term	Explanation
HAV	Hepatitis A virus	Etiologic agent of hepatitis A
Anti-HAV	Hepatitis A antibody	Indicates past infection of hepatitis A; provides immunity
HBV	Hepatitis B virus	Etiologic agent of hepatitis B
HBsAg	Hepatitis B surface antigen (Australia antigen)	Antigenic particle found on surface of virus; persistence identifies carrier of hepatitis B
Anti-HBs	Hepatitis B surface antibody	Indicates past infection of hepatitis B; provides immunity
HBeAg	Hepatitis B e antigen	Antigenic particle whose presence is associated with increased infectivity
Anti-HBe	Hepatitis B e antibody	Presence is a favorable sign in carriers; suggests low degree of infectiousness
HBcAg	Hepatitis B core antigen	Core of Dane particle; no test available yet
Anti-HBc	Hepatitis B core antibody	Indicates past infection of hepatitis B
NANB	Non-A, non-B hepatitis	Diagnosis of exclusion; similar to hepatitis B

TABLE 10-5. Comparison of viral hepatitis: types A, B, and NANB

	Type A	Type B	Type NANB
Etiologic agent	HAV	HBV	Not yet defined
Antigen-antibody systems	HAV; anti-HA	HBsAg; anti-HBs HBcAg; anti-HBc HBeAg; anti-HBe	Not yet defined
Principal transmission route	Predominantly fecal-oral	Predominantly parenteral	Predominantly parenteral via transfusions
Incubation period	2 to 5 weeks	2 to 6 months	Similar to type B
Age preference	Predominantly children and young adults	Any age but uncommon under age 15 years	Probably similar to type B
Seasonal incidence	Fall and winter	None	None
Severity	Usually mild	Occasionally severe	Occasionally severe
Complications	Rare	Yes	Yes
Immunity conferred following infection	Probably lifetime	Probably lifetime	Probably lifetime
Immune globulin (IG) prophylaxis	IG usually effective	IG has variable effectiveness; hepatitis B IG usually effective	Unknown
Vaccine available	No	Yes	No
Carrier state	No	Yes, in 5% to 10% of patients	Probably, but not yet defined

Epidemiology

In the past, type A hepatitis and type B hepatitis were identified and described on a clinical and epidemiologic basis. Type A hepatitis was classically described as having an exclusively fecal-oral route of transmission, a short incubation period, and a benign course and as being highly contagious. In contrast, type B hepatitis was classically described as having an exclusively parenteral route of transmission, a longer incubation period, and a more serious clinical course than type A and as not being as contagious as type A. These distinctions are now recognized as being more apparent than real. In reality, the various types of viral hepatitis cannot be readily distinguished by clinical expression alone. In fact, serologic differentiation is the only consistently reliable means of identifying the viral agent.

Type A hepatitis has occurred with relative consistency over the past 10 years. In 1966 there were 32,859 cases reported in the United States, and in 1980 there were 29,087 cases reported. In contrast, the incidence of type B hepatitis has increased markedly, from 1497 reported cases in

1966 to 19,015 in 1980.[2,9] This is approximately a 1000% increase in incidence over a 14-year period. This increase may be explained by several factors, including improved detection capabilities, greater awareness of the disease, increased illicit drug use, and immigration of high-risk populations, such as Haitians and Indochinese.

HEPATITIS A

Type A hepatitis is transmitted predominantly by fecal contamination of food or water. Common sources of contamination include wells or water supplies, food sources, and shellfish beds along coastlines. Transmission can theoretically occur by the parenteral route, though this is rare. Since the reservoir of infection is frequently a common source of food or water, hepatitis A may occur as an epidemic. Transmission is also enhanced by poor personal hygiene. This may be especially apparent among schoolage youngsters or food handlers. Hepatitis A may occur sporadically or episodically (no known exposure), and it accounts for 20% to 40% of all cases of sporadic viral hepatitis.[10]

Persons of any age may be infected; however, the disease occurs primarily in children and young adults. In general the disease tends to be of mild severity. Of importance is the fact that no carrier state is known to exist for hepatitis A; therefore once a patient has clinically recovered (i.e., symptoms have subsided), he is no longer considered to be infectious.

HEPATITIS B

Hepatitis B is transmitted in a number of ways, including (1) direct percutaneous inoculation of infected serum or plasma by needle or transfusion of infective blood or blood products; (2) indirect percutaneous introduction of infective serum or plasma, such as through minute skin cuts or abrasions; (3) absorption of infective serum or plasma, such as through mucosal surfaces of the mouth or eye; (4) absorption of other potentially infective secretions, such as saliva or semen, through mucosal surfaces, as might occur following heterosexual or homosexual contact; and (5) transfer of infective serum or plasma via inanimate environmental surfaces or possibly vectors. Experimental data indicate that fecal transmission of HBV does not occur and that airborne spread is not epidemiologically important.[11]

The role of saliva in transmission, except by percutaneous or mucosal routes, does not appear to be significant. Observations reported to the Centers for Disease Control suggest that transmission of hepatitis B to humans after oral contact with HBsAg-positive saliva is unlikely.[14] Another study reported that out of 19 dental professionals who had cutaneous contact with HBsAg- and HBeAg-positive saliva, none developed serologic evidence of hepatitis B.[25] Therefore it would appear that the inoculation of saliva is necessary for the transmission of disease to occur.

The estimated lifetime risk of hepatitis B among the general population is approximately 5%; however, certain groups have a much higher risk.[12] Included among these are health care workers, refugees from Indochina and Haiti, residents of mental institutions and prisons, hemodialysis patients, users of illicit drugs, male homosexuals, and recipients of blood transfusions.[11,12] The incidence among general dentists is approximately 13%, while that among oral surgeons is 27%.[3,17,24]

Of interest is the fact that, although hepatitis B can occur at any age, statistically it is unusual for it to occur in persons under the age of 15. In fact, of the 19,015 cases of type B hepatitis reported in the United States in 1980, only 407 were in patients under age 15 years. This is an incidence rate only of 2.1%.[2]

As opposed to hepatitis A, hepatitis B tends to have greater associated morbidity and mortality, especially in older patients. One of the significant features of hepatitis B is the existence of a carrier state that can persist for variable periods after symptoms of acute disease subside. A carrier is defined as an individual in whom the HBsAg persists in the serum and is detectable for longer than 6 months. It is estimated that up to 10% of hepatitis B viral infections result in a carrier state.[12] All carriers of hepatitis B should be considered potentially infectious; however, it has been shown that not all carriers are equally infectious. There is a positive correlation between infectiousness and the simultaneous existence of HBsAg and HBeAg in the serum. Serum with HBeAg and HBsAg is 10 times more infectious than serum with HBsAg only.[4,9,28]

It is significant to note that most carriers are unaware that they have had hepatitis. An explanation for this is that many cases of hepatitis B are probably mild, subclinical, and nonicteric. These cases may be essentially asymptomatic or may be identical to any mild viral disease and therefore go undetected. Studies on dental school patients who were carriers of hepatitis B found that 50% to 80% gave no history of a past hepatitis infection.[7,26] This is indeed unfortunate, because for the most part these patients are not identifiable by past medical history. It would require routine laboratory screening of every patient to identify these patients; this approach is not practical.

HEPATITIS NANB

Little definite is known about hepatitis NANB; however, it is believed that it accounts for approximately 90% of cases of posttransfusion hepatitis in the United States today.[22] As previously mentioned, hepatitis NANB is essentially a diagnosis of exclusion whenever serologic tests are negative for the antigenic markers of HAV and HBV. Hepatitis NANB is not limited to posttransfusion cases but may be seen in similar settings as hepatitis types A and B. It accounts for approximately 20% of sporadic cases.[10]

Epidemiologically, hepatitis NANB resembles hepatitis B. It is transmitted predominantly by parenteral means. Furthermore, there is evidence that hepatitis NANB may be caused by more than one virus, and it is suspected that a carrier state is probably associated with the disease, which aids in its perpetuation.[22]

Pathophysiology

Although there is no single histopathologic lesion that can be said to be characteristic of viral hepatitis, the appearance of types A, B, and NANB hepatitis is similar. Therefore they will be described together.

Commonly, acute viral hepatitis is characterized by degeneration and necrosis of liver cells with ballooning degeneration of the hepatocytes. The entire liver lobule is inflamed and is composed of lymphocytes and mononuclear phagocytes.[8]

Icterus, or jaundice, is commonly associated with hepatitis and is caused by an accumulation of bilirubin in the skin. Bilirubin is a degradation product of hemoglobin. It is yellowish in color and is one of the major constituents of bile. Bilirubin is normally transported to the liver by way of the plasma. In the liver it conjugates with glucuronic acid and is then excreted into the intestine, where it aids in the emulsification of fats and stimulates peristalsis. When liver disease is present, bilirubin tends to build up in the plasma because of decreased liver metabolism.

Jaundice will become clinically apparent only when the plasma level exceeds 3 mg/100 ml (normal is less than 1 mg/100 ml).[19] Thus if the plasma bilirubin does not approach this level, the patient would be anicteric (without jaundice), and this explains the presence of nonicteric hepatitis.

Sequelae and complications

Most cases of viral hepatitis, especially type A, resolve without any attendant complications. However, with hepatitis B there are occasional chronic problems that develop.

Approximately 3% to 5% of patients who have acute hepatitis B will develop chronic active hepatitis. This form of hepatitis is characterized by the persistence of signs and symptoms of chronic liver disease, persistent hepatic cellular necrosis, and biochemical abnormalities for longer than 6 months.[5] There is also a persistence of HBsAg in the serum. It appears that patients who have HBeAg in their serum have a greater chance of developing this form of hepatitis than those who do not. The chronic liver destruction and resulting fibrosis can lead to cirrhosis in cases of chronic hepatitis, and in fact 11% of deaths from cirrhosis are associated with hepatitis B.[29]

The most serious complication of acute viral hepatitis is fulminant hepatitis. This is, fortunately, a rare entity characterized by massive hepatocellular destruction. The mortality approaches 80%.[29]

The complication of a persistent carrier state, which was previously discussed, is seen in 5% to 10% of cases. There is noteworthy evidence that suggests a positive correlation between chronic HBsAg carriage and the development of hepatocellular carcinoma.[29] This relationship is particularly strong in some Asian countries in which 20% to 40% of the population are carriers of hepatitis B.

CLINICAL PRESENTATION
Signs and symptoms

As previously indicated, it is frequently impossible to differentiate hepatitis A and B by clinical appearance; therefore it is appropriate to describe acute viral hepatitis in general. Many of the signs and symptoms of acute viral hepatitis are common to many viral diseases and may be described as flulike. This is especially true of the early or prodromal phase. There are classically three phases of acute viral hepatitis. The prodromal (preicteric) phase usually precedes the onset of jaundice by 1 or 2 weeks and may consist of anorexia, nausea, vomiting, fatigue, myalgia, malaise, and fever. With hepatitis B, 5% to 10% of patients may demonstrate serum sickness–like manifestations, including arthralgia or arthritis, rash, and angioedema.[5]

The icteric phase is indicated by the onset of clinical jaundice. Many of the nonspecific prodromal symptoms may subside, but gastrointestinal symptoms such as anorexia, nausea, vomiting, and right upper quadrant pain may increase, especially early in the phase. Hepatomegaly and splenomegaly are commonly seen. This phase usually lasts 6 to 8 weeks.

During the convalescent or recovery (posticteric) phase the symptoms disappear, but hepatomegaly and abnormal liver function values may persist for a variable time. This phase may last for weeks or months, with recovery time for hepatitis type B usually being longer. The usual sequence is for recovery (clinical and biochemical) to be complete approximately 4 months after the onset of jaundice.

Laboratory findings

The laboratory studies most useful in making a diagnosis of acute viral hepatitis include the serum transaminase levels (SGOT and SGPT), serum bilirubin level, alkaline phosphatase level, white blood cell count, and prothrombin time. With hepatitis A and B, the antigen-antibody systems are of extreme importance.

The serum transaminase levels will usually become elevated before elevation of the serum bilirubin level. The highest levels usually correspond to the peak of the icteric phase and gradually subside during the convalescent phase.

The rise of serum bilirubin level usually follows the rise of the transaminase levels. Jaundice will become clinically evident when the level approaches 3 mg/100 ml. The rise may be typically as high as 20 mg/100 ml, with higher levels being associated with more severe disease.[5,10] The bilirubin levels may persist after the transaminase levels begin to fall.

The serum alkaline phosphatase level may be mildly elevated or normal. This is a relatively nonspecific test.

There is usually an increase in the white blood cell count, with a relative lymphocytosis. Atypical

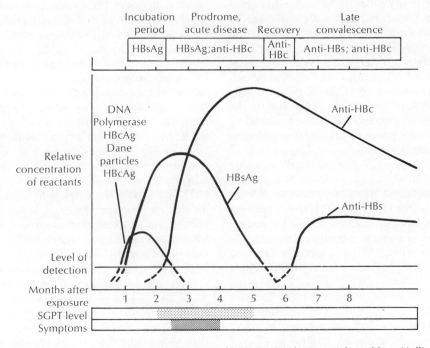

FIG. 10-4. Serologic patterns observed in acute viral hepatitis B infection. (Adapted from Hollinger, F.B., and Graham, D.Y.: Viral hepatitis: types A, B and non A/non B, Drug Ther. 8(9):46, Sept. 1978.)

lymphocytes are seen that are identical to those seen in infectious mononucleosis.

It is important to monitor the prothrombin time, since it may be elevated, especially in more extensive disease that results in hepatic cellular destruction. If the prothrombin time is severely elevated (more than twice normal), an IM injection of vitamin K will correct the problem.

Of particular interest in hepatitis B are the antigen-antibody systems and their relationship to the progress of the disease. Fig. 10-4 demonstrates these serologic relationships. It should be recognized that the appearance of the antibody (anti-HBs) connotes recovery, and permanent immunity is usually conferred. Of the available serologic tests for the detection of HBsAg, the radioimmunoassay (RIA) is the most sensitive. This test is performed by many commercial laboratories.

MEDICAL MANAGEMENT

As is the case with most viral diseases, there is no specific treatment for acute viral hepatitis. Therapy is basically palliative and supportive. Bed rest may be prescribed, especially early in the course of the disease. A nutritious, high-calorie diet is advisable. Drugs metabolized by the liver are to be avoided. The effectiveness of corticosteroids is doubtful in treatment of acute viral hepatitis; they are usually reserved for fulminant hepatitis. Prophylaxis of viral hepatitis is obviously the preferred form of treatment and is accomplished by using either early postexposure immune globulins or the hepatitis B vaccine.

Immune globulin (IG), previously called gamma globulin or immune serum globulin, is a pool of antibodies collected from nonselective human plasma that is free of HBsAg. This sterile solution contains antibodies against both hepatitis A and B. Another type of immune globulin called hepatitis B immune globulin (HBIG) is specially prepared from preselected plasma that is very high in titers of anti-HBs. In terms of effectiveness, HBIG is the better choice; however, it can cost up to 20 times more than IG.[11]

If IG is given very soon after exposure to HAV, the patient will be protected in 80% to 90% of cases, making this very effective therapy.[11] With hepatitis B, however, the effectiveness of IG is variable because of its relatively low titer of anti-HBs. IG may still be the therapy of choice if actual exposure to HBsAg-positive blood is not known to have occurred (i.e., low risk). In high-risk cases, such as a needle stick with HBsAg-positive blood, HBIG is the treatment of choice. It can prevent up to 75% of infections in certain cases.[16] The choice of which IG to use is based on occurrence, exposure, risk, and cost.

Preexposure protection against hepatitis B became available in 1982 in the form of an inactivated hepatitis B vaccine. The vaccine is prepared from pooled human plasma from donors known to be HBsAg positive and is then inactivated and purified through numerous steps. Trials of the vaccine have demonstrated an effectiveness of up to 95% in preventing infection, with no significant side effects reported except local inflammation and soreness.[21] Considerable concern exists as to the possibility of the hepatitis B vaccine being an agent for transmission of acquired immunodeficiency syndrome (AIDS). Evidence continues to accumulate that AIDS is caused by a transmissible agent. However, no evidence yet exists that links the occurrence of AIDS to the hepatitis B vaccine, and the possibility seems unlikely because of the extensive sterilization, testing, and processing of the vaccine before use. The vaccine is not intended for use in mass inoculations but rather in selected target populations who are at high risk of contracting hepatitis B. Table 10-6 is a list of groups who are at substantial risk of contracting hepatitis B and who should receive the vaccine. It should be noted that health care workers (including dentists) are near the top of the list.

The question often arises as to what happens to the dentist who is identified as being a carrier of HBsAg. As previously noted, carriers demonstrate variable degrees of infectivity; that is, not all carriers actually transmit the disease to their contacts. In several cases in which dentists were found to be carriers and had infected patients, their practice was suspended for variable periods of time. Others who had not infected patients were allowed to continue practice. In all instances, however, the dentists were required to use gloves and mask at all times and to inform their patients that they were carriers of hepatitis B.[1] Therefore unless a dentist-

TABLE 10-6. Persons at substantial risk for hepatitis B

Health care workers
 Medical
 Dental
 Laboratory
Hospital staff
 Especially those who have contact with blood and blood products
Clients and staff of institutions for the mentally retarded
Hemodialysis patients
Homosexually active males
Users of illicit, injectable drugs
Recipients of certain blood products
 Factors VIII and IX concentrates
Household and sexual contacts of HBV carriers
Special high-risk populations
 Alaskan Eskimos
 Asian refugees
 African refugees
 Haitian refugees
Inmates of long-term correctional facilities

From Inactivated hepatitis B virus vaccine: recommendation of the Immunization Practices Advisory Committee, Morbidity and Mortality Weekly Report **31**:322, 1982.

carrier is documented as having actually caused an infection in his or her patients, there is no basis for preventing continuation of practice. However, ethics and morals mandate aggressive efforts to prevent potential transmission by adherence to strict aseptic technique and informed consent.

DENTAL MANAGEMENT
Medical considerations (see Table 10-7)

There are five categories of patients with a past history of hepatitis that must be considered by the dentist: patients with active hepatitis, patients with a past history of hepatitis, patients at high risk for HBV infection, patients who are HBV carriers, and patients with signs or symptoms of hepatitis.

PATIENTS WITH ACTIVE HEPATITIS

Under no circumstances should routine, elective dental care be performed for a patient who has active hepatitis. If a patient is seen for routine care

TABLE 10-7. Dental management of patients with history of viral hepatitis

Recommendation: Since more than 50% of carriers of hepatitis B, as well as of many other infectious diseases, are *undetectable by history*, all patients should be treated with a strict aseptic approach, including the use of rubber gloves. In addition, the risk of contracting hepatitis B from an infectious patient can essentially be eliminated by the inoculation of all dental personnel with the hepatitis B vaccine.

I. Patients with active hepatitis
 A. Consult with physician about infectiousness
 B. Give emergency dental care only
II. Patients with past history of hepatitis (selective screening of this type will not reveal many carriers)
 A. Consult with physician regarding type and carrier status
 B. Additional information may be helpful in determining type
  1. Age at time of infection (type B uncommon under age 15)
  2. Source of infection (if contaminated food or water, type A)
 C. If type indeterminate, order RIA for HBsAg
III. Patients in high-risk category
 Order screening RIA for HBsAg
IV. HBsAg-positive patients (carriers)
 A. Consult with physician to discuss status and planned treatment
 B. Employ strict aseptic technique
 C. Use rubber gloves and mask
 D. Use rubber dam when possible
 E. Minimize aerosol production
 F. Scrub and sterilize all equipment after use
 G. Minimize drugs metabolized by liver
 H. Treat normally otherwise
V. Patients with signs or symptoms of hepatitis
 A. Refer to physician and postpone treatment
 B. If treatment necessary, treat as emergency patient only

TABLE 10-8. Emergency dental care for patient with hepatitis

Consult with patient's physician to discuss patient's status and planned dental treatment

Minimize use of drugs metabolized by liver

If surgery is necessary, obtain preoperative prothrombin time and bleeding time and discuss abnormal results with physician

Adhere to strict aseptic technique

Wear rubber gloves, gown, and mask

Use isolated operatory

Use rubber dam when possible to minimize contact with saliva or blood or both

Minimize aerosol production by using slow-speed handpiece when possible and using air syringe judiciously

Scrub and sterilize all equipment, including handpieces, after use

Do only work that is acutely necessary

---

and says in the history that he presently has hepatitis, the physician should be contacted immediately. Unless the patient is clinically and biochemically recovered and considered no longer infectious, no care should be rendered other than emergency care (see Table 10-8).

PATIENTS WITH A PAST HISTORY OF HEPATITIS

A primary concern of the dentist is to identify patients who are or could be hepatitis B carriers. Unfortunately, this is a difficult task, because more than 50% of carriers give no past history of hepatitis and thus are not detectable by history. Since it is estimated that there are between 400,000 and 800,000 carriers in the United States today, this means that there are 200,000 to 400,000 carriers who cannot be detected by history. Routine screening with an RIA for all patients is economically impractical because of its low cost-effectiveness. Therefore the only practical method of protection from these individuals (and other patients with undetected infectious disease) is to adopt a strict program of clinical asepsis, including the wearing of rubber gloves, for all patients. In addition, the availability and effectiveness of the hepatitis B vaccine essentially eliminates this group of patients as a threat. The vaccine is recommended for all dental personnel.

For patients who give a positive history of hepatitis, additional historical information about their disease can occasionally be of some help in determining the type of disease and thus the threat of infection. For instance, if the infection occurred under age 15 years or was caused by contaminated food or water, this would suggest hepatitis A and would probably not necessitate alteration of the dental management plan. Unfortunately, this approach has limited usefulness, since it would not reveal a person who had infections of both types A and B in which the type B infection was subclinical or undiagnosed. This again supports the adoption of strict aseptic technique for all patients and inoculation of dental personnel with hepatitis B vaccine.

An additional consideration in patients with a past history of hepatitis of unknown type is to use the clinical laboratory to screen for the presence of the HBsAg. As previously mentioned, the test of choice is an RIA for HBsAg. This may be indicated even in patients who specifically tell you which type of hepatitis they have had, since studies have shown that information of this type is unreliable 50% of the time.[6]

PATIENTS AT HIGH RISK FOR HBV INFECTION

As indicated in Table 10-6, there are many groups of people who are at unusually high risk for HBV infection. Individuals who fall into these categories should routinely be screened for HBsAg before dental care is provided unless there is laboratory evidence of anti-HBs. The benefits of performing this test are twofold. First, the dentist can better manage the patient with knowledge of the test results, and second, the patient will know his serologic status for future reference.

PATIENTS WHO ARE HBV CARRIERS

If a patient is found to be a carrier (HBsAg positive), the following management approach should be employed:

1. Consult with patient's physician to discuss patient's current status and planned dental treatment
2. Employ strict aseptic technique
3. Use rubber gloves and mask
4. Use rubber dam when possible to minimize contact with saliva and blood

5. Minimize aerosol production by using slow-speed handpiece when possible and using air syringe judiciously
6. Scrub and sterilize all equipment after use, including handpieces*; Sanger et al. have reviewed all commercially available handpieces that can be sterilized[23]

If the results of the RIA are reported as "negative for hepatitis," the patient is assumed to be free of HBsAg and is treated as a normal patient, with no special precautions.

PATIENTS WITH SIGNS OR SYMPTOMS OF HEPATITIS

Any patient who has signs or symptoms that suggest hepatitis should not be treated but referred immediately to a physician. Should emergency care be necessary, it should be provided as for the patient with acute disease (see Table 10-8).

Drug administration

In a completely recovered patient there are no special drug considerations. However, if a patient has chronic hepatitis or is a carrier of HBsAg, drugs metabolized by the liver should be avoided if possible, or the dosage should be adjusted downward. As can be seen from Table 10-3, many drugs commonly used in dentistry are metabolized principally by the liver. However, in other than the most severe cases of hepatic disease, these drugs could be used, but should be used in limited amounts. For example, the maximum amount of lidocaine used should empirically be limited to approximately 100 mg (three carpules of 2%).

Treatment planning modifications

No treatment planning modifications are required for completely recovered patients.

Oral complications

The only oral complication associated with hepatitis is the potential for abnormal bleeding in cases of significant liver damage. Before any surgery the prothrombin time should be checked to ensure that it is less than twice normal (28 seconds). If it is greater than 28 seconds, the potential for severe bleeding exists. In this case, should surgery be necessary, an injection of vitamin K will usually correct the problem. It is also advisable to monitor the bleeding time to check platelet function, since liver damage can also result in a decreased platelet count. The Ivy bleeding time should be less than 6 minutes. Values greater than this may require platelet replacement before surgery and should be discussed with the patient's physician.

EMERGENCY DENTAL CARE

Should it be determined that dental care is necessary for a patient who has active or suspected hepatitis, the management scheme in Table 10-8 should be employed.

REFERENCES

1. Ahtone, J., and Goodman, R.A.: Hepatitis B and dental personnel: transmission to patients and prevention issues, J. Am. Dent. Assoc. 106:2119-2222, 1983.
2. Annual Summary 1980, Morbidity and Mortality Weekly Report 29:10, 1981.
3. Bass, B.D., et al.: Quantitation of hepatitis B viral maskers in a dental school population, J. Am. Dent. Assoc. 104: 629-632, 1982.
4. Crawford, J.J.: New light on the transmissability of viral hepatitis in dental practice and its control, J. Am. Dent. Assoc. 91:829-835, 1975.
5. Dienstag, J.L., et al.: Acute hepatitis. In Isselbacher, K.J., et al., editors: Harrison's principles of internal medicine, ed. 9, New York, 1980, McGraw-Hill Book Co., pp. 1459-1467.
6. Galili, D., et al.: A modern approach to prevention and treatment of oral bleeding in patients with hepatocellular disease, Oral Surg. 54:277-280, 1982.
7. Goebel, W.M.: Reliability of the medical history in identifying patients likely to place dentists at an increased hepatitis risk, J. Am. Dent. Assoc. 98:907-913, 1979.
8. Golden, A.: Pathology: understanding human disease, Baltimore, 1982, The Williams & Wilkins Co., pp. 258-278.
9. Hepatitis: United States, 1975, 1976, Morbidity and Mortality Weekly Report 26:177, 1977.
10. Hollinger, F.B., and Graham, D.Y.: Viral hepatitis: types A, B and non A/non B, Drug Ther. 8(9):39-55, Sept. 1978.
11. Immune globulins for protection against viral hepatitis, Morbidity and Mortality Weekly Report 30:423-435, 1981.
12. Inactivated hepatitis B virus vaccine: recommendation of the Immunization Practices Advisory Committee, Morbidity and Mortality Weekly Report 31:318-328, 1982.

---

*The use of "cold sterilization" is unacceptable, since germicides cannot guarantee sterilization of instruments and provide only varying degrees of disinfection.[2]

13. Kwann, H.C.: Disorders of fibrinolysis, Med. Clin. North Am. **56:**163-176, 1972.

14. Lack of transmission of hepatitis B to humans after oral exposure to hepatitis B surface antigen-positive saliva, Morbidity and Mortality Weekly Report **27:**247, 1978.

15. Lamont, J.T., et al.: Cirrhosis. In Isselbacher, K.J., et al., editors: Harrison's principles of internal medicine, ed. 9, New York, 1980, McGraw-Hill Book Co., pp. 1473-1484.

16. Lieber, C.S., and Rubin, E.: Ethanol: a hepatotoxic drug, Gastroenterology **54:**642-646, 1968.

17. Mosley, J.W., et al.: Hepatitis B virus infection in dentists, N. Engl. J. Med. **293:**729-734, 1975.

18. Nichols, C., et al.: Gingival bleeding: the only sign in a case of fibrinolysis, Oral Surg. **38:**681-690, 1974.

19. Ostrow, J.D.: Jaundice. In Brooks, F.P., editor: Gastrointestinal pathophysiology, New York, 1978, Oxford University Press, pp. 163-186.

20. Pises, P., et al.: Hyperfibrinolysis in cirrhosis, Am. J. Gastroenterol. **60:**280-288, 1972.

21. Rauch, S., and Gorlin, R.J.: Diseases of the salivary glands. In Gorlin, R.J., and Goldman, H.M., editors: Thomas' oral pathology, vol. 2, ed. 6, St. Louis, 1970, The C.V. Mosby Co., pp. 962-1003.

22. Recovery of virus-like particles associated with non A, non B hepatitis, Morbidity and Mortality Weekly Report **27:** 199, 1978.

23. Sanger, R.G., Bradford, B.A., and Delaney, J.M.: An inquiry into the sterilization of dental handpieces relative to transmission of hepatitis B virus, J. Am. Dent. Assoc. **96:**621-624, 1978.

24. Smith, J.L., et al.: Comparative risk of hepatitis B among physicians and dentists, J. Infect. Dis. **13:**705-706, 1976.

25. Sywassink, J.M., and Lutwick, L.I.: Risk of hepatitis B in dental care providers: a contact study, J. Am. Dent. Assoc. **106:**182-184, 1983.

26. Tullman, M.J., et al.: The threat of hepatitis B from dental school patients: a one year study, Oral Surg. **49:**214-216, 1980.

27. Tumen, H.J.: Alcoholic liver disease, Hosp. Med. **10**(9):6-27, 1974.

28. Werner, B.G. and Grady, G.F.: Accidental hepatitis B surface antigen positive innoculations: Use of e antigen to estimate infectivity, Ann. Intern. Med. **97:**367-369, 1982.

29. Zuckerman, A.J.: Hepatitis B: its prevention by vaccine, J. Infect. Dis. **143:**301-304, 1981.

11

END-STAGE
RENAL DISEASE

There are 8 million people in the United States today with some form of kidney disease. Of these, 60,000 die annually as a result of chronic, progressive, and irreversible kidney failure (end-stage renal disease [ESRD] or chronic renal failure), and half of these are over age 55 years.

The early phase of ESRD, which is usually clinically asymptomatic except for some mild laboratory abnormalities, is called renal insufficiency. Progressively, however, more damage occurs, resulting in decreased ability of the kidney to perform its excretory, endocrine, and metabolic functions beyond compensatory mechanisms. The disease then becomes frank renal failure. This indicates inability of the kidneys to maintain normal homeostasis. The resulting syndrome caused by kidney failure, retention of excretory products, and interference with endocrine and metabolic functions is called uremia. The manifestations of uremia are seen in many organ systems, including the cardiovascular, gastrointestinal, neuromuscular, hematologic, and dermatologic systems.

As the disease progresses, conservative medical management becomes inadequate, and either artificial filtration of the blood by dialysis or transplantation of a kidney is required. Patients in both of these categories pose significant management considerations for the dentist.

GENERAL DESCRIPTION
Etiology

ESRD is a bilateral, progressive, and chronic deterioration of nephrons that results in uremia and ultimately leads to death. The rate of the destruction and the severity of the disease depend on the underlying causative factors; however, in many cases the cause remains unknown.

Some of the more common among the known causes of ESRD are nephrosclerosis, pyelonephritis, glomerulonephritis, diabetic nephropathy, congenital disorders, drug-induced nephropathy, obstructive uropathy, and hypertension.[2,3]

Pathophysiology

Deterioration and destruction of functioning nephrons are the underlying pathologic processes of renal failure. The nephron includes the glomerulus, renal tubules, and renal vasculature. Various diseases affect different segments of the nephron first, but eventually the entire nephron is affected. For example, hypertension affects the vasculature first, while glomerulonephritis first affects the glomerulus.

Once nephrons are lost, they are not replaced. However, because of a compensatory hypertrophy of the remaining nephrons, renal function is well maintained for a time.[3] This is a period of relative renal insufficiency, during which homeostasis is preserved. The patient remains asymptomatic and demonstrates only a few laboratory abnormalities that reflect a diminished glomerular filtration rate.[6]

Normal function is maintained until 70% to 80% of the nephrons are destroyed. At this point compensatory mechanisms are overwhelmed, and the signs and symptoms of uremia appear.[3,6] Morpho-

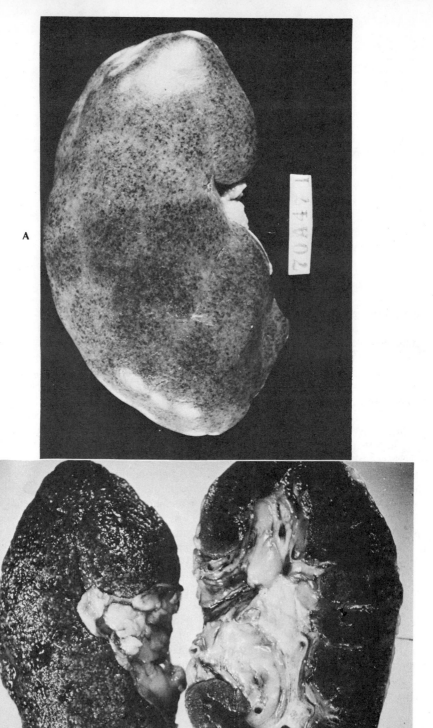

FIG. 11-1. A, Morphology of normal kidney. **B,** Morphology in ESRD. (Courtesy A. Golden, M.D., Lexington, Ky.)

logically the end-stage kidney is markedly reduced in size, scarred, and nodular (Fig. 11-1).

Sequelae and complications

Although a patient with early renal failure may remain asymptomatic, physiologic changes invariably occur as the disease progresses. These changes occur because of the loss of nephrons, which results in loss of overall renal function. Because of the tubular malfunction, the sodium pump loses its effectiveness, and excretion of sodium occurs. Along with sodium, excess amounts of dilute urine are excreted.[2] This accounts for the polyuria that is commonly encountered. Two of the hallmarks of ESRD are excretion of urine of a relatively fixed specific gravity or osmolality and inflexibility of the kidneys in response to sudden changes in water intake.[6]

With the loss of glomerular filtration function there is a buildup of nonprotein nitrogen compounds in the blood, mainly in the form of urea.[3,12] This is termed *azotemia*. In addition to the nitrogenous waste products, other acids accumulate because of tubular impairment, resulting in loss of bicarbonate ions and inability to synthesize ammonium for excretion.[12] The combination of waste products causes acidosis, the major factor of which is decreased ammonia excretion. In the later stages of renal failure, acidosis causes nausea, anorexia, and fatigue. Patients may tend to hyperventilate to attempt a respiratory compensation for the metabolic acidosis.

In the patient with acidosis of ESRD, adaptive mechanisms are already taxed beyond normal, and any increase can lead to serious consequences. For example, sepsis or a febrile illness can lead to profound acidosis and can be fatal.[6]

As would be expected, there are severe electrolyte disturbances in renal failure. Sodium depletion has already been mentioned. With the progressive azotemia of the later stages, hyperkalemia may develop.[2] This becomes particularly evident as urine output falls.

Patients with ESRD demonstrate several hematologic abnormalities. Anemia is one of the more familiar manifestations of chronic renal failure. It is caused by decreased erythropoietin production by the kidney, inhibition of red blood cell production by uremic serum, and red blood cell hemoly-

sis, which probably results from unidentified substances in uremic plasma as well as from other factors.[6,10]

There are also changes that occur in the production and function of white blood cells and lead to alteration of the immune response, inflammation, and an enhanced susceptibility to infection.[2]

Hemorrhagic tendencies are common in patients with ESRD and are attributed primarily to abnormal platelet aggregation and decreased platelet factor III.[2] A possible defect in factor VIII has also been implicated.[5]

The cardiovascular system is affected by a tendency to develop congestive heart failure or pulmonary edema or both. There is also hypertrophy of the left ventricle that may compromise blood supply via the coronary vessels. This is worsened by anemia. There is also a tendency for accelerated

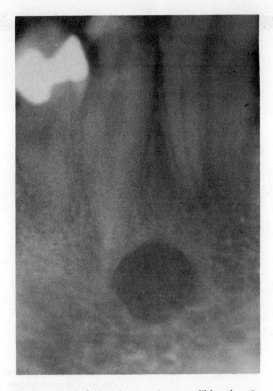

FIG. 11-2. Lytic lesion in anterior mandible of patient with hyperparathyroidism. (Courtesy L.R. Bean, D.D.S., Lexington, Ky.)

atherosclerosis in patients with ESRD. Pericarditis is common.[2,6]

A variety of bone disorders is seen in ESRD, but the most common term used to describe these changes is *renal osteodystrophy*. Briefly, with decreasing nephron function there is decreased glomerular filtration, which results in an increased serum level of phosphate. Since phosphate is a driving force of bone mineralization, the excess phosphate tends to cause serum calcium to be deposited in bone, resulting in a decreased serum calcium level. In response to low serum calcium, the parathyroid glands secrete parathyroid hormone (PTH), causing a secondary hyperparathyroidism. PTH then (1) inhibits the tubular reabsorption of phosphate, (2) stimulates renal produc-

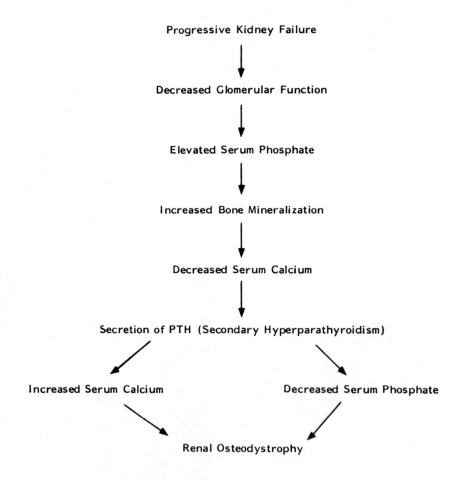

FIG. 11-3. Summary of changes that result in renal osteodystrophy.

tion of vitamin D, which is necessary for calcium metabolism, and (3) enhances vitamin D absorption from the intestine. These actions cause a mobilization of calcium from the bones and elevate the serum calcium, in addition to causing the excretion of phosphate to lower the serum phosphate. The result of these activities leads to osteomalacia (increased unmineralized bone matrix), osteitis fibrosa (bone resorption and lytic lesions) (Fig. 11-2), and osteosclerosis (enhanced bone density) in varying degrees[2,4,12] (Fig. 11-3).

With renal osteodystrophy there is a tendency for spontaneous fractures, myopathy, aseptic necrosis of the hip, and extraosseous calcification.[2]

CLINICAL PRESENTATION
Signs and symptoms

The signs and symptoms of uremia may be manifested in any of a number of organ systems, several of which have already been mentioned.

Patients with the uremic syndrome may demonstrate mental slowness or depression. They may become psychotic in the later stages. They may also show muscular hyperactivity. Convulsion is a late finding that is directly correlated with the level of azotemia.

Patients with renal failure demonstrate a variety of gastrointestinal signs. Anorexia and vomiting are common, especially later in the disease. Stomatitis manifested by oral ulceration is not unusual, and candidiasis also occurs (Fig. 11-4). Parotitis may be seen, and there may be an ammonia-like odor to the breath. These patients commonly suffer from malnutrition and diarrhea.

Hyperpigmentation of the skin is common. It is characterized by a brownish yellow color caused by the retention of carotene-like pigments that are normally excreted by the kidney. These pigments also may produce a profound pruritus. An interesting occasional finding is a whitish coating of the skin of the trunk and arms called uremic frost. It is caused by residual urea crystals left on the skin when perspiration evaporates.

Because of the bleeding diatheses that accompany ESRD, hemorrhagic episodes are not uncommon, especially in the gastrointestinal tract. In addition, ecchymosis or petechiae may be noted on the skin or mucous membranes (Fig. 11-5).

Cardiovascular manifestations of ESRD include hypertension, congestive heart failure (shortness of breath, orthopnea, dyspnea on exertion, peripheral edema), and pericarditis.

Laboratory findings

There are several tests used to monitor the progress of ESRD. These include urinalysis, serum creatinine, creatinine clearance, and electrolyte measurements. The most basic test of kidney function is the urinalysis, with special emphasis placed on the specific gravity (normally 1.003 to 1.035) and the presence of protein (normally none present).[8]

Creatinine is an excellent measure of glomerular filtration and tubular excretion and is commonly used as the index of clearance in a 24-hour urine collection. Serum creatinine level is relatively con-

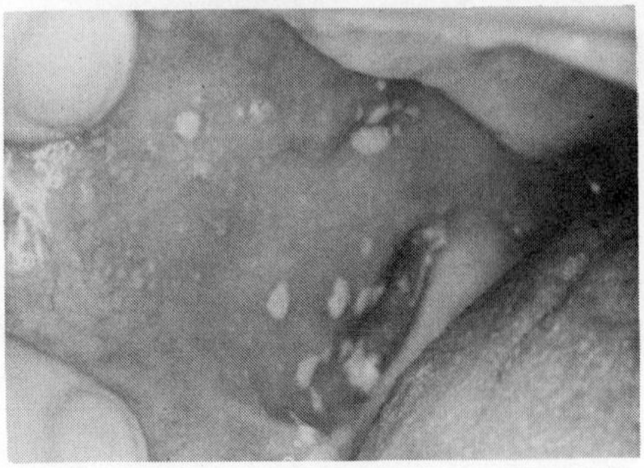

FIG. 11-4. Oral candidiasis in patient with ESRD. This patient also has diabetes.

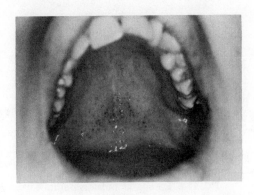

FIG. 11-5. Palatal petechiae in patient with ESRD.

stant, with normal of 0.5 to 1.0 mg/100 ml.[8]

The blood urea nitrogen (BUN) is a common indicator of kidney function but is not as specific as the serum creatinine. Normal range for BUN is 8 to 26 mg/100 ml.[8]

Serum sodium level ranges between 135 and 148 mmol/liter, serum potassium between 3.8 and 5.5 mmol/liter, serum chloride between 98 and 106 mmol/liter, and total carbon dioxide between 23 and 30 mmol/liter for venous blood.[8]

MEDICAL MANAGEMENT
CONSERVATIVE CARE

Once the diagnosis of ESRD is made, the goals of treatment are to retard the progress of disease and to preserve the quality and quantity of life. A conservative approach to treatment is the first step and may be adequate for a prolonged period.

Conservative care is based on an attempt to decrease the retention of nitrogenous waste products and to control fluids and electrolyte imbalances. This is accomplished by dietary modification and protein restriction as well as closely monitored fluid sodium, and potassium levels.[2] Also, any treatable associated conditions, such as hypertension, congestive heart failure, infection, volume depletion, urinary tract obstruction, hypercalcemia, and hyperuricemia, are corrected. Additionally, it is most important to avoid any nephrotoxic drugs or drugs that are metabolized principally by the kidney.

The anemia that occurs in renal failure is usually refractive to conservative tretment but is well tolerated by most patients.[10] No treatment is indicated unless the patient becomes severely symptomatic, develops an infection, or requires surgery. Even in that event, a hematocrit between 25 and 30 vol.% is usually adequate. Infusion of packed red blood cells is the treatment of choice if replacement becomes necessary.

DIALYSIS

As more and more nephrons are destroyed, attempts at medical management become inadequate

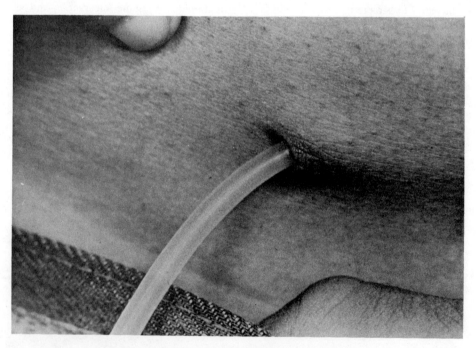

FIG. 11-6. Chronic ambulatory peritoneal dialysis catheter site on abdominal wall. (Courtesy Dialysis Center, Lexington, Ky.)

to prevent or control azotemia. At this point, artificial filtration of the blood is required in the form of peritoneal dialysis or hemodialysis.

Peritoneal dialysis is accomplished by injecting a hypertonic solution into the peritoneal cavity. Time is allowed to elapse, and then the solution is drawn out. Dissolved solutes, such as urea, are drawn out with the solution. The advantages of peritoneal dialysis are its relatively low cost and ease of performance. Disadvantages include the need for frequent sessions and significantly lower effectiveness than hemodialysis. Its principal use is for patients who are in acute renal failure or who require only occasional dialysis.

A newer method of peritoneal dialysis is chronic ambulatory peritoneal dialysis. This is a method of continuous peritoneal dialysis that is performed by the patient. Dialysate is emptied into the peritoneal cavity and then allowed to drain into a bag strapped to the patient (Fig. 11-6). This method allows the patient more freedom than older methods. A disadvantage of this method is the high risk of peritonitis.

When dialysis is used as a chronic treatment, hemodialysis is usually the method of choice. Approximately 26,000 patients are currently being maintained by hemodialysis in the United States.[2] Hemodialysis treatments are performed every 2 to 3 days depending on need. Usually 3 to 5 hours are required for each session (Fig. 11-7). Obviously, this consumes an enormous amount of the patient's time and is extremely confining.

The technique requires the surgical creation of a subcutaneous arteriovenous fistula that is readily accessible to venipuncture (Fig. 11-8). The patient is "plugged in" to the hemodialysis machine at the fistula site, and blood is then passed through the machine, filtered, and returned to the patient. Heparin is administered during the procedure to prevent clotting.

While hemodialysis is a lifesaving technique, there are complications associated with it. In addition to the problems attendant to ESRD, the risk of hepatitis B is significant, because these patients have usually had multiple blood transfusions. It is estimated that about 17% of patients receiving chronic hemodialysis are carriers of hepatitis B (positive for hepatitis B surface antigen [HBsAg])

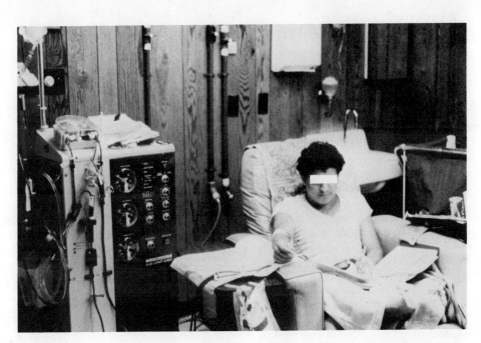

FIG. 11-7. Patient undergoing hemodialysis. (Courtesy Dialysis Center, Lexington, Ky.)

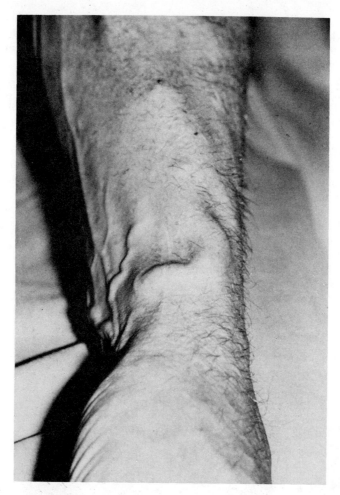

FIG. 11-8. Site of surgically created arteriovenous fistula with subsequent dilation and hypertrophy of veins. (Courtesy Dialysis Center, Lexington, Ky.)

and thus constitute a reservoir of potential infection.[2]

Infection of the arteriovenous fistula is an ongoing concern and can result in infective endarteritis or endocarditis. The incidence or risk of fistula infection from surgical procedures (e.g., urogenital or oral surgery procedures) is not precisely known, but it is felt to be low. However, should an infection occur, the results could be fatal.

As with all patients with ESRD, drugs that are metabolized primarily by the kidney or are nephrotoxic are to be avoided.

A final problem associated with hemodialysis is that of bleeding tendencies. As previously mentioned, patients with ESRD have bleeding tendencies because of altered platelet aggregation, decreased platelet factor III, and possibly defective factor VIII. With hemodialysis, there is the additional problem of platelet destruction by the treatment. Also, recent evidence suggests that hemodialysis may cause activation of prostaglandin I_2, which reduces platelet aggregation. It is significant to note that since the half-life of this compound is 1 to 3 minutes, its adverse effects may not be demonstrable by routine laboratory tests.[7] It should be noted, however, that these hemorrhagic tendencies are not usually clinically significant, and in most cases they will not prevent surgical procedures.

KIDNEY TRANSPLANTATION

An alternative to dialysis is transplantation of a kidney from either a living donor or a cadaver. The obvious advantage to this approach is that the individual gains freedom in his life and no longer is "married" to the dialysis machine. Also, if the transplant is successful, all of the consequences of the metabolic abnormalities of ESRD tend to be completely reversed.[2]

Transplantation of a kidney has become standard surgical procedure in most large medical centers and is no longer considered an experimental oddity. The success and safety of the procedure continue to improve, and more kidneys are transplanted each year. A survey of experiences with kidney transplants in seven centers between the years of 1977 and 1978 revealed with 881 transplants were performed in 879 patients in these centers. Of these, there was a 1-year survival rate of over 90% and a 1-year graft success rate between 55% and 78%, depending on whether the graft was from a cadaver or a living donor, respectively.[11] It is felt that these statistics are representative of the state of the art nationwide.

Kidney transplantation, however successful, is not without problems. As with all organ transplants, the major problem is graft rejection. Numerous methods have been attempted to suppress rejection, including immunosuppressive chemotherapy with cytotoxins and steroids, local radiation therapy, and antilymphocyte globulin. Chemotherapy seems to be the most widely accepted mode of therapy and commonly includes prednisone and azathioprine in varying degrees. With these medications the patient is extremely susceptible to infection and poor wound healing. Sepsis is one of the major complications in transplant patients. In fact, despite advances in decreasing the effects of antirejection therapy, more than 80% of transplant recipients develop infections.[9] The large dosages of steroids also serve to suppress markedly adrenal function and thus depress endogenous cortisol production.

TABLE 11-1. Dental management of ESRD (including emergency dental care)

Patient under conservative care

Consultation with physician

Avoid dental treatment if disease is poorly controlled or patient is in advanced failure

Presurgical screening for bleeding disorder (bleeding time, partial thromboplastin time, paltelet count, hematocrit, hemoglobin count)

Close monitoring of blood pressure

Meticulous attention to good surgical technique

Avoidance of drugs metabolized by kidney or nephrotoxic drugs (see Table 11-2)

Aggressive management of orofacial infections with culture and sensitivity test

Consideration of hospitalization for severe infection or major procedures

Patient receiving hemodialysis

Same as conservative care recommendations, *as well as*

Antibiotic prophylaxis for all dental work to prevent infective endarteritis

Avoidance of dental care on day of treatment (especially within first 4 hours afterward); best treated on day after

Screening for HBsAg before any treatment—treat as potential carrier

Consideration of hospitalization for severe infection or major procedures

Patient with renal transplant

Same as conservative care recommendations, *as well as*

Consideration of corticosteroid supplementation

Consideration of prophylactic antibiotics to prevent oral infection in surgical patient (e.g., extractions)

Aggressive management of orofacial infection with culture and sensitivity test and antibiotics

Consideration of hospitalization for severe infection or major procedures

DENTAL MANAGEMENT
PATIENT UNDER CONSERVATIVE CARE
(See Table 11-1)
Medical considerations

Consultation with the physician is mandatory before dental care is provided to patients under conservative care for ESRD. If the patient's disease is well controlled, there is generally no problem in providing outpatient care. However, if the patient is in the advanced stages of failure, dental care is best provided in a hospital setting. This decision should be made in concert with the physician and the patient.

If it is decided to treat the patient as an outpatient, the blood pressure should be closely monitored before and during treatment. Any excessive readings should be reported to the physician. Because of the potential for bleeding problems, these patients should receive pretreatment screening for bleeding disorders, including bleeding time, platelet count, and partial thromboplastin time. A hematocrit and a hemoglobin count should also be ordered to assess the status of anemia. The values, if abnormal, should be discussed with the physician. Few problems are encountered if the hematocrit is above 25 vol.%. Prophylactic antibiotics are not required unless infection is present (e.g., incision and drainage of an abscess). If there is an orofacial infection, aggressive management with culture and sensitivity tests and appropriate antibiotics is necessary.

When surgical procedures are undertaken, meticulous attention to good surgical technique is necessary to decrease the risks of excessive bleeding and infection.

One of the major problems in treating patients with ESRD is drug therapy.[1] Of special concern are drugs that are excreted by the kidney or that are nephrotoxic. Tetracycline, for example, is contra-indicated in a patient with renal dysfunction, since it is excreted by the kidneys and may result in untoward toxic effects. This is true for any drug that is primarily excreted by the kidney. Table 11-2 is a list of some of the more commonly used drugs in dental practice and recommendations for their use in patients who have renal failure.

Treatment planning modifications

The goal of dental care for patients under conservative care for ESRD should be to restore the mouth to the healthiest condition possible and to eliminate all possible sources of infection. Oral physiotherapy training is very important for the maintenance of long-term oral health. It is important to remember that ESRD is a progressive disease that may ultimately necessitate hemodialysis or a transplant. From a dental standpoint it is much easier to manage the medically treated patient than either the hemodialysis patient or the patient who has had a transplant. Once an acceptable level of oral hygiene has been established, there is no contraindication to routine dental care.

Oral complications

The stomatitis that results in oral ulceration can usually be treated symptomatically. A solution of bicarbonate and water rinsed in the mouth, followed by a teaspoon of promethazine hydrochlo-

TABLE 11-2. Drug therapy in renal disease

Drug	Normal dosage OK	Decrease frequency	Do not give
Lidocaine (dental)	Yes		
Aspirin	Every 4 hours in mild renal failure	Every 6 to 12 hours in moderate to severe renal failure	
Phenacetin			Avoid
Acetaminophen	Yes in mild to moderate renal failure		Avoid in severe renal failure
Codeine	Yes		
Propoxyphene	Yes		
Meperidine	Yes		
Penicillin	Yes in mild to moderate renal failure	Every 12 to 16 hours in severe renal failure	
Erythromycin	Yes		
Tetracycline			Best to avoid if possible
Diazepam (Valium)	Yes		

Adapted from Bennett, W.M., Singer, I., and Coggins, C.J.: A guide to drug therapy in renal failure, JAMA **230:**1544-1553, 1974. Copyright 1974, American Medical Association.

ride syrup, provides topical anesthesia for short periods. It is important to rule out candidiasis as a source of oral infection in these individuals. This may be confirmed clinically by scraping the lesion and submitting the specimen for cytologic examination. The treatment of choice for oral candidiasis is nystatin.

Emergency dental care

Essentially the same rationale should be used for emergency care as for routine dental care; however, with severe infection or major procedures, hospitalization may be required.

PATIENT RECEIVING HEMODIALYSIS
(See Table 11-1)

The recommendations applying to management of the patient receiving hemodialysis are the same as those for the patient under conservative care, with a few exceptions. Peritoneal dialysis really presents no additional considerations; however, this is not the case with hemodialysis. The surgically created arteriovenous fistula is susceptible to infection (endarteritis) resulting from a bacteremia. Endarteritis in the hemodialysis patient is similar to infective endocarditis in the patient with rheumatic heart disease in terms of threat to the patient. Therefore patients who have the fistula require prophylactic antibiotic coverage for dental procedures, as do rheumatic heart disease patients, to prevent infection from occurring.

Since hemodialysis tends to aggravate bleeding tendencies through destruction of platelets, it is important to determine the status of hemostasis before any surgery is performed. A battery of screening tests, including bleeding time, platelet count, prothrombin time, and partial thromboplastin time should be ordered. Heparinization during dialysis will not produce significant residual bleeding tendencies, since heparin's peak activity lasts only 3 to 4 hours after infusion. Patients who have just had a hemodialysis session, however, could have bleeding tendencies; therefore it is best to avoid dental care the day of a treatment. If immediate care is necessary, protamine sulfate will block the anticoagulant effect of heparin. Probably the best time for dental treatment is the day following hemodialysis.

All hemodialysis patients should have periodic testing for HBsAg, because a significant percent-age of them are or will become carriers. However, even if the test has been negative in the past, all hemodialysis patients should be treated as potential carriers, because they may have acquired the disease since last tested. (See Chapter 10 for management of hepatitis B carriers.)

In planning treatment for hemodialysis patients it seems prudent to discourage extensive restorative or reconstructive procedures. Instead, a long-term maintenance program that would not generally include replacement of missing teeth should be emphasized. However, if the patient is very motivated about tooth replacement, this should certainly be considered as reasonable treatment.

Patients with emergency dental needs may be managed in a way similar to those with routine needs; however, in cases of severe infection or major procedures, hospitalization may be required.

PATIENT WITH RENAL TRANSPLANT
(Table 11-1)

If the patient with renal failure becomes a candidate for transplantation, the dentist should critically examine the condition of the patient's teeth for potential problems. It should be kept in mind that any dental care may require treatment modification and drug alteration.

It is advisable to remove any seriously questionable teeth, even though they may be presently functional. These teeth may represent a serious future problem if they are not removed before the surgery. Extensive reconstructive work or other time-consuming invasive procedures should be discouraged. The treatment of choice is maintenance of the present dentition in a sound, healthy state, although in many cases the patient's future needs may be better served with complete or partial dentures.

If the transplant patient is receiving high-dose steroid therapy, adrenal suppression will have occurred. The patient may require additional steroid supplementation, although many patients will already be taking sufficient steroids. The additional steroids will enable the patient to handle the stress created by the dental appointment or procedures. This is usually an individual modification that should be managed in cooperation with the physician (see Chapter 16).

In addition to steroids, cytotoxic drugs are frequently standard therapy. This combination of drugs greatly predisposes the patient to infection, sepsis, and poor wound healing. Therefore antibiotics should be given prophylactically to minimize bacteremia and to avoid postoperative infection at the site of treatment. The infective endocarditis prophylaxis schedule may be adequate, but consultation with the physician is advisable (see Chapter 2). Oral infections should be managed aggressively with a culture and sensitivity test and appropriate antibiotics.

Transplant patients also have a high incidence of hepatitis B and therefore should be screened for HBsAg.

Transplant patients with emergency dental needs may be managed in a way similar to those with routine needs; however, in cases of severe infection or major procedures, hospitalization may be required.

REFERENCES

1. Bennett, W.M., Singer, I., and Coggins, C.J.: A guide to drug therapy in renal failure, JAMA **230:**1544-1553, 1974.
2. Brenner, B.M., and Lazarus, J.M.: Chronic renal failure. In Isselbacher, K.J., et al., editors: Harrison's principles of internal medicine, ed. 9, New York, 1980, McGraw-Hill Book Co.
3. Golden, A: Pathology: understanding human disease, Baltimore, 1982, The Williams & Wilkins Co.
4. Kanis, J.A.: Osteomalacia and chronic renal failure, J. Clin. Pathol. **34:**1295-1307, 1981.
5. Kaztchkine, M., et al.: Bleeding in renal failure: a possible cause, Br. Med. J. **2:**612-615, 1976.
6. Kurtzman, N.A.: Chronic renal failure: metabolic and clinical consequences, Hosp. Pract. **17:**107-122, 1982.
7. Milam, S.B., and Cooper, R.L.: Extensive bleeding following extraction in a patient undergoing chronic hemodialysis, Oral Surg. **55:**14-16, 1983.
8. Murphy, J.E., and Henry, J.B.: Evaluation of renal function and water, electrolyte, and acid-base balance. In Henry, J.B., editor: Todd, Sanford and Davidsohn's clinical diagnosis and management by laboratory methods, vol. 1, ed. 16, Philadelphia, 1979, W.B. Saunders Co.
9. Rubin, R.H., et al.: Infection in the renal transplant recipient, Am. J. Med. **70:**405-411, 1981.
10. Sexauer, C.L., and Matson, J.R.: Anemia of chronic renal failure, Ann. Clin. Lab. Sci. **11:**484-487, 1981.
11. Standards Committee of the American Society of Transplant Surgeons: Current results and expectations of renal transplantation, JAMA **246:**1330-1331, 1981.
12. Woo, J., et al.: Metabolic intermediates and inorganic ions. In Henry, J.B., editor: Todd, Sanford and Davidsohn's clinical diagnosis and management by laboratory methods, vol. 1, ed. 16, Philadelphia, 1979, W.B. Saunders Co.

12

SEXUALLY TRANSMITTED DISEASES

Sexually transmitted diseases (STDs) are major health problems in the United States today and are considered epidemic in many parts of the world. There are at least 14 recognized STDs, five of which are epidemic in the United States.[9]

Since STDs are communicable, they are of interest to the dentist from three vantage points. First, the dentist is at risk to contract an STD from an infected patient, or conversely, the dentist may have a disease and transmit it to patients by means of contaminated hands or instruments. Second, an STD can occasionally be present in or around the oral cavity, either as a primary or disseminated site of infection, and the dentist must be alert to include STDs in the differential diagnosis of suspicious oral lesions that have no obvious cause. Finally, the dentist can act as a case finder of previously undetected disease. This is accomplished through the history, pertinent review of systems, and physical evaluation.

Although there are many STDs, only the three that are most commonly encountered—gonorrhea, syphilis, and genital herpes—will be considered in this chapter.

Gonorrhea

GENERAL DESCRIPTION
Incidence and epidemiology

Gonorrhea is the most frequently reported infectious disease in the United States today. The incidence has grown steadily over the past two decades; in 1980 there were 1,004,029 cases reported as compared to 404,836 cases reported in 1967.[1] This represents an increase of over 100% in 14 years (Fig. 12-1). It is believed that the number of cases reported represents only a small percentage of the actual number of cases, which is estimated to be over 3 million. The reported incidence is equivalent to 443.27 cases per 100,000 population.[1] Thus it is apparent that this disease is one of staggering proportions.

Humans are the only natural host for this disease, and its occurrence is worldwide. The transmission of gonorrhea is almost exclusively via sexual contact, whether it be genital-genital, oral-genital, or rectal-genital. The primary sites of infection are the genitalia, anal canal, and pharynx.

Gonorrhea can occur at any age; however, it occurs most commonly in the 15- to 24-year-old age group.[1] This group includes many single people who have a high potential for multiple sexual partners. High-risk factors other than age include low socioeconomic standing and being an urban dweller. Cases are reported more commonly in men than in women, at a ratio of 3:1. This difference is probably more apparent than real, however, because many women are unaware that they have the disease.

Etiology

Gonorrhea is caused by *Neisseria gonorrhoeae*, which is a gram-negative diplococcus commonly

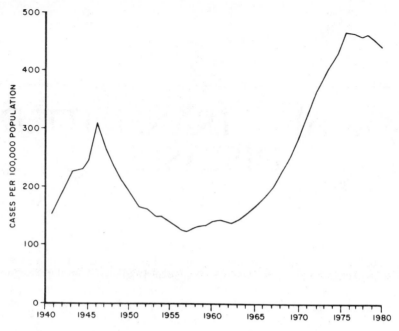

FIG. 12-1. Reported cases of gonorrhea per 100,000 population in United States from 1940 to 1980. (Adapted from Annual Summary, 1980, Morbidity and Mortality Weekly Report, 29(54), 1981.)

found within polymorphonuclear leukocytes. *N. gonorrhoeae* is an aerobe that requires high humidity and specific temperature and pH for optimum growth. It is a fragile bacterium that is readily killed by drying, so it is not easily transmitted by fomites.[13,22] It develops resistance to antibiotics rather easily, and many strains have developed resistance to penicillin as well as to other antibiotics.

Pathophysiology

The pathophysiology of gonorrhea is significant in that the type of host epithelium influences the invasiveness of the bacterium. Columnar epithelium, such as that found in the mucosal lining of the urethra and cervix, is susceptible to infection, while stratified squamous epithelium, such as that found on the skin and mucosal lining of the oral cavity, is highly resistant to infection.[13,14,22,28] It should be noted that transitional epithelium, such as that found in the oropharynx, is also susceptible to infection.[22] This explains the occurrence of pharyngeal and tonsillar infection and the relative infrequency of oral infection. Fig. 12-2 indicates

the areas of relative epithelial susceptibility to *N. gonorrhoeae* infection in the oral cavity and oropharynx. It is noteworthy that there are no recorded cases of gonorrhea infection of the fingers caused by direct contact with infected genital, anal, or oral secretions.

Infection in men usually begins in the anterior urethra. The bacteria establish a subepithelial infection and produce a purulent exudate. The infection may remain localized or may extend to the posterior urethra, bladder, epididymis, prostrate gland, or seminal vesicles. It is spread by means of lymphatics and blood vessels. Gonococcemia may occur, resulting in expression of the disease at distant body sites, including the oral cavity.

Infection in women occurs most commonly in the cervix and urethra. The same subepithelial invasion with production of purulent exudate occurs. The infection tends to be less severe in women but may spread to the endometrium, fallopian tubes, ovaries, and pelvic peritoneum. Gonococcemia can also occur.

In either sex, gonorrhea of the rectum may occur

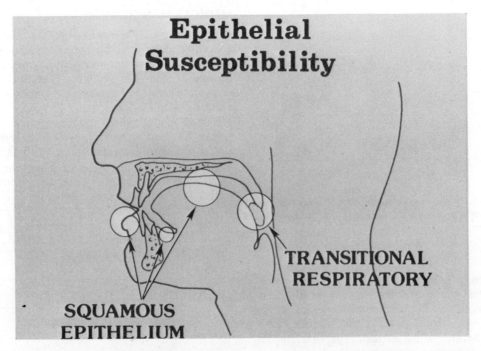

FIG. 12-2. Areas of relative epithelial susceptibility to infection by *N. gonorrhoea* within oral cavity.

following rectal-genital intercourse. Infection of the pharynx and oral cavity may follow oral-genital relations, resulting in a primary infection, or may occur secondary to genital infection. Primary infection at either site can result in gonococcemia.

Gonococcemia can lead to widespread dissemination and may result in a variety of disorders, including migratory arthritis, skin and mucous membrane lesions, endocarditis, meningitis, and pericarditis.

CLINICAL PRESENTATION
Signs and symptoms

In men, symptoms usually occur after an incubation period of about 1 week. The most common findings include urethral discharge, pain on urination, and urinary urgency and frequency. Tenderness and swelling may also occur.

In women, a significant percentage of cases may be asymptomatic or only minimally symptomatic. Women who have a symptomatic infection may demonstrate a vaginal or urethral discharge and dysuria with frequency and urgency. Backache and abdominal pain may also be present.

Approximately 50% of women and 5% to 10% of men are asymptomatic or only mildly symptomatic. This is unfortunate, because these patients may not seek medical care for their problem.[14,28] As a result, a reservoir of infection goes undetected.

Gonococcal infection of the anal canal is commonly less intense than genital infection, but similar symptoms can be noted, including discharge and pain.

Within the oral cavity, the pharynx is the area most commonly affected. Pharyngeal infection is found in up to 20% of patients with gonorrhea.[7,12,16] It may be an asymptomatic infection with diffuse, nonspecific inflammation or as a mild sore throat. Pharyngeal gonorrhea is most commonly found in homosexual men. It is probably the result of fellatio with an infected partner. The incidence of transmission of pharyngeal gonorrhea to the genitalia seems to be much less than that of genital-genital transmission.[7,16]

Gonococcal stomatitis or oral gonorrhea is un-

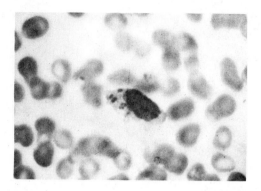

FIG. 12-3. Smear demonstrating gram-negative diplococci within leukocyte. (Courtesy H.D. Wilson, M.D., Lexington, Ky.)

common; however, persistent case reports verify its existence.[15,17,20,31] Chue[5] has presented an excellent review of the manifestations of oral gonorrhea. These include acute ulceration, diffuse erythema, necrosis of the interdental papillae, lingual edema, edematous tissues that bleed easily, and vesiculations. A prominent feature is the presence of a pseudomembrane that is nonadherent and leaves a bleeding surface on removal. Lesions may be solitary or widely disseminated. Symptoms include a burning or itching sensation, dryness, increased salivation, bad taste, fetid odor, fever, and submandibular lymphadenopathy. The lesions of oral gonorrhea may closely resemble the lesions of erythema multiforme, bullous or erosive lichen planus, or herpetic gingivostomatitis.

In a separate report, Chue[4] describes an acute temporomandibular joint arthritis that was caused by disseminated gonococcal infection from a genital site.

Laboratory findings

Laboratory diagnosis of *N. gonorrhoeae* infection can be made presumptively from the findings of gram-negative intracellular diplococci in a smear of purulent discharge (Fig. 12-3). Statistically, most men with a mucopurulent urethral discharge have gonorrhea.[18] Confirmation of the findings is made by culture. This is especially important in suspected cases of oral gonorrhea, since other species of *Neisseria* are normal inhabitants of the oral cavity.

MEDICAL MANAGEMENT

Current medical management of uncomplicated gonorrhea includes the use of oral tetracycline or parenteral amoxicillin or ampicillin with oral probenecid or the use of parenteral penicillin G with oral probenicid.[32] An alternative drug for use against penicillinase-producing *N. gonorrhoeae* is spectinomycin, although spectinomycin is not effective for treatment of pharyngeal infection. A follow-up culture is recommended 4 to 7 days after completion of treatment. There is a very low treatment failure rate with gonorrhea, though this may well change with the increased prevalence of penicillinase-producing bacterial strains.[13,22,28] Following the initiation of medical treatment of gonorrhea, infectiousness is rapidly diminished, probably within a matter of hours.[26]

Syphilis

GENERAL DESCRIPTION
Incidence and epidemiology

Syphilis is the third most frequently reported infectious disease in the United States today, surpassed only by gonorrhea and chickenpox. In 1980 the reported incidence of this disease was approximately 27,204 cases, which represented a 34% increase over 1977[1] (Fig. 12-4). The true incidence of the disease, however, is probably much higher.

As with gonorrhea, humans are the only known natural host for syphilis, although many different animal models have been experimentally infected.

The transmission of syphilis is predominantly sexual, including the oral-genital and rectal-genital routes; however, transmission also occurs through nonsexual means, such as kissing, transfusion, or accidental inoculation with a contaminated needle.[14,30] Indirect transmission by fomites is possible but uncommon.[30] Congenital syphilis occurs when the fetus is infected in utero by the infected mother.

The primary site of syphilitic infection is most commonly the genitalia, although primary lesions also occur extragenitally, at the lips, tongue, fingers, nipples, and anal orifice.[30] Syphilis is most common in those in their early 20s, followed by those in their late teens. There does not seem to be any significant difference in reported incidence between men and women.

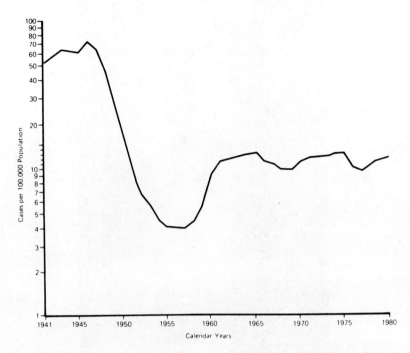

FIG. 12-4. Reported cases of syphilis (primary and secondary) per 100,000 population in United States from 1941-1980. (Adapted from Annual Summary, 1980, Morbidity and Mortality Weekly Report, **29**(54), Sept. 1981.)

Etiology

The etiologic agent of syphilis is *Treponema pallidum,* which is a slender, fragile anaerobic spirochete. It is easily killed by heat, drying, exposure to oxygen, and soap and water.[28,30] The organism is difficult to stain, except with certain silver-impregnation methods. Demonstration is best done using dark-field microscopy with a fresh specimen.

Pathophysiology

It is believed that *T. pallidum* probably does not invade completely intact epithelium or mucosa but rather enters through minute abrasions or hair follicles.

Within a few hours after invasion, bacterial spread to the lymphatics and bloodstream occurs, resulting in early widespread dissemination of the disease. The early basic lesion of syphilis is granulomatous and results in obliteration of arterioles with necrosis and subsequent healing with fibrosis

and scarring. The degree of scarring is variable and ranges from imperceptible to disfiguring.

CLINICAL PRESENTATION
Signs and symptoms

The manifestations and descriptions of syphilis are classically divided into stages of occurrence, with each stage having its own peculiar signs and symptoms that are related to time and antigen-antibody responses. The stages are primary, secondary, latent or tertiary, and congenital. Each will be briefly described.

PRIMARY SYPHILIS

The classical lesion of primary syphilis is the chancre, which is a solitary granulomatous lesion. Accompanying the chancre are enlarged regional lymph nodes. The chancre usually occurs within 2 to 3 weeks after exposure (Fig. 12-5). Patients are infectious, however, before appearance of the chancre.[14] The lesion begins as a small papule and

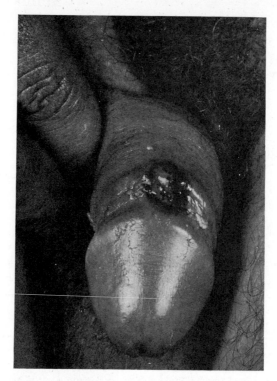

FIG. 12-5. Primary syphilis: chancre of penis. (From Rudolph, A.W.: Syphilis. In Top, F.H., and Wehrle P.F., editors: Communicable and infectious disease, ed. 8, St. Louis, 1976, The C.V. Mosby Co., p. 674.)

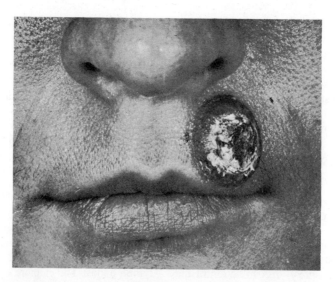

FIG. 12-6. Primary syphilis: extragenital chancre of lip. (From Rudolph, A.W.: Syphilis. In Top, F.H., and Wehrle, P.F., editors: Communicable and infectious diseases, ed. 8, St. Louis, 1976, The C.V. Mosby Co., p. 674.)

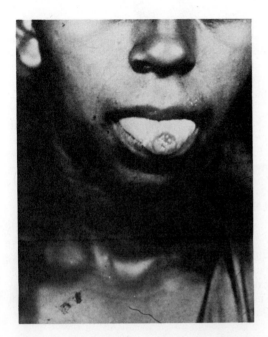

FIG. 12-7. Primary syphilis: extragenital chancre of tongue.

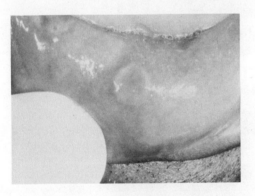

FIG. 12-8. Secondary syphilis: mucous patch of lower lip.

enlarges to form a chancre with surface erosion or ulceration. It is commonly covered with a yellowish, hemorrhagic crust and teems with *T. pallidum*. The chancre is most commonly asymptomatic. Associated with the chancre are enlarged, painless, hard regional lymph nodes. The chancre usually subsides in 3 to 5 weeks, leaving variable scarring in the form of a healed papule. The lymph node involvement resolves somewhat later. The genitalia, oral cavity, and anus are common sites for chancres. Fig. 12-6 and 12-7 are examples of syphilitic chancres of the lip and tongue.

SECONDARY SYPHILIS

The manifestations of secondary syphilis appear 6 to 8 weeks after the initial exposure. The chancre may or may not be completely resolved at this time. The symptoms and signs of secondary syphilis include a flulike syndrome, generalized lymphadenopathy, and generalized eruption of the skin and mucous membrane. These manifestations may occur singly or in combination. The associated oral manifestations of secondary syphilis include a pharyngitis and mucous patch.[14,23,30] Papular lesions have also been described.[10] Mucous patches may be seen in approximately 4% of cases.[3] The mucous patch, which typically appears as a painless raised lesion with central erosion covered by a grayish plaque, is highly infectious (Fig. 12-8). Secondary syphilis remains for a variable period of time, ranging from days to as long as a year.

LATENT OR TERTIARY SYPHILIS

An intermediate stage of syphilis is the latent stage, which follows untreated secondary syphilis and during which a person remains completely asymptomatic. This latent stage may last for many years or in fact for the remainder of the person's life. Without treatment, about two thirds of patients remain in this asymptomatic stage. However, in the other third of untreated patients, late manifestations of tertiary syphilis appear.

The gumma—the classical localized lesion of tertiary syphilis—involves numerous tissues, including skin, mucous membranes, bone, nervous tissue, and viscera. It is believed that the gumma represents the end result of a hypersensitivity reaction. It is basically an inflammatory granulomatous lesion with a central zone of necrosis. It is not infectious.

All of the other manifestations of tertiary syphilis are essentially vascular in nature and result from an obliterating endarteritis. Cardiovascular syphilis is most commonly seen as an aneurysm of the ascending aorta. Neurosyphilis can result in a meningitis-like syndrome, Argyll Robertson pupils (reaction to accommodation but not to light), altered tendon reflexes, general paresis (incomplete paralysis), or tabes dorsalis (degeneration of dorsal columns of the spinal cord and sensory nerve trunks).[14,23]

The oral lesions of tertiary syphilis are the gumma and a diffuse interstitial glossitis. Interstitial glossitis is considered a premalignant condition, and the tongue may appear lobulated and fissured with atopic papillae, resulting in a bald, wrinkled surface. Leukoplakia is frequently present. The oral gumma is a rare lesion that involves the tongue and palate most commonly. It appears as a firm tissue mass with central necrosis. Palatal gummas may perforate into the nasal cavity or maxillary sinus.

CONGENITAL SYPHILIS

Syphilis or its sequelae will be present in the newborn if the mother is infected while carrying the child. The disease is transmitted to the fetus in utero. Physical manifestations will vary depending on the time of infection. Sequelae of early infection include osteochondritis, periostitis, rhinitis, rash, and ectodermal changes. Syphilis contracted during late pregnancy can involve bones, teeth, eyes, cranial nerves, viscera, skin, and mucous membranes.

Oral manifestations of congenital syphilis include peg-shaped permanent central incisors with notching of the incisal edge (Hutchinson incisors) (Fig. 12-9), defective molars with multiple supernumerary cusps (mulberry molars), and perioral rhagades (skin fissures).

Laboratory findings

T. pallidum has never been cultured successfully on any kind of medium; therefore the definitive diagnosis of syphilis must be made from a positive dark-field microscopic examination. Dark-field examination is performed on fresh exudate from suspected lesions and is consistently positive only during primary and early secondary stages.

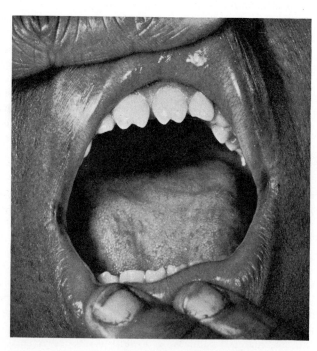

FIG. 12-9. Congenital syphilis: hutchinsonian teeth. (From Rudolph, A.W.: Syphilis. In Top, F.H., and Wehrle, P.F., editors: Communicable and infectious diseases, ed. 8, St. Louis, 1976, The C.V. Mosby Co., p. 681.)

Although the dark-field examination is the only way to make the definitive diagnosis of syphilis, serologic tests for syphilis (STS) provide presumptive evidence of syphilis. These tests are of two basic types and are differentiated by the type of antibodies they investigate.

REAGINIC TESTS

Reaginic tests are designed to detect the presence of an antibody-like substance called reagin that is thought to be produced when *T. pallidum* reacts with various body tissues. The Venereal Disease Research Laboratories (VDRL) and rapid plasma reagin (RPR) tests are examples of this kind of test and are essentially flocculation tests. A disadvantage of these tests is the occasional biologic false-positive result that can occur with other disease processes, such as infectious mononucleosis, leprosy, malaria, lupus erythematosus, vaccinia, and viral pneumonia.[28]

These tests are only consistently positive 3 or 4 weeks after the appearance of the primary chancre. The highest titer (concentration) occurs during secondary syphilis. Positive results are variable during tertiary syphilis.

ANTITREPONEMAL TESTS

Antitreponemal tests are designed to detect the specific antibody produced against *T. pallidum*. They are more specific than the reaginic tests but less sensitive. The *Treponema pallidum* immobilization (TPI) test, fluorescent treponemal antibody (FTA) test, and fluorescent treponemal antibody-absorption (FTA-ABS) test are examples of this type of test. The test in most common use today is the FTA-ABS test, which is considered to be the standard treponemal test in most laboratories.

In primary syphilis, all STS usually revert to negative within 6 to 9 months after successful treatment. In secondary syphilis, 12 to 24 months are required for the patient to become seronegative.[32] Occasionally, a patient may remain seropositive for the rest of his life. With tertiary syphilis, many patients remain seropositive for life.

MEDICAL MANAGEMENT

The current medical management of syphilis includes the use of parenteral long-acting penicillin. Alternative drugs for patients allergic to penicillin include oral tetracycline and erythromycin.[32] Following treatment, patients should be periodically retested serologically to monitor their conversion to negative. This conversion will usually occur within a year. There is a very low failure rate in the treatment of syphilis. An important aspect to note in the management of syphilis is that, as with gonorrhea, infectiousness is rapidly reversed, probably within a matter of hours on the initiation of medical treatment.[26]

Genital herpes

GENERAL DESCRIPTION
Incidence and epidemiology

Genital herpes (herpes simplex type 2) is an important sexually transmitted disease in the United States as well as the world. The exact incidence of the infection is unknown at present, because it is not yet a reportable disease. The awareness and occurrence of the disease are rapidly increasing, however, as evidence by the coverage in the lay press as well as in the scientific literature. The Centers for Disease Control[11] estimate that the number of patient consultations in the United States for genital herpes increased from 29,560 in 1966 to 260,890 in 1979. As with other STDs, this official estimate is probably grossly understated.

The herpes simplex virus (HSV) has been called the "virus of love," because the usual mode of transmission is by direct contact. Airborne droplet infection is not well demonstrated, although it is possible.[25] Autoinoculation via face, fingers, eyes, and genitalia is a clinical problem. HSV is an extremely common virus, as evidenced by the fact that most adults have antibodies to herpes simplex.

Etiology

HSV is a member of the herpesvirus group, which also includes cytomegalovirus, Epstein-Barr virus, and varicella-zoster virus.[24] HSV is classified into two closely related types, 1 and 2 (HSV-1 and HSV-2).

HSV-1 is the causative agent of most herpetic infections that occur above the waist, especially of the mucosa of the mouth (herpetic gingivostomatitis; herpes labialis), nose, eyes, brain, and skin. Infection with HSV-1 is extremely common; more than 70% of adults demonstrate antibodies to this virus.[24] It is thought that many primary infections with HSV-1 are subclinical and thus never known to the infected person. Transmission is usually by close contact, such as touching or kissing, via transfer of infective saliva. HSV-1 may also be transmitted via sexual contact.

HSV-2 is the causative agent of most herpes infections that occur below the waist, such as in or around the genitalia (genital herpes). HSV-2 is transmitted predominantly by sexual contact but may also be transmitted nonsexually. It can be transmitted to a neonate from an infected mother. There is a positive epidemiologic association between genital herpes and cervical carcinoma. There also seems to be a relationship to socioeconomic status, because only 10% of persons in the upper socioeconomic group demonstrate antibodies to HSV-2, while 20% to 60% of persons in the lower socioeconomic group have antibodies.[25]

Although the primary site of occurrence of HSV-1 is above the waist and of HSV-2 below the waist, each infection may occur in either site and in fact can be inoculated from one site to the other[6,8] (Fig. 12-10).

Pathophysiology

The pathologic processes of herpesvirus infections of HSV-1 and HSV-2 are essentially identical, and as such the lesions of skin and mucous membranes are identical. The infection begins with intimate contact with a lesion or infective fluid (e.g., saliva). Cells are invaded, and viral replication occurs. Characteristic cellular changes include ballooning degeneration, intranuclear inclusion bodies, and the formation of multinucleated giant cells. With cellular destruction come inflammation and increasing edema, which result in a papular formation that progresses to fluid-filled vesicles. The vesicles rupture, leaving an ulcerated or crusted surface. Lymphadenopathy and viremia are prominent features. In normal individuals, the infection is contained by usual host defenses and immunologic systems; however, in

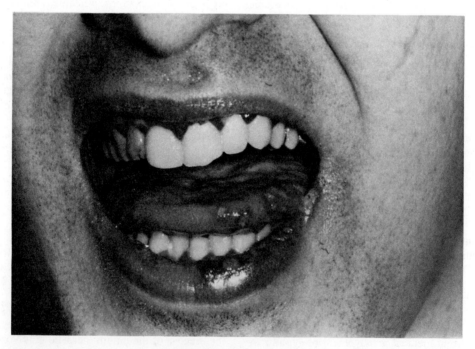

FIG. 12-10. Primary type II herpes simplex occurring in oral cavity documented by laboratory testing. (Courtesy R.C. Noble, M.D., Lexington, Ky.)

an immunosuppressed person or infant, an infection of this type may become systemic, widespread, and fatal.

When the infection has run its course, usually in 10 to 14 days, the viruses then enter the ends of peripheral neurons and migrate up the axonal sheath to the regional ganglion (HSV-1 in the trigeminal, HSV-2 in the sacral), where they reside. Then on adequate stimulation, such as trauma, sunlight, menses, or intercourse, the virus reactivates, migrates back down the axon, and produces a recurrent infection with lesions identical to the primary. However, the lesions of recurrent infection are generally of a less severe nature.

CLINICAL PRESENTATION
Signs and symptoms

After an incubation period of 2 to 7 days, the lesions of primary genital herpes appear. In women both internal and external genitalia may be involved, as may the perineal region and the skin of the thighs and buttocks. In men the external genitalia may be involved, as may the skin. Lesions in moist areas tend to ulcerate early and are very painful. Lesions on exposed, dry areas tend to remain pustular or vesicular and then crust over (Fig. 12-11). Regional, painful lymphadenopathy accompanies the infection along with headache, malaise, and symptoms of fever. Symptoms subside in about 2 weeks, with healing in 3 to 5 weeks.[19,27]

As previously stated, recurrent genital herpes is generally a less severe infection that is frequently precipitated by menses or intercourse. A prodrome of localized itching, tingling, pain, and burning is noted and is followed by a vesicular eruption. Healing occurs in 10 to 14 days. Constitutional symptoms are generally absent.

Whether the virus is HSV-1 or HSV-2, the lesions are highly infectious and therefore can be transmitted to other individuals or to other sites on the patient. The infectious period of herpetic lesions is uncertain, therefore one should assume that all herpetic lesions are infectious, regard-

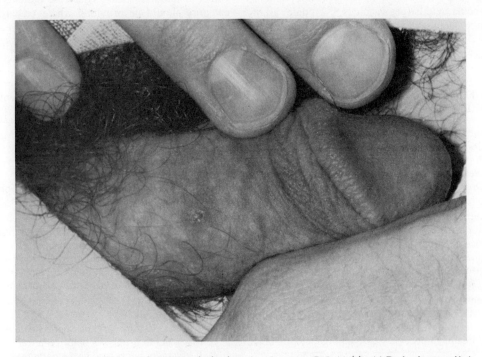

FIG. 12-11. Solitary herpetic lesion on shaft of penis. (Courtesy R.C. Noble, M.D., Lexington, Ky.)

less of stage (papular, vesicular, ulcerative, or crusted).

Laboratory findings

Cytologic examination of a smear taken from the base of a herpetic lesion will reveal the typical features of viral lesions, including ballooning degeneration of cells, intranuclear inclusion bodies, and multinucleated giant cells.

Viral typing can be performed by using tissue cultures, isolation of viruses, and then specific type identification by a number of methods, including restriction endonuclease, immunofluorescence, and immunoperoxidase.[2,27]

MEDICAL MANAGEMENT

The management of primary and recurrent genital herpes continues to be of a symptomatic and palliative nature, because no definitive treatment or cure yet exists. Many forms of therapy, both topical and systemic, have been tried. These include iododeoxyuridine, photodynamic inactivation with vital dyes, adenine arabinoside, lysine, bacillus Calmette-Guérin (BCG) vaccine, smallpox vaccine, and herpes vaccines.[27] To date, all of these approaches have proven to be of little or no value.

A recently introduced drug, acyclovir, has been approved for use both topically and IV. The effectiveness of the drug is greatest when used very early in the course of a primary infection. Acyclovir has been shown to decrease pain and duration of viral shedding and to reduce healing times. It is ineffective in treating recurrent infections.[33]

DENTAL MANAGEMENT
Medical considerations (see Tables 12-1 to 12-3)

Dental patients can be categorized into three groups for the purpose of management description—patients currently receiving treatment for an STD, patients with a past history of an STD, and patients with signs, symptoms, or oral lesions suggestive of an STD.

PATIENTS CURRENTLY RECEIVING TREATMENT FOR STD

Gonorrhea. In all likelihood the patient under treatment for gonorrhea poses little threat of disease transmission to the dentist. This is because of the mode of transmission as well as the early reversal of infectiousness. Therefore patients in this category should be provided whatever care is required. However, it would be prudent to contact the physician before beginning work as well as to wear disposable gloves during all treatment.

TABLE 12-1. Dental management of patient with history of gonorrhea

1. Patients currently receiving treatment for gonorrhea
   a. Consult with physician before treatment
   b. Provide required dental care
   c. Wear disposable gloves
   d. Oral lesions of gonorrhea can resemble many other lesions—use caution
2. Patients with past history of gonorrhea
   a. Approach with caution; obtain good history of disease, its treatment, and follow-up culture
   b. If no culture after treatment, consult with physician
   c. If free of disease, treat as normal patient
3. Patients with signs, symptoms, or oral lesions suggestive of gonorrhea
   a. Refer to physician and postpone treatment
   b. If treatment necessary, give emergency care only

TABLE 12-2. Dental management of patient with history of syphilis

1. Patients currently receiving treatment for syphilis
   a. Consult with physician before treatment
   b. Give emergency care only
   c. Wear disposable gloves
   d. Oral lesions of primary and secondary syphilis are infectious—treat cautiously
2. Patients with past history of syphilis
   a. Approach with caution; obtain good history of disease, its treatment, and negative STS
   b. If no follow-up STS, order STS, and, if positive, consult with physician before treatment
   c. If free of disease, treat as normal patient
3. Patients with signs, symptoms, or oral lesions suggestive of syphilis
   a. Refer to physician and postpone treatment
   b. May elect to order STS before referral
   c. If treatment necessary, give emergency care only

Syphilis. Absolute effectiveness of therapy for syphilis cannot be determined except by conversion of the positive STS to negative. The time required for this conversion varies from a few months to over a year; therefore patients who are currently being treated or who have a positive STS following treatment should be treated as potentially infectious until consultation with the physician. Patients determined to be infectious or potentially infectious should receive only emergency care until they are found to be noninfectious. The oral lesions of primary and secondary syphilis are infectious and should require only palliative care. The gumma is noninfectious.

Genital herpes. The localized, uncomplicated genital herpes infection poses little or no problem for the dentist; however, because of the possibility of autoinoculation by the patient to the oral cavity or adjacent skin, it is advisable to wear disposable gloves when providing dental treatment during this stage. Also, in a severe primary infection, a consultation with the physician is advisable.

TABLE 12-3. Dental management of patient with history of genital herpes

---

1. Patient currently receiving treatment for genital herpes
    a. With severe primary infection, consult with physician
    b. Provide required dental care
    c. Wear disposable gloves
    d. Be sure to examine for autoinoculated oral or skin lesions
2. Patient with past history of genital herpes
    a. Approach with caution; obtain good history of disease, its treatment, and progress
    b. Perform good examination of soft tissues
    c. If free of lesions, provide routine dental care
3. Patient with signs, symptoms, or oral lesions suggestive of herpes
    a. Attempt to relate past and present history to appearance of oral herpetic lesions
    b. Postpone elective dental care until lesions have disappeared
    c. For severe primary oral infection, consider referral to physician

---

PATIENTS WITH PAST HISTORY OF STD

Patients with a past history of an STD should be approached with a measure of caution, because they have been identified as being in a high-risk group for a disease. This can include risk from the inadequate treatment of the previous infection or from a new infection. Special effort should be made in the examination of oral, pharyngeal, and perioral tissues for unexplained lesions. Also, a thorough review of systems may reveal urogenital symptomatology of an STD. Patients with a history of gonorrhea should have produced a negative culture at the termination of their therapy. Patients treated for syphilis should receive periodic STS for 1 year to monitor their conversion from positive to negative. In the absence of follow-up medical supervision for these disorders, consultation and referral to a physician should be considered. An alternative for a history of syphilis would be for the dentist to order STS. If results of examination or history give reason for suspicion, dental treatment should be delayed and the patient referred to a physician.

PATIENTS WITH SIGNS, SYMPTOMS, OR ORAL LESIONS SUGGESTIVE OF STD

Patients who have symptoms or signs suggestive of an STD or who have unexplained oral or pharyngeal lesions should be viewed with suspicion. The index of suspicion should be even higher if the patient is between 15 and 24 years of age, male, an urban dweller, single, and from a lower socioeconomic group. Any patient who has these findings should be advised to seek medical care, and dental treatment should be postponed. An alternative procedure, if syphilis is suspected, would be to order STS before referral. Herpetic lesions in or around the oral cavity, combined with a history of past involvement, should be recognizable. Patients with acute oral herpes lesions should not receive routine dental care but emergency care only. For a severe primary oral infection, the patient may require referral to a physician.

Drug administration

There are no adverse interactions between the usual antibiotics used to treat STDs and the drugs commonly used in dentistry. No drugs are contraindicated.

Treatment planning modifications

No modifications in the treatment plan are required for these patients.

Oral complications

GONORRHEA

As previously mentioned, the presentation of oral gonorrhea is varied and may range from slight erythema to severe ulceration with a pseudomembranous coating. The patient may be essentially asymptomatic or may be incapacitated, with limitations of oral function including eating, drinking, and talking.

The initial step in treatment is to ensure that the patient is under the care of a physician and receiving proper chemotherapy. After this, treatment of the oral lesions is symptomatic and may include frequent oral lavage with a bland mouthwash, such as sodium bicarbonate in water or 3% peroxide in water. This can be followed by topical application of Orabase, viscous lidocaine (Xylocaine), or promethazine hydrochloride syrup. These preparations afford some temporary pain relief. The patient should be assured that the lesions will regress as the systemic infection resolves.

SYPHILIS

Syphilitic chancres and mucous patches are usually painless unless they become secondarily infected. These lesions are infectious. They regress spontaneously with or without antibiotic therapy, although chemotherapy is required to eradicate the systemic infection. As with gonorrhea, any oral treatment rendered is essentially symptomatic. The gumma is a painless lesion, but it may also become secondarily infected. It is noninfectious. Interstitial glossitis is viewed as a premalignant lesion.

GENITAL HERPES

Since it is impossible to differentiate clinically between lesions caused by HSV-1 and HSV-2, all herpetic lesions of the oral cavity should be treated in the same way. All oral and perioral herpetic lesions should be considered infectious, regardless

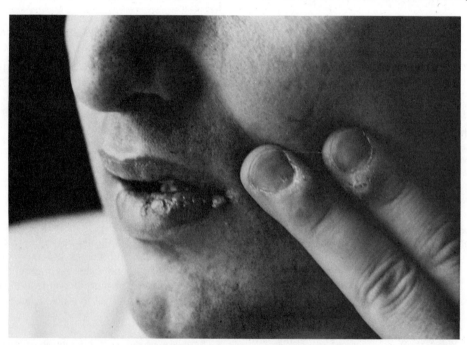

FIG. 12-12. Herpes simplex type I infection of nailbeds (herpetic whitlow, herpetic paronychia) as result of autoinoculation. (Courtesy R.C. Noble, M.D., Lexington, Ky.)

of stage (papular, vesicular, ulcerative, or crusted). It is recommended that elective dental treatment be delayed until the herpetic lesion is completely healed. This is because of the dangers of autoinoculation to a new site on the patient, of infection to the dentist (i.e., herpetic paronychia), and of aerosol or droplet inoculation of the conjunctiva of either patient or dental personnel. If dental treatment does become necessary, the dentist should wear disposable gloves and protective eyeglasses.

A problem of particular concern to dentists is herpetic infection of the nail beds contracted by finger contact with a herpetic lesion of the lip or oral cavity of a patient (Fig. 12-12). The infection is called herpetic whitlow or herpetic paronychia and is a serious, debilitating problem. It is a well-documented entity that is probably more common than realized.[21,29,34]

Emergency dental care

In some instances it may be necessary to provide emergency care to a patient who has recently been diagnosed as having or is suspected of having an STD. If analgesics will not suffice, treatment should be accomplished by carrying out the recommendations in Table 12-4.

TABLE 12-4. Emergency dental care for patient with STD

Consult with physician before treatment
Use strict aseptic procedure
Use gloves and mask
Use rubber dam when possible
Scrub and sterilize all equipment after use
Do only acutely required work

REFERENCES

1. Annual Summary 1980, Morbidity and Mortality Weekly Report **29:**34, 78, 1981.
2. Burns, J.C.: Diagnostic methods for herpes simplex infection: a review, Oral Surg. **50:**346-349, 1980.
3. Chapel, T.A.: The signs and symptoms of secondary syphilis, Sex. Transm. Dis. **7:**161-164, 1980.
4. Chue, P.W.Y.: Gonococcal arthritis of the temporomandibular joint, Oral Surg. **39:**572-577, 1975.
5. Chue, P.W.Y.: Gonorrhea: its natural history, oral manifestations, diagnosis, treatment and prevention, J. Am. Dent. Assoc. **90:**1297-1301, 1975.

6. Embil, J.A., et al.: Concurrent oral and genital infection with an identical strain of herpes simplex virus type 1, Sex. Transm. Dis. **8:**70-72, 1981.
7. Feldman, Y.M., and Nikitas, J.A.: Pharyngeal gonorrhea, N.Y. State J. Med. **80:**957-959, 1980.
8. Fife, K.H.: Primary and recurrent concomitant genital infection with herpes simplex virus types 1 and 2, J. Infect. Dis. **147:**163, 1983.
9. Fiumara, N.J.: Venereal diseases of the oral cavity, J. Oral Med. **31:**36-40, 1976.
10. Fiumara, N.J., Grande, D.J., and Giunta, J.L.: Papular secondary syphilis of the tongue, Oral Surg. **45:**540-542, 1978.
11. Genital herpes infection—United States, 1966-1979, Morbidity and Mortality Weekly Report **31:**137, 1982.
12. Golden, A.: Pathology: understanding human disease, Baltimore, 1982, The Williams & Wilkins Co., pp. 44-45.
13. Hart, G., and Rein, M.: Gonococcal infection. In Top, F.H., and Wehrle, P.F., editors: Communicable and infectious diseases, St. Louis, 1976, The C.V. Mosby Co., pp. 299-310.
14. Holmes, K.K.: Gonococcal infections and syphilis. In Isselbacher, K.J., et al., editors: Harrison's principles of internal medicine, ed. 9, New York, 1980, McGraw-Hill Book Co., pp. 624-629.
15. Jamsky, R.J., and Christen, A.G.: Oral gonococcal infections: report of two cases, Oral Surg. **53:**358-362, 1982.
16. Karus, S.J.: Incidence and therapy of gonococcal pharyngitis, Sex. Transm. Dis. **6:**143-147, 1979.
17. Kohn, S.R., Shaffer, J.F., and Chomenko, A.G.: Primary gonococcal stomatitis, JAMA **219:**86, 1972.
18. Krugman, S., et al.: Infectious diseases of children and adults, ed. 6, St. Louis, 1977, The C.V. Mosby Co., pp. 83-89.
19. Lerner, A.M.: Infections with herpes simplex virus. In Isselbacher, K.J., et al., editors: Harrison's principles of internal medicine, ed. 9, New York, 1980, McGraw-Hill Book Co., pp. 847-851.
20. Merchant, H.W., and Schuster, G.S.: Oral gonococcal infection, J. Am. Dent. Assoc. **95:**807-809, 1977.
21. Miller, J.B.: Herpes simplex virus infection of the fingers of a dentist, J. Dent. Child. **43:**99-102, 1976.
22. Morse, S.A.: Neisseria. In Braude, A.I., editor: Medical microbiology and infectious diseases, Philadelphia, 1981, W.B. Saunders Co., pp. 326-333.
23. Musher, D.M.: Syphilis of the genital tract. In Braude, A.I., editor: Medical microbiology and infectious diseases, Philadelphia, 1981, W.B. Saunders Co., pp. 1210-1217.
24. Nahmias, A.J., et al.: The human herpesviruses: an interdisciplinary approach, New York, 1980, Elsevier North-Holland, Inc.
25. Nahmias, A.J., and Roizman, B.: Infection with herpes-simplex viruses 1 and 2. III, N. Engl. J. Med. **289:**781-789, 1973.
26. Noble, R.C.: Personal communication, Aug. 1981.
27. Pagano, J.S., and Lemon, S.M.: The herpesviruses. In Braude, A.I., editor: Medical microbiology and infectious

diseases, Philadelphia, 1981, W.B. Saunders Co., pp. 541-549.

28. Robbins, S.L., and Cotran, R.S.: Pathologic basis of disease, Philadelphia, 1979, W.B. Saunders Co., p. 440.
29. Rowe, N.H., Heine, C.S., and Kowalski, C.J.: Herpetic whitlow: an occupational disease of practicing dentists, J. Am. Dent. Assoc. **105:**471-473, 1982.
30. Rudolph, A.H.: Syphilis. In Top, F.H., and Wehrle, P.F., editors: Communicable and infectious diseases, St. Louis, 1976, The C.V. Mosby Co., pp. 672-687.
31. Schmidt, H., et al.: Gonococcal stomatitis, Acta Derm. Venereol. **41:**324-327, 1961.
32. Sexually transmitted diseases treatment guidelines, 1982, Morbidity and Mortality Weekly Report Supplement **31:** 375, 1982.
33. Two dosage forms of acyclovir available, FDA Drug Bull. **13:**5, 1983.
34. Watkinson, A.C.: Primary herpes simplex in a dentist, Br. Dent. J. **153:**190-191, 1982.

13

ARTHRITIS AND
JOINT PROSTHESES

Arthritis is a nonspecific term that denotes inflammation of the joints but does not indicate type of inflammation or cause. It is commonly used interchangeably with the term *rheumatism;* however, this is a nonclinical lay term used to describe unexplained aches, pains, and stiffness in the joints and muscles and therefore is not a particularly helpful term. However, *rheumatic disease* is accepted terminology descriptive of a group of related disorders. As a group, the rheumatic diseases all have inflammation of connective tissue as a common denominator. Included within this group of related diseases are rheumatoid arthritis, degenerative joint disease (osteoarthritis), juvenile rheumatoid arthritis, ankylosing spondylitis, gout, psoriatic arthritis, systemic lupus erythematosus, and rheumatic fever. Although this is a large group of important diseases, this discussion will be limited for illustrative purposes to rheumatoid arthritis, because it is one of the more severe forms of arthritis. Recommendations for patients with rheumatoid arthritis would apply in varying degrees to patients with other forms of arthritis as well.

Rheumatoid arthritis

GENERAL DESCRIPTION

Rheumatoid arthritis is one of the most serious forms of arthritis and can result in severe crippling and disability. It is characterized by symmetric inflammation of peripheral joints with a preference for the wrists and hands. In addition, there are various systemic manifestations that include pulmonary, hematologic, neurologic, and cardiovascular abnormalities.

Incidence and epidemiology

According to estimates made in 1975 by the Arthritis Foundation[1], there are 20,000,000 Americans who suffer with some form of severe arthritis. Of these, some 5,000,000 have rheumatoid arthritis. It is obvious that this is a disease of significant magnitude.

In terms of economic impact, all forms of arthritis are estimated to cost directly and indirectly well in excess of $13 billion per year. In addition, there are approximately 15 million workdays lost per year to arthritis.[1]

Rheumatoid arthritis can appear at any age but usually develops between the ages of 30 and 60 years. It is primarily a disease of women, affecting them three times more commonly than it does men.[9]

Etiology

The exact cause of rheumatoid arthritis is unknown; however, there are a number of possible causative or contributing factors. Chief among these is infection, either bacterial or viral.[3,10] There is also evidence of biochemical and physiologic abnormalities in many patients. One of the most active areas of research at present is that of immunologic disorders, and this field implicates rheumatoid arthritis as an autoimmune disease. In addition, it appears that in many patients there is a genetic predisposition to the disease. Stress also may play a contributing role. It would appear at present that the most likely cause of rheumatoid arthritis is the exposure of individuals who have a particular genetic constitution to an infectious agent.[10] Of importance is the fact that there is no evidence that a nutritional deficiency leads to rheumatoid arthritis or that certain foods or vitamins affect its outcome.[3]

Pathophysiology

In rheumatoid arthritis primary changes occur in the synovium, which is the inner lining of the joint capsule. There is edema of the synovium, followed by thickening and folding. This excessive tissue is called pannus. There is a marked infiltration of lymphocytes and plasma cells into the capsule. Gradually, granulation tissue covers articular sur-

faces and destroys them through enzymatic activity (Fig. 13-1). The process also extends to the capsule and ligaments. New bone or fibrous tissue is then deposited, and this results in fusion or loss of mobility.[3,4,10]

A likely sequence of events begins with a synovitis, perhaps of viral origin, that stimulates immunoglobulin G (IgG) antibodies. These antibodies form antigenic aggregates in the joint space and result in production of rheumatoid factor. Rheumatoid factor then complexes with IgG complement and produces an inflammatory reaction that injures the joint space.[4]

An associated finding in 20% to 25% of patients with rheumatoid arthritis is subcutaneous nodules, usually found around the elbow.[3,4] These nodules are thought to arise from the same antigen-antibody complexing that is found in the joint.[4] A vasculitis confined to small- to medium-sized vessels also may occur in rheumatoid arthritis and is probably caused by the same complexing.[3]

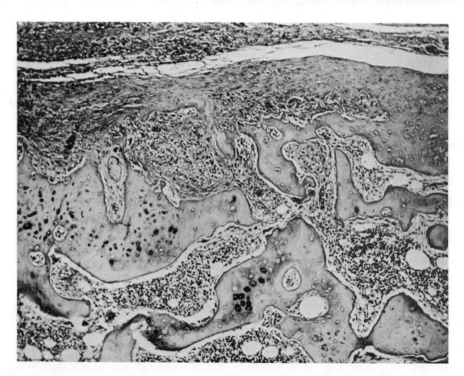

FIG. 13-1. Photomicrograph of joint space and articular surface of joint involved with rheumatoid arthritis. (Courtesy A. Golden, M.D., Lexington, Ky.)

Sequelae and complications

The course and severity of rheumatoid arthritis are unpredictable but characterized by remissions and exacerbations. Approximately 10% to 20% of patients will undergo permanent remission of disease while another 10% will experience relentless crippling, leading to nearly complete disability.[3] For the majority of patients, however, the disease can be successfully controlled or modified to allow a normal or nearly normal life.

Many complications may accompany rheumatoid arthritis. Included among these are temporomandibular joint involvement, digital gangrene, skin ulcers, keratoconjunctivitis sicca (Sjögren's syndrome), pulmonary interstitial fibrosis, pericarditis, splenomegaly, amyloidosis, anemia, neutropenia, and thrombocytopenia.[3]

CLINICAL PRESENTATION
Signs and symptoms

The usual presentation of rheumatoid arthritis is a process with an onset that is gradual and subtle. It is commonly preceded by a prodromal phase of fatigue and weakness with joint and muscle achiness. Characteristically, these symptoms come and go over a period of time. Then painful joint swelling, especially of the hands and feet, occurs in several joints and progresses to other joints in a

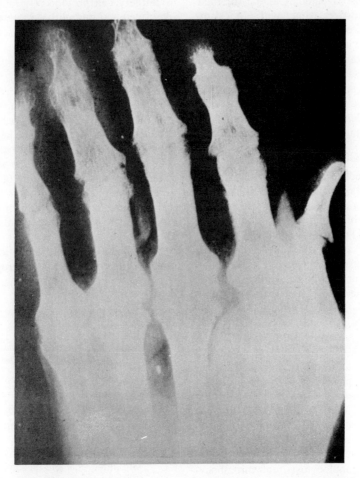

FIG. 13-2. Typical radiographic appearance of hand of patient with rheumatoid arthritis. (Courtesy A. Golden, M.D., Lexington, Ky.)

symmetric fashion. The joint involvement persists and progresses to immobility, contractures, subluxation, deviation, and other deformities to varying degrees (Fig. 13-2). Morning stiffness in affected joints is characteristic. The joints most commonly affected are fingers, wrists, feet, ankles, knees, and elbows. The temporomandibular joint is also affected in many individuals.[3,10]

Rheumatoid nodules are seen in 20% to 25% of patients with rheumatoid arthritis and are most commonly found around the elbows, fingers, back of the head, and sacrum.[3,4,10]

Laboratory findings

No laboratory test is pathognomonic for rheumatoid arthritis; however, along with clinical examination and radiographs, laboratory tests are confirmatory of the diagnosis.

Some of the more common test results obtained include an increased erythrocyte sedimentation rate, anemia, and a positive rheumatoid factor.[10] In patients with Felty's syndrome (a triad of rheumatoid arthritis, splenomegaly and neutropenia) thrombocytopenia may also be demonstrated.[3]

MEDICAL MANAGEMENT

Conservative medical management of rheumatoid arthritis consists of patient education, rest, and physical therapy, in addition to drug therapy.

The cornerstone of drug therapy continues to be aspirin, usually in high doses. A common dose is 3 to 6 g (9 to 18 5-grain aspirin tablets) daily.[3] Patients who cannot take aspirin may be given one of the many new nonsteroidal antiinflammatory (NSA) drugs. Some of the more commonly prescribed drugs in this group are ibuprofen (Motrin), naproxen (Naprosyn), tolmetin sodium (Tolectin), sylindac (Clinoril), and diflunisal (Dolobid). Both aspirin and the NSA drugs can cause a qualitative platelet defect that can result in a bleeding diathesis, especially after prolonged use in high doses.

Gold salts are beneficial when used to treat rheumatoid arthritis and suppress the disease in some patients. The medication is given intramuscularly. Gold salts can have serious side effects, including dermatitis, stomatitis, bone marrow suppression, aplastic anemia, agranulocytosis, and thrombocytopenia.[3,10]

Chloroquine and penicillamine are two additional drugs that may be prescribed for treatment, but both are limited by side effects. Chloroquine use can result in blindness, and penicillamine can cause bone marrow suppression and kidney damage.

When the just-described drugs are not adequate for control of the disease, corticosteroids may be used. They are usually effective in controlling symptoms; however, their use is limited by side effects, especially adrenal suppression.

A number of cytotoxic drugs, such as azathioprine and methotrexate, are being investigated for chemotherapy of rheumatoid arthritis. However, because of their severe side effects, these drugs are very limited in use.

Surgery can provide restoration of function to deformed and immobilized joints and may include the total replacement of a diseased joint with a prosthesis.

DENTAL MANAGEMENT
Medical considerations (see Table 13-1)

Since patients may have multiple joint involvement with varying degrees of pain and immobility, dental appointments should be kept as short as possible, and the patient should be allowed to make frequent position changes. The patient may also be more comfortable in a sitting or semisupine position as opposed to a completely supine one. Physical supports, such as a pillow or rolled towel, may be needed to provide support for deformed limbs or joints.

The most significant complications associated with rheumatoid arthritis are drug related. Aspirin

TABLE 13-1. Dental management of patient with rheumatoid arthritis

1. Short appointments
2. Ensure physical comfort
   a. Frequent position changes
   b. Most comfortable chair position
   c. Physical supports as needed
3. Management of drug complications
   a. Aspirin/NSA drugs—pretreatment bleeding time
   b. Gold salts/penicillamine—complete blood count with differential and bleeding time
   c. Corticosteroids—if recent use of longer than 1 month, consult physician and plan steroid supplement for treatment (see Chapter 16)

and NSA drugs can cause decreased platelet adhesiveness and result in abnormal bleeding. Because of this, patients taking these drugs should have a pretreatment bleeding time performed. Abnormal results should be discussed with the patient's physician. Even if the bleeding time is moderately prolonged (6 to 20 minutes), patients can usually be treated, as long as curettage or surgery is performed conservatively and in small segments.

Patients taking gold salts or penicillamine are susceptible to bone marrow suppression that results in anemia, agranulocytosis, and thrombocytopenia. As a rule, these patients should be followed closely by their physician to detect this problem. If a patient has not had recent laboratory tests, it is advisable to order a complete blood count with a differential and a bleeding time. Abnormal results should be discussed with the physician.

If corticosteroids are used for prolonged periods, the potential problem of adrenal suppression always exists. Management of this problem is discussed in Chapter 16.

Treatment planning modifications

Treatment planning modifications are dictated by the patient's physical disabilities. A patient with marked disability or limited jaw function caused by temporomandibular joint involvement should not be subjected to prolonged, extensive treatment, such as complicated crown and bridge procedures. If replacement of missing teeth is desired, consideration should be given to a removable prosthesis because of the decreased chair time needed for preparation and the easy cleansability of the appliance. If a fixed prosthesis is elected, cleansability must be a significant factor in design.

The disabled patient may have significant difficulty cleaning his teeth. Cleaning aids such as floss holders, toothpicks, irrigating devices, and mechanical toothbrushes may be recommended. Manual toothbrushes can be modified by placing acrylic or a rubber ball on the handle to improve the grip.

It should be remembered that rheumatoid arthritis is a progressive disease that can ultimately lead to severe disability and crippling, which can make providing dental care difficult. Therefore the dentist should be aggressive in providing good preventive care and should attempt to identify and treat or eliminate potential problems.

Oral complications

The major maxillofacial complication of rheumatoid arthritis is temporomandibular joint involvement leading to fibrosis, adhesions, and ankylosis (Fig. 13-3). This problem can be surgically corrected with excellent results.

Another significant oral complication is a sto-

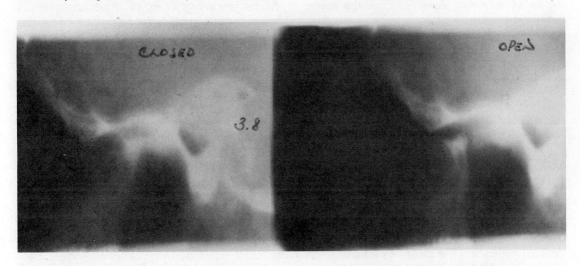

FIG. 13-3. Lateral laminograms of patient with rheumatoid arthritis demonstrating osseous changes of temporomandibular joints. (Courtesy L.R. Bean, D.D.S., Lexington, Ky.)

matitis that may be seen with the administration of gold salts. This is an indication of drug toxicity and should be reported to the physician. Treatment is palliative.

Emergency dental care

No special approaches or cautions are necessary for emergency dental care. The standard recommendations should be followed.

Joint prostheses

In the patient with arthritis, the goal of treatment is to prevent deformity and loss of function. Unfortunately, this is not always possible, and function is lost. At this point, surgical correction may become necessary for a small percentage of patients. Of the various surgical procedures, one that presents potential problems for the dentist is the replacement of a diseased joint with a prosthesis.

There are other indications for a joint prosthesis besides arthritis, including nonunion of a fracture, avascular necrosis of the bone of the femoral head, and, occasionally, acute trauma. Most experience to date has been with total hip replacement and knee replacement, although other joints have been replaced, including shoulders, elbows, wrists, and metacarpophalangeal joints (Fig. 13-4). It is estimated that more than 80,000 total hip prostheses are placed annually.[5] From this figure, it is evident that these patients will be among those seen by the dental practitioner.

One of the biggest problems that faces the recipient of a prosthetic joint is that of infection around the prosthesis. If unchecked, the infection can result in a need for replacement of the unit or total loss of the joint. It is evident that this complication could have catastrophic effects physically, emotionally, and economically. Current estimates of the rate of prosthesis infection place the figure at 1.3%.[7]

The infection of the prosthesis may occur either early or late, the early infection (within 3 months of surgery) usually being related to the surgery itself. The source of late infection (more than 3 months after surgery) is not as clear; however, most authorities feel it is caused by a latent infection resulting from the original surgery, hematogenous spread from distant infection, or from tran-

sient bacteremias secondary to trauma or surgical, dental, or urinary tract procedures.[7]

Dental procedures or manipulations as a source of late infection of prostheses have been variably implicated; however, the true incidence of infection from transient bacteremia is unknown. On an experimental basis, Blomgren[2] has demonstrated in rabbits that transient bacteremias can infect joint replacements. From a clinical standpoint, however, the association is not as clear. Peterson[8] reviewed 90 cases of prosthetic joint infection secondary to hematogenous spread of bacteria and concluded that none could be clearly related to transient bacteremia from dental treatment. There were, however, cases associated with established infections from the teeth and salivary glands.

Jacobsen and Murray[6] reviewed 33 cases of prosthetic joint infection out of 1,855 hip prosthesis replacements and found only one case that could be associated with dental treatment; however, the treatment was necessitated by a dental abscess that required prolonged care. The incidence of dentally related infection of prosthetic joints in this series was 0.05%. These authors further found that, based on the type of infecting organisms in their series, erythromycin, clindamycin, or a penicillinase-resistant penicillin would be the drug of choice for prophylaxis.

After an extensive review of the literature and analysis of the problem, Little[7] concluded that the current practice of using prophylactic antibiotics before and after most dental procedures on patients with prosthetic joints is questionable. He bases this skepticism primarily on the apparently low risk of occurrence (0.04% to 0.05%) and secondarily on the fact that the complications of antibiotic exposure may well outweigh any benefits of protection against an extremely low risk.

It seems obvious that additional investigation of this question is required to establish risk and, if prophylaxis is determined to be necessary, to establish a uniform regimen of antibiotic prophylaxis. Presently, since little uniformity of opinion exists on this question, each patient must be managed individually in consultation with the orthopedic surgeon, keeping in mind risk, dental condition, and antibiotic sensitivity of the most common infecting organisms.

The overall goal of dental treatment of these patients should be the maintenance of a disease-

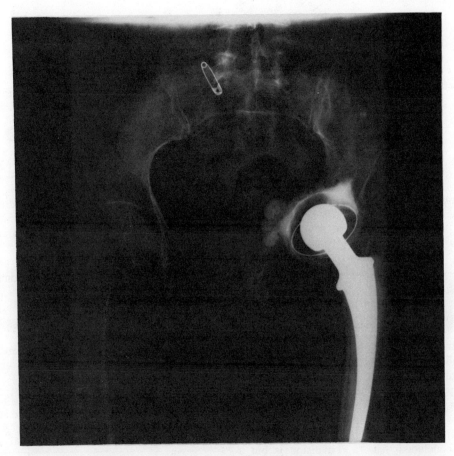

FIG. 13-4. Radiograph of prosthetic hip joint. (Safety pin was on patient's clothing.)

free oral cavity. Preventive measures should be aggressive and may require frequent recall appointments to reinforce home-care procedures. Any acute infections that may arise should be managed immediately and aggressively with antibiotics and medical consultation.

REFERENCES

1. The Arthritis Foundation: Arthritis: the basic facts, Atlanta, 1976, The Foundation.
2. Blomgren, G.: Hematogenous infection of total joint replacement: an experimental study in the rabbit, Acta. Orthop. Scand. (Suppl.) **187:**1-64, 1981.
3. Gilliland, B.C., and Mannik, M.: Rheumatoid arthritis. In Isselbacher, K.J., et al., editors: Harrison's principles of internal medicine, ed. 9, New York, 1980, McGraw-Hill Book Co., pp. 1872-1880.
4. Golden, A.: Pathology: understanding human disease, Baltimore, 1982, The Williams & Wilkins Co., pp. 435-436.
5. Hori, R.Y.: The number of total joint replacements in the United States, Clin. Orthop. **132:**46-52, 1978.
6. Jacobsen, P.L., and Murray, W.: Prophylactic coverage of dental patients with artificial joints: a retrospective analysis of thirty-three infections in hip prostheses, Oral Surg. **50:** 130-133, 1980.
7. Little, J.W.: The need for antibiotic coverage for dental treatment of patients with joint replacements, Oral Surg. **55:**20-23, 1983.
8. Peterson, L.J.: Prosthetic joint infection and dental procedures, J. Am. Dent. Assoc. **101:** 598-600, 1980.
9. Scott, J.T.: Arthritis and rheumatism: the facts, New York, 1980, Oxford University Press, Inc.
10. Znaifler, N.J.: Etiology and pathogenesis of rheumatoid arthritis. In McCarty, D.J., editor: Arthritis and allied conditions, ed. 9, Philadelphia, 1979, Lea & Febiger, pp. 417-428.

14

NEUROLOGIC DISORDERS

Although there is a myriad of neurologic diseases, two of the more common and significant disorders, epilepsy and stroke, will be discussed in this chapter.

Epilepsy

Epilepsy is an emotionally charged term that historically has had rather negative connotations. Many times a social stigma was attached to any person who was an "epileptic," and that person was shunned by society. Fortunately, there is better appreciation and understanding of the disorder today, although much confusion still exists, especially regarding terminology.

In the 1800s Hughlings Jackson's discourse on epilepsy concluded that "a convulsion is but a symptom, and implies only that there is an occasional, an excessive and a disorderly discharge of nerve tissue." This has proven to be accurate; however, it is too limited. This is because there are many other forms of epilepsy (or seizures) besides the classic convulsion, many of which are focal, limited, and nonconvulsive. Therefore to redefine an expanded group of related seizure disorders, Sutherland and Eadie[11] have proposed the following definition:

Epilepsy should be regarded as a symptom due to excessive temporary neuronal discharging which results from intracranial or extracranial causes: epilepsy is characterized by discrete episodes, which tend to be recurrent, in which there is a disturbance of movement, sensation, behavior, perception and/or consciousness.

The cause of epilepsy is known in many patients. Possible causes include trauma, intracranial neoplasm, hypoglycemia, drug withdrawal, and febrile illnesses. However, many patients have epilepsy for which there is no known cause, and this is termed *idiopathic epilepsy*.

Further help in understanding the spectrum of epilepsy is afforded by the International League Against Epilepsy[2], which provided a revised classification of epilepsy in 1981 (Table 14-1). This classification is based on clinical behavior and electroencephalographic changes.

From the foregoing it is clear that there are many forms of epilepsy or seizures. However, the dis-

---

TABLE 14-1. Classification of epileptic seizures based on clinical behavior and electroencephalographic phenomena

Partial seizures (focal, local)

Simple partial seizures
Complex partial seizures
Partial seizures evolving to generalized tonic-clonic convulsion

Generalized seizures (convulsive or nonconvulsive)

Absence seizures (petit mal)
Atypical absence seizures
Myoclonic seizures
Clonic seizures
Tonic-clonic seizures (grand mal)
Tonic seizures
Atonic seizures
Unclassified epileptic seizures

From Commission on Classification and Terminology of the International League Against Epilepsy: Proposal for revised clinical and electroencephalographic classification of epileptic seizures, Epilepsia 22:489-501, 1981.

cussion in this chapter will be limited to the generalized tonic-clonic seizures (idiopathic grand mal seizures), because these represent the most common and severe form of generalized epilepsy that the dentist will encounter.

GENERAL DESCRIPTION
Etiology and incidence

It is estimated that 10,000,000 people in the United States have consulted with a physician at some time in their lives because of a seizure and that about 1,000,000 presently suffer from recurrent seizures.[10] The overall incidence of idiopathic epilepsy is between 0.3% and 0.7% per year, with a prevalence rate of 2%. In the United States, the approximate range of new cases is from 23,000 to 147,000 per year.[8]

The prevalence rate is highest in childhood, because idiopathic epilepsy tends to express itself with maximum frequency in those between the ages of 2 and 5 years and around the age of puberty.[10]

Although the underlying cause of idiopathic generalized epilepsy is unknown, seizures can sometimes be evoked by a specific stimulus. Approximately 1 out of 15 patients reports that his seizures follow exposure to a specific circumstance, such as flickering lights, monotonous sounds, music, or a loud noise.[10] Of interest are reports of epileptic seizures in youngsters who are exposed to flickering lights and geometric patterns while playing video games.[2]

Pathophysiology

The basic pathophysiologic event underlying an epileptic seizure is an excessive focal neuronal discharge that spreads to thalamic and brainstem nuclei.[11] The cause of this abnormal electrical activity is not precisely known; however, a number of theories have been proposed as explanations. These include altered neuronal membrane potentials, altered synaptic transmission, diminution of inhibitory neurons, increased neuronal excitability, and decreased electrical threshold for epileptic activity.[10,11]

A significant feature is that no specific type of brain lesion is absolutely correlated with epileptic seizures. That is, the same lesion in the same location of the brain may be epileptogenic in one patient and not in another. In fact in many cases there is no identifiable lesion at all. This would seem to suggest an abnormality on a biochemical level.

Sequelae and complications

Approximately 50% of patients with epilepsy will achieve complete to 90% control over their seizures, while an additional 35% will achieve control adequate to maintain a normal life.[8] The remaining 15% are not able to maintain a normal life-style.

A significant problem with epileptic patients is one of compliance, that is, making sure that patients take their anticonvulsant medication as directed.[14] This problem is common to many chronic disorders, such as hypertension, because the patients may have to take medication for the rest of their lives even though they may remain asymptomatic.

Another common problem relating to anticonvulsant drugs is toxicity. Common examples of this are phenytoin-induced ataxia and phenobarbital-induced drowsiness.[14] If a patient has frequent, severe seizures there may also be altered mental function resulting in dullness, confusion, or argumentativeness. Mental deterioration, fortunately, is a rare occurrence, and if it does occur may be indicative of a disorder other than epilepsy.[10]

A common complication associated with phenytoin is gingival hyperplasia. This may occur in varying degrees and may become extensive enough to require surgical reduction. It is most common in children and adolescents. (See "Oral Complications," p. 188.)

The most serious acute complication of epilepsy is the occurrence of repeated seizures over a short time. This is called status epilepticus, and it constitutes a medical emergency. Patients may become seriously hypoxic and acidotic during this occurrence and may suffer permanent brain damage or death.

CLINICAL PRESENTATION
Signs and symptoms

The clinical manifestations of a grand mal seizure are classic and well known. The seizure is initiated by a sudden cry, caused by spasm of the diaphragmatic muscles. Then loss of consciousness with a fall to the ground occurs. The tonic phase consists of generalized muscle rigidity, followed by clonic activity that consists of uncoordinated beating and movement of the limbs and head. Incontinence of urine or feces may occur. All movement soon ceases, and the person becomes comatose. Then, generally within a few minutes, the person gradually regains consciousness with stupor, headache, and confusion. Once the seizure has begun, the jaws and teeth are clamped tightly and cannot be pried apart. Relaxation occurs with termination of the seizure.

Laboratory findings

Once the diagnosis of idiopathic epilepsy has been established, laboratory analysis is of little help. There are no characteristic findings associated with the disorder except for changes seen on the electroencephalogram (EEG). Each phase of the convulsion is associated with characteristic spike and wave patterns on the EEG. Even during intervals between seizures, many patients will demonstrate an abnormal EEG. It should be noted, however, that the EEG is not absolutely conclusive in making the diagnosis.

MEDICAL MANAGEMENT

The medical management of epilepsy is based on drug therapy, which is very successful in up to 85% of patients. Phenytoin (Dilantin) is the anticonvulsant drug that is still the most commonly used as a first line of treatment; however, there are several other drugs in common use. Table 14-2 is a list of the more common drugs in use today for the control of grand mal seizures. Attempts are made to use single-drug therapy to avoid adverse drug interactions and facilitate compliance. Unfortu-

nately, it is frequently necessary to use combination therapy.

In selected instances of complex partial epilepsy, neurosurgical intervention may be indicated; however, there is controversy regarding this technique.

DENTAL MANAGEMENT
Medical considerations (see Table 14-3)

The first step in the management of the epileptic dental patient is identification. This is best accomplished by the medical history and discussion with the patient or family members. Once an epileptic patient is identified, it is important to learn as much as possible about his seizure history. This includes type of seizures, age at onset, cause if

---

TABLE 14-3. Dental management of epileptic patient

1. Identification of epileptic patient by history
   a. Type of seizure
   b. Age at time of onset
   c. Cause of seizures (if known)
   d. Medications
   e. Frequency of physician visits (name and phone number)
   f. Degree of seizure control
   g. Frequency of seizures
   h. Date of last seizure
   i. Known precipitating factors
   j. History of seizure-related injuries
2. Well-controlled seizures pose no management problems—provide normal care
3. If questionable history or poorly controlled seizures, consult with physician before dental treatment—may require modification of medications
4. Be alert to adverse effects of anticonvulsants
   a. Drowsiness
   b. Slow mentation
   c. Dizziness
   d. Ataxis
   e. Gastrointestinal upset
   f. Allergic signs (rash, erythema multiforme)
5. Patients taking valproic acid may have bleeding tendencies because of platelet interference—order pretreatment bleeding time; if abnormal, consult with physician
6. Be prepared to manage grand mal seizure

TABLE 14-2. Drugs in common use for management of grand mal seizures

Generic name	Trade name	Usual adult dose
Phenytoin	Dilantin	200 to 500 mg
Phenobarbital	Luminal	60 to 200 mg
Primidone	Mysoline	750 to 1500 mg
Mephenytoin	Mesantoin	300 to 600 mg
Carbamazepine	Tegretol	1000 to 1200 mg
Valproic acid	Depakene	400 mg

known, current medications, frequency of physician visits, degree of seizure control, frequency of seizures, date of last seizure, and any known precipitating factors. In addition, a history of previous injuries associated with seizure and their treatment may be helpful.

Fortunately, most epileptic patients are able to attain good control of their seizures with anticonvulsants and are therefore able to receive normal, routine dental care. In some instances, however, the history may reveal a degree of seizure activity that suggests noncompliance or a severe seizure disorder that does not respond to anticonvulsants. For these patients, a consultation with the physician is indicated before any dental treatment is rendered. A patient with poorly controlled disease may require additional anticonvulsant or sedative medication, as directed by the physician.

Patients who are taking anticonvulsants may suffer from the toxic or side effects of these drugs, and the dentist must always be sensitive to these manifestations. Among the more common adverse effects are drowsiness, slow mentation, dizziness, ataxia, and gastrointestinal upset.[3,14] Occasionally, allergy to these drugs may be seen as a rash or an erythema multiforme–like reaction.

A recently introduced anticonvulsant, valproic acid (Depakene), is associated with spontaneous hemorrhage and multiple petechiae.[7] This bleeding tendency is apparently related to valproic acid's effect on platelet aggregation, which is similar to that of aspirin. Patients taking this medication should have their bleeding time checked before receiving dental treatment. If the bleeding time is elevated, consultation with the physician should be sought.

SEIZURE MANAGEMENT

In spite of all the appropriate preventive measures taken by the dentist and patient, there is always the possibility that an epileptic patient may have a grand mal seizure in the dental office. The dentist and staff should always anticipate this occurrence and be prepared to deal with it.

The primary task in seizure management is to protect the patient and try to keep him from injury. If the patient has a seizure while in the dental chair, no attempt should be made to move him to the floor. Instead, the chair should be placed in a supported supine position (Fig. 14-1), and the patient should, if possible, be turned to the side to control the airway and minimize aspiration of secretions. No attempt should be made to tightly restrain or hold the patient down. Passive restraint should be used to prevent injury from hitting nearby objects or from falling out of the chair.

One often is counselled to place a padded tongue blade between the teeth to prevent tongue biting. In reality, this is nearly an impossible task once the seizure has begun, and it may damage the teeth or mouth. Therefore this is not advised. An exception to this would be if the patient sensed a pending seizure and could cooperate. In this case, a padded tongue blade or folded towel may be placed between the teeth before they are clenched.

Seizures generally do not last more than a few minutes. After the seizure the patient will fall into a deep sleep from which he cannot be aroused. Then in a few minutes the patient will gradually regain consciousness, but he may be confused, disoriented, and embarrassed. Headache is a prominent feature of this period.

No further treatment should be attempted. Any injuries sustained, such as lacerations or fractures, should receive immediate attention (Fig. 14-2). In the event of avulsed or fractured teeth or fractured appliances, an attempt should be made to locate the tooth or fragments to rule out aspiration. A chest x-ray film may be required to locate missing fragments or teeth.

Treatment planning considerations

Because of the gingival hyperplasia associated with phenytoin, every effort should be made to bring the patient to an optimum level of oral hygiene and to keep him there. This may require frequent visits for monitoring progress.

If significant hyperplasia exists, surgical reduction will be necessary; however, this must be accompanied by an increased awareness of oral hygiene needs and a positive commitment by the patient to maintain oral cleanliness.

Missing teeth should be replaced if possible to prevent the tongue from being caught in the edentulous spaces during seizures, as commonly happens. As a general rule, fixed prostheses are more desirable than removable prostheses for epileptic patients. The removable prostheses are obviously

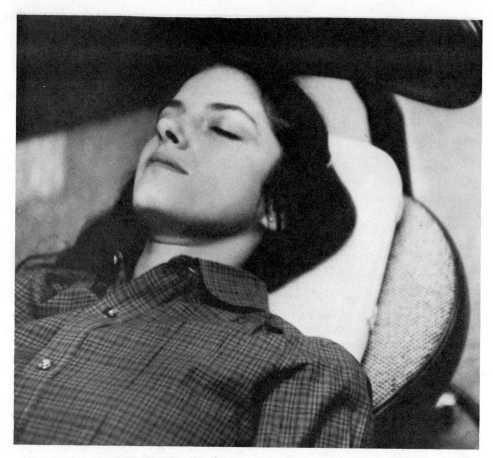

FIG. 14-1. Dental chair in supine position with back supported by operator or assistant's stool.

more easily dislodged during a seizure. For fixed prostheses, all-metal units should be considered when possible to minimize the chance of fracture. When placing anterior castings, the dentist may wish to consider using three-quarter crowns or retentive acrylic facings in lieu of porcelain to facilitate repair if fracture occurs.

Removable prostheses may be constructed for epileptic patients. Metallic palates and bases are preferable to all-acrylic ones. If acrylic is used, it should be reinforced with a wire mesh.

Oral complications

The most significant oral complication seen in epileptic patients is gingival hyperplasia associated with phenytoin (Fig. 14-3). The incidence of this problem in epileptics is difficult to ascertain be-

cause of the variable criteria used in studies; however, reported incidences range from 0% to 100%, with an average of approximately 42%.[6] There seems to be a greater tendency for youngsters to develop hyperplasia than adults. The anterior labia of both the maxillary and mandibular gingiva are most commonly and severely affected in most individuals.

Some disagreement exists in the literature as to the relationship between drug dosage and severity of hyperplasia, but the majority of studies do not support a statistically valid relationship between them.[6]

Another area of controversy is the effectiveness of oral hygiene in preventing hyperplasia; however, the preponderance of studies suggests that meticulous oral hygiene will prevent or at least

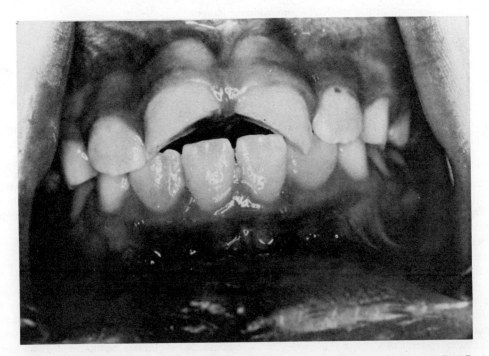

FIG. 14-2. Fractured teeth sustained during grand mal seizure. (Courtesy G. Ferretti, D.M.D., Lexington, Ky.)

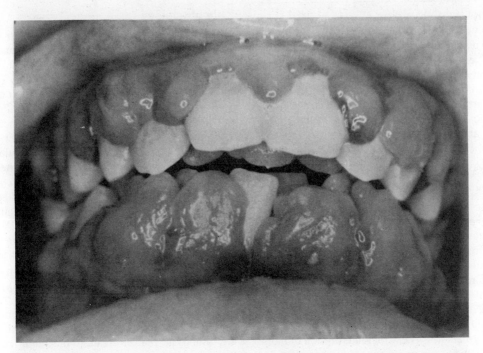

FIG. 14-3. Phenytoin (Dilantin)-induced gingival hyperplasia. (Courtesy H. Abrams, D.D.S., Lexington, Ky.)

decrease the severity of gingival hyperplasia.[6] Good home care must always be combined with removal of all irritants, such as overhanging restorations and calculus. Frequently, hyperplastic tissues will become large enough to interfere with function or appearance, and surgical reduction will become necessary.

Emergency dental care

Emergency dental care for a patient with well-controlled epilepsy should pose no specific problems, provided the patient is continuing normal medication.

Patients with poorly controlled epilepsy should be managed in consultation with their physician. It is advisable to start an IV drip (5% dextrose in water) to maintain an open line, and preoperative sedative doses of diazepam should be considered. If a seizure does occur, no drug therapy is indicated unless the seizure becomes prolonged or is repeated (status epilepticus).

Stroke

A stroke (cerebrovascular accident [CVA] or apoplexy) is a serious and often fatal event that is the end result of long-standing cerebrovascular disease. Even if the stroke is not fatal, the survivor is frequently severely debilitated in motor function, speech, or mentation. The scope and gravity of stroke are reflected in the facts that stroke is the third most common cause of death in the United States, and its annual estimated cost in terms of medical care and lost income is $9.5 billion.[12]

GENERAL DESCRIPTION
Etiology and incidence

Stroke is a generic term used to refer to the acute occurrence of signs and symptoms of neurologic deficit caused by cerebrovascular disease. A stroke results from a focal necrosis of brain tissue, which is caused by interruption of the cerebral blood supply. There are many forms of cerebrovascular disease that may result in a stroke, but the most common are atherosclerosis, hypertensive vascular disease, and cardiac pathosis (myocardial infarction, atrial fibrillation).[9] The actual interruption of blood supply is most commonly caused by thrombosis of

a cerebral vessel. This type accounts for 75% of strokes in the United States.[15] Other common causes of the interruption of cerebral blood flow include intracranial hemorrhage and cerebral embolism.

Although the incidence of stroke has declined by nearly one quarter over the past three decades, it still remains as one of the most significant health problems in the United States today.[4] Every year more than 400,000 Americans suffer a stroke. Of these, 40% die within 1 month, and two thirds of the survivors suffer some degree of permanent disability.[12]

Epidemiology

Epidemiologic investigations have identified susceptible individuals and associated risk factors that predispose to stroke. Included among these risk factors are the occurrence of transient ischemic attacks or a previous stroke, hypertension, cardiac abnormalities, atherosclerosis, diabetes mellitus, and elevated blood lipid levels. Other, less well-documented possible risk factors include cigarette smoking, inactivity, and stress.[13]

Pathophysiology

The pathologic changes associated with stroke are infarction, intracerebral hemorrhage, and subarachnoid hemorrhage.

Cerebral infarctions are most commonly caused by either atherosclerotic thrombi or emboli of cardiac origin (Fig. 14-4). The extent of an infarction is determined by a number of factors, including site of occlusion, size of the occluded vessel, duration of the occlusion, and collateral circulation.[5] Neurologic abnormalities depend on the artery involved and its area of supply.

The most common cause of intracerebral hemorrhage is hypertensive arteriosclerosis, which results in microaneurysms of the arterioles.[13] Rupture of these microaneurysms within brain tissue results in extravasation of blood, which displaces brain tissue and causes increased intracranial volume until the resulting tissue compression halts bleeding[9] (Fig. 14-5).

Subarachnoid hemorrhage is most commonly caused by rupture of saccular aneurysms that are found at the bifurcation of major cerebral arteries.

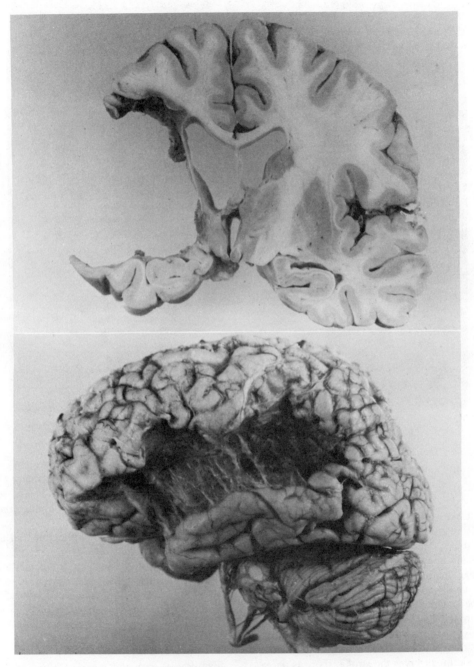

FIG. 14-4. Old cerebral infarction.

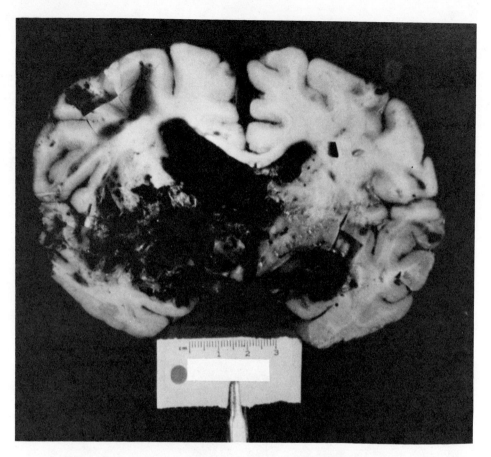

FIG. 14-5. Cerebral hemorrhage caused by hypertensive vascular disease.

Sequelae and complications

The most serious sequela of stroke is death, which, as previously noted, occurs in more than 40% of stroke victims in the first month. Mortality is directly related to type of stroke. The mortality is about 80% following an intracerebral hemorrhage of any appreciable size, about 50% following a subarachnoid hemorrhage, and about 30% if a major vessel is occluded by a thrombus.[13] It should be noted that death from a stroke is not usually immediate (sudden death) but rather occurs hours, days, or some weeks after the initial stroke episode.

If the victim survives the stroke, there is an excellent chance that there will be a significant neurologic deficit or disability of varying degree and duration. The deficit is directly dependent on size and location of the infarct or hemorrhage. Deficits include unilateral paralysis, numbness, sensory deficit, dysphasia, blindness, diplopia, dizziness, and dysarthria[9] (Fig. 14-6).

Return of function is unpredictable and usually takes place slowly, over several months. Even with improvement, patients are frequently left with some permanent residual problem, such as difficulty in walking, in using the hands or performing skilled acts, and in speaking.[13]

CLINICAL PRESENTATION
Signs and symptoms

Familiarity with the warning signs and symptoms of stroke can lead to appropriate action that may be lifesaving.

In many cases, strokes are preceded by "minor

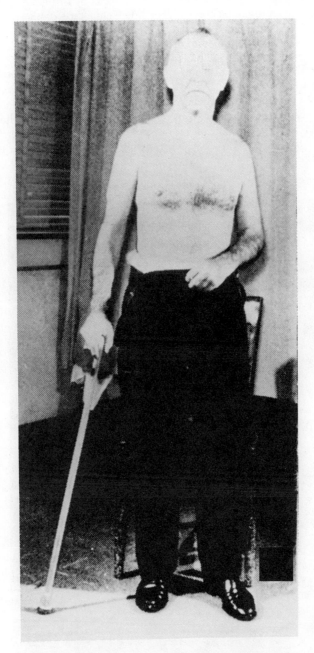

FIG. 14-6. Typical habitus of hemiplegia following stroke.

strokes'' called transient ischemic attacks (TIAs). These attacks reflect an ongoing thrombotic process and herald a severe cerebrovascular event. The attacks usually last less than 10 minutes and may present as dizziness, diplopia, hemiplegia, or speech disturbances. Most commonly a major stroke is preceded by one or two TIAs within a day to a week of the first attack.[9]

Warning signs of stroke include the following:

1. Sudden, temporary weakness or numbness of the face, arm, and leg on one side of the body

2. Temporary loss of speech or trouble in speaking or understanding speech

3. Temporary dimness or loss of vision, particularly in one eye

4. Unexplained dizziness, unsteadiness, or sudden falls

Although these are classic manifestations of stroke, they are not pathognomonic. A differential diagnosis would include diabetes mellitus, uremia, abscess, tumor, acute alcoholism, drug poisoning, and extradural hemorrhage.[13] History and physical examination serve to make the correct diagnosis.

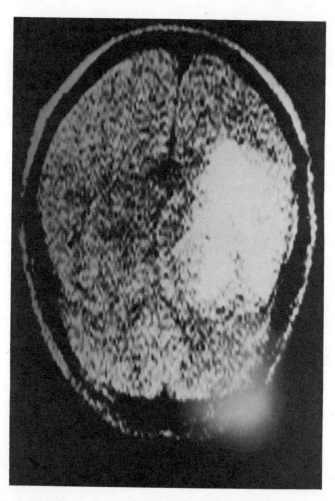

FIG. 14-7. NMR scan of brain, demonstrating edema. (Courtesy L.R. Bean, D.D.S., Lexington, Ky.)

Laboratory findings

Patients suspected of having had a stroke are usually submitted to a variety of laboratory tests, including urinalysis, blood sugar level, complete blood count, erythrocyte sedimentation rate, serologic tests for syphilis, blood cholesterol and lipid levels, chest x-ray examination, and electrocardiogram.[10,12] Variable abnormalities may exist in these test results, depending on type and severity of stroke as well as causative factors. A lumbar puncture may also be done to check for blood, protein, and altered cerebrospinal fluid pressure.[9]

Various neuroradiologic procedures may be performed, including arteriography and computed tomography (CT scan) and nuclear magnetic resonance (NMR) examination of the brain[10] (Fig. 14-7).

MEDICAL MANAGEMENT

The first aspect of stroke management is prevention. This is accomplished by identifying risk factors in individuals, such as hypertension, diabetes, atherosclerosis, and cigarette smoking, and then attempting to reduce or eliminate as many risk factors as possible.

If a patient has a stroke, treatment is generally in three parts. The primary task is sustaining life during the period immediately after the stroke by means of life-support measures. Second, efforts are made to prevent further thrombosis or hemorrhage. It is important to note that no therapy has been proven to reverse or restore damage already done by stroke; therefore treatment is by necessity of a prophylactic nature.[9]

Prophylactic approaches include anticoagulant therapy in cases of thrombosis or embolism. Medications such as heparin, coumarin drugs, and aspirin are commonly used. Heparin is used acutely, while coumarin drugs and aspirin are used for prolonged periods. Coumarin drugs are only used for a few months after the stroke, while aspirin may be used on a more long-term basis.[13] Dipyridamole (Persantine), an antiplatelet drug, may also be used along or in combination with aspirin.[9]

Corticosteroids may be used in the acute period after the stroke to reduce the cerebral edema that accompanies cerebral infarction. This can markedly reduce complications.[9,13]

Surgical intervention may be indicated in certain instances. Removal of a superficial hematoma is a lifesaving measure. Management of obstruction is commonly accomplished by thromboendarterectomy or bypass grafts in the neck or thorax.[9]

If the patient survives and prevention therapy is instituted, the third and final step in stroke management is rehabilitation. This is generally accomplished by intense physical therapy and speech therapy, if indicated. Although marked improvement is common, many patients are left with some degree of permanent deficit.

DENTAL MANAGEMENT
Medical considerations (see Table 14-4)

Some primary tasks of the dentist are stroke prevention and identification of the stroke-prone individual. Patients with a history of hypertension, diabetes mellitus, coronary atherosclerosis, elevated blood cholesterol or lipid levels, or cigarette smoking are predisposed to stroke as well as to myocardial infarction. The dentist should encourage the patient to seek medical care and to eliminate or control all possible risk factors.

TABLE 14-4. Dental management of stroke patient

I. Identification of stroke-prone patient
  A. Hypertension
  B. Diabetes mellitus
  C. Coronary atherosclerosis
  D. Elevated blood cholesterol or lipid levels
  E. Cigarette smoking

II. Encourage patient to control risk factors for stroke and refer to physician if appropriate

III. History of stroke
  A. Previous history places at high risk for another stroke
  B. Patient with TIAs—no elective care
  C. Anticoagulant drugs predispose to bleeding problems
    1. Aspirin/dipyridamole—pretreatment bleeding time
    2. Coumarin drugs—pretreatment prothrombin time less than 28 seconds
  D. Short, morning appointments
  E. Monitor blood pressure
  F. Avoid vasoconstrictor in anesthetic if possible; otherwise use mimimum amount
  G. Avoid epinephrine in retraction cord

A patient with a past history of stroke is at greater risk for stroke than a person who has not had one.[9,13] These individuals should be approached with a degree of caution. A patient suffering from TIAs should not receive elective dental care. Medical consultation and referral to a physician are mandatory.

Patients who are taking coumarin drugs or antiplatelet drugs are at risk for abnormal bleeding. The status of coumarin anticoagulation may be monitored by the prothrombin time. A level of twice normal or less (normal being 11 to 14 seconds) is acceptable for performing surgical procedures. If the prothrombin time is greater than 28 seconds, the physician should be consulted to modify the dosage of anticoagulant downward.

The effect of aspirin or dipyridamole on platelet aggregation is monitored by the bleeding time. A result of greater than 6 minutes can result in excessive bleeding, and abnormal results should be discussed with the physician.

Management of stroke-prone patients or patients with a history of stroke includes short, morning appointments that are as stress free as possible. Blood pressure should be monitored to ensure good control. Pain control is especially important. Nitrous oxide may be used if good oxygenation is maintained at all times. A local anesthetic with epinephrine 1:100,000 or 1:200,000 may be used in judicious amounts (6 ml or less) if required for lengthy procedures; however, for procedures that will take 45 minutes or less, it is recommended that a local anesthetic without a vasoconstrictor be used.

Gingival retraction cord impregnated with epinephrine should not be used. Instead, the use of cord impregnated with ferrous sulfate or aluminum chloride is recommended.

Treatment planning modifications

Technical modifications may be required for patients with residual physical deficits that make adequate oral hygiene difficult if not impossible. For these patients, extensive bridgework is not a good choice. All restorations should be placed with ease of cleansability in mind. Hygiene may be facilitated by an electric toothbrush, a large-handled toothbrush, or a water irrigation device. Flossing aids should also be prescribed. Frequent professional prophylaxis is advisable.

Oral complications

No specific oral findings are associated with stroke.

Emergency dental care

The same management recommendations apply to the provision of emergency dental care.

REFERENCES

1. Commission on Classification and Terminology of the International League Against Epilepsy: Proposal for revised clinical and electroencephalographic classification of epileptic seizures, Epilepsia 22:489-501, 1981.
2. Dahlquist, N.R., Mellinger, J.F., and Klass, D.W.: Hazard of video games in patients with light-sensitive epilepsy, JAMA 249:776-777, 1983.
3. Engel, J., et al.: Recent developments in the diagnosis and therapy of epilepsy, Ann. Intern. Med. 97:584-598, 1982.
4. Furlan, A.J., et al.: Decreasing incidence of primary intracerebral hemorrhage: a population study, Ann. Neurol. 5: 367-373, 1979.
5. Golden, A.: Pathology: understanding human disease, Baltimore, 1982, The William & Wilkins Co., pp. 234-240.
6. Hassell, T.M.: Epilepsy and the oral manifestations of phenytoin therapy. In Myers, H.M., editor: Monographs in oral science, vol. 9, Basel, Switzerland, 1981, S. Karger, pp. 116-177.
7. Hassell, T.M., et al.: Valproic acid: a new antiepileptic drug with potential side effects of dental concern, J. Am. Dent. Assoc. 99:983-987, 1979.
8. McIntyre, H.B.: The primary care of seizure disorders: a practical guide to the evaluation and comprehensive management of seizure disorders, Woburn, Mass., 1982, Butterworth Publishers, Inc, pp. 1-66.
9. Mohr, J.P., et al.: Cerebrovascular disease. In Isselbacher, K.J., et al., editors: Harrison's principles of internal medicine, ed. 9, New York, 1980, McGraw-Hill Book Co, pp. 1911-1942.
10. Salam-Adams, M., and Adams, R.D.: The convulsive state and idiopathic epilepsy. In Isselbacher, K.J., et al., editors: Harrison's principles of internal medicine, ed. 9, New York, 1980, McGraw-Hill Book Co, pp. 131-139.
11. Sutherland, J.M., and Eadie, M.J.: The epilepsies; modern diagnosis and treatment, ed. 3, Edinburgh, 1980, Churchill Livingstone.
12. Toole, J.F.: Diagnosis and management of stroke, pub. no. 70-004-B, Dallas, 1979, American Heart Association.
13. Toole, J.F., and Merritt, H.H.: Vascular diseases of brain and spinal cord. In Merritt, H.H., editor: A textbook of neurology, ed. 6, Philadelphia, 1979, Lea & Febiger, pp. 152-185.
14. Wannsamaker, B.B.: Problems in seizure management, Res. Staff Phys. 27:43-48, 1981.

15

DIABETES

Diabetes mellitus is a disease complex with metabolic and vascular components. The metabolic component involves elevation of blood glucose associated with alterations in lipid protein metabolism resulting from a relative or absolute lack of insulin. The vascular component includes an accelerated onset of nonspecific atherosclerosis and a more specific microangiopathy that particularly affects the eyes and kidneys.

This disease is of great importance to the dentist, because he or she is in a position as a member of the health team to detect new cases of diabetes. The dentist must also be able to render dental care to patients who are already being treated for diabetes without endangering their lives.

The purpose of this chapter is to review the following: the pathogenesis of diabetes, the detection of the patient with undiagnosed diabetes, the referral of these patients to a physician for medical diagnosis and treatment, and the management of the diabetic patient receiving dental treatment.

GENERAL DESCRIPTION
Incidence

There are over 200 million people in the world with diabetes mellitus. In the United States there are about 4 million people with diabetes, which represents about 2% of the population. One half of these people are unaware that they are diabetic. The greatest prevalence is found in individuals over the age of 45 years; 4 of every 5 diabetic persons are over this age. A breakdown according to age shows that the number of cases in the United States is 1.3 per 1000 from birth to the age of 17 years, 17 per 1000 from ages 25 to 40 years, and 79 per 1000 over the age of 65 years.[3,11]

The number of cases of diabetes in the United States will increase, because the population is increasing, the life expectancy is increasing, the number of people with obesity is increasing, people with diabetes are living longer because of better medical management, and these individuals are having more children who will pass on the disease. Based on this information, it is plain to see that diabetes is a common disease and that the rate of new cases will most likely increase in the near future.

A dental practice serving a population of 2000 could expect to encounter about 40 persons with diabetes, about 20 of whom will be unaware of their condition.

Etiology

Diabetes mellitus may occur as a result of (1) a genetic disorder, (2) the primary destruction of the islets of Langerhans of the pancreas caused by inflammation, cancer, or surgery, (3) an endocrine condition such as hyperpituitarism or hyperthyroidism, or (4) an iatrogenic disease following administration of steroids.[3,11] In this chapter the discussion will be limited to the genetic type of diabetes, which also has been called primary, hereditary, or essential diabetes.

Although the most common form of diabetes is referred to as the genetic or hereditary type, its genetic marker is not known at present; thus the mode of transfer remains to be established. It is known that if one identical twin develops diabetes the other will become diabetic if he lives long enough. In addition, if both parents have diabetes

TABLE 15-1. Hereditary probability of developing diabetes in members of families

Chance of developing diabetes mellitus	Family A	Family B
85%	Parent	Parent
60%	Parent	Grandparent, aunt, uncle
40%	Parent	First cousin
20%	Parent	
14%	1 grandparent	
9%	1 first cousin	

From Saadoun, A.P.: Diabetes and periodontal disease: a review and update, J. Western Soc. Periodontol. **28:**116-139, 1980.

TABLE 15-2. Classification of diabetes by the American Diabetic Association, 1975

1. Hereditary, primary, or idiopathic diabetes
   a. Prediabetes
   b. Subclinical, latent, or stress diabetes
   c. Chemical diabetes
   d. Overt or clinical diabetes
      Juvenile or early onset
      Maturity, adult, or late onset
2. Nonhereditary-secondary diabetes
   a. Damage to or removal of pancreatic islet tissue
   b. Disorders of other endocrine glands
   c. Drugs or chemicals

From National Diabetes Data Group: Classification and diagnosis of diabetes mellitus and other categories of glucose intolerance, Diabetes **28:**1039-1057, 1979. Reproduced with permission from the American Diabetes Association, Inc.

TABLE 15-3. Classification of diabetes by the National Diabetes Data Group, 1979

1. Diabetes mellitus
   a. Type I—insulin-dependent diabetes mellitus (IDDM)
   b. Type II—non-insulin-dependent diabetes mellitus (NIDDM)
   c. Type III—Other types of diabetes
      Pancreatic disease
      Hormonal
      Drugs—thiazide diuretics, lithium salts
      Others
2. Impaired glucose tolerance (IGT)
   a. Nonobese IGT
   b. Obese IGT
   c. IGT associated with other conditions
      Pancreatic disease
      Hormonal
      Drugs
3. Gestational diabetes mellitus (GDM)
4. Previous abnormality of glucose tolerance (Pre AGT)
5. Potential abnormalities of glucose tolerance (Pot AGT)

From National Diabetes Data Group: Classification and diagnosis of diabetes mellitus and other categories of glucose intolerance, Diabetes **28:**1039-1057, 1979. Reproduced with permission of the American Diabetes Association, Inc.

chromosome 6 in most cases of type I diabetes mellitus. Non-insulin-dependent diabetes mellitus (NIDDM), or type II diabetes, has a stronger genetic basis than type I diabetes. In a mild form of type II diabetes found in children, adolescents, and adults, autosomal dominant inheritance has been established.[7]

The chance of various family members for developing diabetes is shown in Table 15-1. If both parents are diabetic, the offspring have about an 85% chance of developing diabetes mellitus.[9]

Diabetes mellitus appears to have multiple causes and several mechanisms of transmission. It can be thought of as several diseases that have in common the cardinal clinical feature of glucose intolerance.[8]

In 1975, the American Diabetic Association classified diabetes as shown in Table 15-2.[11] There were problems with this classification from several standpoints. The primary problem involved the fact that juvenile, or early-onset, diabetes could be

the offspring has nearly a 100% chance of developing the disease. Susceptibility to diabetes appears to be inherited in many other cases, but the chance of it showing up in the offspring is far less predictable. One problem in establishing patterns of transmission is that the susceptible individual may not develop the disease until very late in life.

Recent studies have shown that the frequency of insulin-dependent diabetes mellitus (IDDM), or type I diabetes, is linked to the presence or absence of certain genetically determined cell surface antigens found on lymphocytes. These antigens are not considered to be direct markers or the only determinants for type I diabetes mellitus.[8]

Histocompatibility (HLA) antigens are found on

found in both children and adults. Also, the adult, or late-onset, diabetes could be found in children.

In 1979, The National Diabetes Data Group proposed a new classification for diabetes mellitus and related conditions.[7] This classification is shown in Table 15-3 and is now in general use in the United States. This terminology will be used for this chapter.

It is estimated that about 1% to 5% of individuals with impaired glucose tolerance (IGT) will develop clinical diabetes per year.

The onset of IGT or clinical diabetes during pregnancy is termed *gestational diabetes*. These patients were usually found to return to "normal" following the birth of the child. However, they have an increased risk to develop diabetes in 5 to 10 years. Gestational diabetes carries an increased risk for loss of the fetus.

Several groups of patients are found in the previous abnormality of glucose tolerance classification; patients who had gestational diabetes, obese individuals who had lost weight, patients with hyperglycemia following myocardial infarction, and patients with posttraumatic hyperglycemia are all under this classification.

Patients who have never had an abnormal glucose tolerance test but who by genetic background are at increased risk to develop diabetes mellitus are placed in the potential abnormalities of glucose tolerance classification.

Patients with clinical signs and symptoms of diabetes mellitus may have type I, type II, or type III diabetes. These patients will show an elevation of the fasting blood glucose, abnormal glucose tolerance test, and microangiopathy.

Type I diabetes usually has a sudden onset of clinical symptoms and is usually found in individuals under 40 years of age. It may, however, occur at any age. These patients are dependent on exogenous insulin to maintain life. They have associated HLA antigen types and abnormal autoimmune reaction, including islet cell antibodies.[8]

Type II diabetes usually has a slow onset of clinical symptoms and is most commonly found in individuals over 40 years of age, though it can occur in younger people. These patients are not dependent on exogenous insulin to maintain life. Some patients under stress may need transient exogenous insulin. Patients with type II diabetes are often obese. There is a very strong inheritance tendency, and HLA antigen types or autoimmune reactions are not associated with this type of diabetes. Insulin receptor or postreceptor defects have been found to be associated with type II diabetes.[8]

The onset of diabetes mellitus in children is usually preceded by a sudden growth spurt. In fact, at the time of the onset of the disease, these children have advanced height, bone age, and dental age when compared to their nondiabetic siblings. Puberty also appears earlier in the diabetic child. In about 30% of patients with type I diabetes, a short period of remission follows a case; however, the remission rarely exceeds 1 year.[1]

Pathophysiology

The metabolic alterations found in diabetes result from an absolute or relative lack of insulin. In some cases it appears that the insulin produced by the pancreas is abnormal in some way; in others antagonizing factors to insulin, such as antibodies, may be involved; and in still others end-organ refractoriness develops.

In most cases there is an abnormality in the amount of insulin secreted and in its actions. Most individuals go through a stage of hyperinsulinism, which may last from a few weeks to years. The basic defect may be quantitative, in which an abnormal amount of insulin is produced, or qualitative, in which increased amounts are secreted to compensate for relative or absolute deficiency in insulin activity. The overworked beta cells in the islets of Langerhans may then become exhausted and undergo degeneration, leading to insulin deprivation. Persons with a predisposition to diabetes may develop clinical diabetes if they are obese, have a prolonged high caloric intake, develop infection, or become pregnant.

There appears to be a good correlation between the status of the beta cells and the clinical severity of the diabetes. In the early stage of type I diabetes the islets of Langerhans may be enlarged, and some may show a lymphocytic infiltrate, which suggests the possibility of an autoimmune response. Later, the islets become smaller, and essentially no insulin is produced. In contrast, most individuals with type II diabetes are able to produce some insulin.[3,11]

The patient with uncontrolled diabetes is deprived of insulin or its action. These patients will continue to use carbohydrate at the usual rates in the brain and nervous system, because insulin is not required by these tissues. However, other tissues in the body will be unable to take glucose into the cells or to use it at a normal rate. Increased production of glucose may occur from glycogen and from protein; thus the rise in blood glucose in the diabetic person results from a combination of underuse and overproduction.

Hyperglycemia leads to glucose excretion in the urine, which results in an increase in urinary volume. The increased fluid lost through urine may lead to dehydration and loss of electrolytes.

The lack of glucose use by many of the cells of the body leads to cellular starvation. The patient will increase the intake of food but still lose weight in many cases.

Cortisol secretion is often increased in the diabetic person in response to the stress of the disease. This leads to protein breakdown and difficulty in incorporating amino acids into proteins. The result is conversion of amino acids to glucose and loss of body nitrogen in the urine.

As the inability to use glucose progresses, the diabetic person shifts to fat metabolism. Body fat stores are mobilized, and the glycerol portion of the triglyceride is separated and converted to glucose. The fatty acids are metabolized through the Krebs cycle. However, if excessive fat breakdown continues, the ability of the breakdown product, acetyl-CoA, to be processed through the Krebs cycle fails. The excess acetyl-CoA is then converted to acetoacetic acid, acetone, and beta-hydroxybutyric acid. These products then build up in concentration in body fluids and are excreted in the urine.[3,11]

If these events continue to progress, the diabetic person will develop metabolic acidosis. The acidosis results from the increased loss of electrolytes in the urine, the accumulation of acetoacetic acid and beta-hydroxybutyric acid in body fluids, and the alteration of the bicarbonate and other buffer systems. For a time the body may be able to maintain the pH near normal levels, but as the buffer system and respiratory and renal regulators fail to compensate, the body fluids become more acidic and the pH falls. Severe acidosis will lead to coma and death if it is not identified and treated.

The prime manifestations of diabetes—hyperglycemia, ketoacidosis, and vascular wall disease—contribute to the inability of the patient with uncontrolled diabetes to manage infection and heal wounds.[3,11] The effect of the hyperglycemia may reduce the phagocytic function of granulocytes and facilitate the growth of certain microorganisms. Ketoacidosis appears to delay the migration of granulocytes in the area of injury and to decrease phagocytic activity. The vascular wall changes may lead to vascular insufficiency, which can result in decreased blood flow to an area of injury. This could hamper granulocytic mobilization and reduce oxygen tension. The end results of the preceding effects and others yet to be identified are to render the patient with uncontrolled diabetes much more susceptible to infection, to reduce ability to deal with an infection once it is established, and to delay the healing of traumatic and surgical wounds.

Complications

The complications of diabetes are associated with the vascular system and the peripheral nervous system. The vascular complications result from two different pathologic changes—microangiopathy and atherosclerosis. In fact, there is some evidence that suggests that the microangiopathies seen in diabetic persons may be a basic part of the disease process and not a later complication. In any case, the vessel changes seen in microangiopathy include thickening of the intima, endothelial proliferation, lipid deposition, and accumulation of para-aminosalicylic acid–positive material. These changes can be seen throughout the body but have particular clinical importance when they occur in the retina and small vessels of the kidney.[3,11]

The changes in the retina result in microaneurysms, hemorrhage, exudation, and proliferation of retinal vessels. This diabetic retinopathy is the second most common cause of blindness in the United States.

The microangiopathy involving the kidney may lead to renal failure but does not usually result in hypertension unless another form of vascular complication that consists of an accelerated onset of atherosclerosis and arteriosclerosis occurs. In arteriosclerosis the small vessels show fibrosis of the

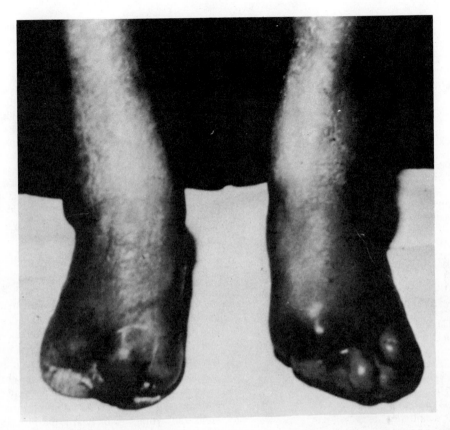

FIG. 15-1. Diabetic gangrene of both feet. (From Falace, D.A.: Medical considerations. In Wood, N.A., editor: Treatment planning: a pragmatic approach, St. Louis, 1978, The C.V. The Mosby Co., p. 63.)

intima and hypertrophy of the media but no para-aminosalicylic acid–positive material or endothelial hyperplasia. These vascular changes may result in ulceration and gangrene of the feet (Fig. 15-1), hypertension, renal failure, myocardial infarction, and coronary insufficiency.

The most common cause of death in patients with type I diabetes is renal failure. In patients with type II diabetes the most common cause of death is myocardial infarction.

Neuropathies may be seen as a complication of diabetes. In the lower extremities they may be manifested as muscle weakness, muscle cramps, deep burning pain, or tingling paresthesia. These symptoms may be seen elsewhere; some cases of oral paresthesia and burning tongue are caused by this complication. These changes may be a result of segmental demyelination and abnormalities of Schwann cells associated with peripheral nerves.

Other complications that may be found in diabetic persons are cataracts, skin rash, and skin deposits of fat (xanthoma diabeticorum). In persons with diabetes in whom the disease has been diagnosed early and has been well controlled, these complications may not develop as quickly or to as great an extent as in those in whom the disease was detected late or was poorly managed.

CLINICAL PRESENTATION
Signs and symptoms

In type I diabetes, the onset of symptoms is sudden. The symptoms include polydipsia (increased thirst), polyuria (increased frequency of urination), polyphagia (increased appetite and eat-

TABLE 15-4. Comparison between clinical picture of type I (IDDM) and type II (NIDDM) diabetes

	Type I (IDDM)	Type II (NIDDM)
Frequency (percentage of diabetic persons)	5%	85%
Age at onset (years)	15	40 and over
Body build	Normal or thin	Obese
Severity	Severe	Mild
Insulin	Almost all	25% to 30%
Oral hypoglycemic agents	Very few respond	50% respond
Ketoacidosis	Common	Uncommon
Complications	90% in 20 years	Less common
Rate of clinical onset	Rapid	Slow
Stability	Unstable	Stable
Family history	Common	More common
HLA antigen and abnormal autoimmune reactions	Present	Not present
Insulin receptor defects	Usually not found	

TABLE 15-5. Symptoms of diabetes

I. Type I diabetes
  A. Cardinal symptoms—common
    1. Polydipsia
    2. Polyuria
    3. Polyphagia
    4. Weight loss
    5. Loss of strength
  B. Other symptoms
    1. Recurrence of bed-wetting
    2. Repeated skin infections
    3. Marked irritability
    4. Headache
    5. Drowsiness
    6. Malaise
    7. Dry mouth
II. Type II diabetes
  A. Cardinal symptoms much less common
  B. Usual symptoms
    1. Slight weight loss or gain
    2. Urination at night
    3. Vulvar pruritus (females)
    4. Blurred vision
    5. Decreased vision
    6. Paresthesias
    7. Loss of sensation
    8. Impotence
    9. Postural hypotension

ing), loss of weight, loss of strength, marked irritability, recurrence of bed-wetting, drowsiness, and malaise. Patients with severe ketoacidosis may complain of vomiting, abdominal pain, nausea, tachypnea (increased respiratory rate), paralysis, and loss of consciousness.[3,11] The onset of symptoms in type II diabetes is usually slow, and the cardinal symptoms are less commonly seen. The signs and symptoms of type I and type II diabetes are summarized in Tables 15-4 and 15-5.

Other signs and symptoms relating to the complications of diabetes may be present. These could include skin lesions, cataracts, blindness, hypertension, chest pain, anemia, etc.

Laboratory findings

Two groups of patients should be examined for diabetes mellitus. First among these are patients with signs and symptoms of diabetes or its complications. Second, individuals who have diabetic relatives, who are obese, who are over age 40, who delivered large babies, or who have had spontaneous abortions or stillbirths should be screened for diabetes at periodic intervals.[3,11]

The diagnosis of diabetes is established by the symptom complex of microangiopathy involving the retina with demonstration of abnormal glucose metabolism by clinical laboratory tests.

Clinical laboratory tests that are used to establish abnormality of glucose metabolism are tests for glucose and acetone in the urine, fasting blood glucose level, 2-hour postprandial blood glucose level, and oral glucose tolerance test.

The use of laboratory tests for the diagnosis of diabetes mellitus has changed since 1979. Before that date the glucose tolerance test was considered to be the diagnostic laboratory test. Since then, the fasting glucose level and/or the 2-hour postprandial blood glucose level measurement have become the standard laboratory tests for the diagnosis of diabetes.[7]

The use and interpretation of the various clinical laboratory tests used to evaluate and diagnose diabetes will be described here in general terms.

URINARY GLUCOSE AND ACETONE

Determination of urinary glucose and acetone is of limited value in detecting overt diabetes. In addition, the finding of glucose in the urine is not diagnostic of diabetes. A few people have a low renal threshold for glucose and may "spill" sugar into the urine on that basis. Other conditions may lead to glucose in the urine, such as renal disease and the administration of steroids. More important is the fact that the failure to find glucose or acetone or both in the urine of a patient suspected of being diabetic does not rule out diabetes. Many studies have demonstrated that some persons with overt diabetes at times may not spill glucose into the urine. Many more may not show any evidence of acetone in the urine. Cases have been reported with blood glucose levels of 300 to 400 mg/100 ml without any evidence of urinary glucose. With the possible exception of the patient who has the classical symptoms of diabetes along with glucose and acetone in the urine, most physicians depend on blood chemistry to establish the diagnosis of diabetes.

BLOOD GLUCOSE DETERMINATION

In interpreting the blood glucose level it is important to keep in mind that the source of blood, age of the patient, nature of the diet, and physical activity of the patient will often affect the results. Also of great importance is the method used to measure the amount of sugar in the blood sample.

Most clinical laboratories collect venous blood from the arm for analysis of blood glucose level. Venous glucose levels are lower than arterial glucose levels. The greatest difference occurs about 1 hour after the ingestion of carbohydrates. Following an overnight fast, the arterial glucose levels are usually only 2 or 3 mg/100 ml higher than the venous glucose levels.

The capillary blood glucose values are closer to the arterial values than are the venous levels. However, methods that use capillary blood are subject to a greater variation in results because of dilution of the blood sample with lymph. Normal fasting blood glucose levels range from 60 to 100 mg/100 ml for venous blood.

In one study of 2983 "normal" persons from 16 to 70 years of age, venous blood glucose levels were measured 1 hour after the ingestion of 100 mg of glucose.[6] It was found that the blood glucose level increased by about 13 mg/100 ml per decade of age. In a study of faculty members who had no familial history of diabetes, the venous blood glucose levels 2 hours after the ingestion of 100 mg of glucose were found to be, on the average, 130 mg/100 ml for persons 50 to 60 years of age and 144 mg/100 ml for persons 60 to 70 years of age.

If the diet has been low in the amount of carbohydrates for several days and the person is given 100 mg of glucose just before the blood glucose level is measured, it is possible to produce a condition termed *starvation hyperglycemia,* which could be misdiagnosed as diabetes mellitus. To prevent this from occurring, the diet should contain at least 250 to 300 g of carbohydrates on each of the 3 days before testing.

Physical activity tends to lower the blood glucose level. Excessive physical activity should be avoided by patients who are going to be tested for blood glucose level.

The most accurate technique for determining the blood glucose level is one that measures only glucose. The Folin and Wu method gives higher results, because it also measures other blood sugars, such as fructose and lactose. Methods that use glucose oxidase give the lowest blood sugar value, because this method is specific for glucose. Most autoanalyzers use a ferricyanide method, which gives values a little higher than methods that use glucose oxidase.

Fasting venous blood glucose. The 1979 international criteria for the diagnosis of diabetes mellitus[7] define diabetes as being present if the fasting blood glucose level is 140 mg/100 ml on two or more occasions.

Two-hour postprandial blood sugar. For the 2-hour postprandial blood sugar test the patient is given a 75 or 100 g glucose load after a night of fasting. The glucose can be given in the form of Glucola or in a meal containing about 100 g of carbohydrate. Glucola works very well, because it gives a measured amount of glucose and can be given in the dental office. Blood glucose levels taken at 2 hours that are higher than 200 mg/100 ml on two or more occasions are diagnostic of diabetes mellitus.[7]

ORAL GLUCOSE TOLERANCE TEST

Glucose taken orally is absorbed from the small intestine. The maximum normal rate of absorption is 0.8 g per kg of body weight per hour. The glucose tolerance test reflects the rate of absorption, uptake by tissues, and excretion in urine of glucose. The glucose load can be given in Glucola, which contains 75 g of glucose in each 7-fluid-ounce bottle. Some laboratories use a 75 g glucose load, while others use a 100 g glucose load following a night of fasting. Venous blood samples are drawn from the arm at ½, 1, 2, and 3 hours after the ingestion of glucose. Urine samples are also collected at each interval.

The following are considered to be representative of the upper level of normal for fasting blood glucose concentration (using an autoanalyzer).

Time (hours)	Amount (mg/100 ml)
½	170
1	170
2	120
3	110

The most characteristic alterations seen in diabetes are an increase in fasting blood glucose, an increase in peak value, and/or a delayed return to normal at the 2- and 3-hour samples. Hypoglycemia may occur in the person with early, mild diabetes 3 to 5 hours after ingestion of glucose. For this reason some physicians will extend the glucose tolerance test to 5 hours for certain patients.

TABLE 15-6. Glycohemoglobin measurement as laboratory test for evaluation of diabetic patient

Glycohemoglobin level (% of total hemoglobin)	Clinical interpretation
4 to 8%	Normal range in adult
Less than 7.5%	Good control of diabetes
7.6% to 8.9%	Fair control of diabetes
9% to 20%	Poor control of diabetes

The urine samples should not contain glucose at any point during the test.

As previously mentioned, the glucose tolerance test is no longer the standard test for the diagnosis of diabetes mellitus. This test is used to identify patients with impaired glucose tolerance and gestational diabetes and is used on those with previous abnormality of glucose tolerance.

GLYCOHEMOGLOBIN

The measurement of the blood concentration of glycohemoglobin has been described as being of value in detecting and evaluating the diabetic patient (Table 15-6). It appears to reflect the glucose level over the past 6 to 8 weeks. The patient does not have to fast before the test, and it can be of value in following the progress of the diabetic patient. However, at present this test is not generally used for the diagnosis of diabetes mellitus.[7]

MEDICAL MANAGEMENT

The patient with diabetes may be treated by control of diet and physical activity and the administration of oral hypoglycemic agents and/or insulin. In many cases of type II diabetes the disease can be controlled by weight loss, diet, and physical activity. Total calories taken must be balanced with physical activity and body weight. A balanced diet with rigid control of total caloric content is indicated. Some physicians will place the diabetic patient on a diet that has a certain balance of carbohydrate, protein, and fat. Others will allow the patient much more freedom and only control total caloric content.[3,11]

If control of diet and physical activity fail to control the blood glucose level, hypoglycemic agents are used. Many cases of type II diabetes can

TABLE 15-7. Signs and symptoms of insulin reaction

Mild stage
Hunger
Weakness
Tachycardia
Pallor
Sweating
Paresthesias

Moderate stage
Incoherence
Uncooperativeness
Belligerence
Lack of judgment
Poor orientation

Severe stage
Unconsciousness
Tonic or clonic movements
Hypotension
Hypothermia
Rapid, thready pulse

be controlled with oral hypoglycemic agents. Certain oral hypoglycemic agents, specifically tolbutamide and related sulfonylurea drugs, were implicated by a report from the University Group Diabetes Program as being ineffective and increasing the risk of cardiovascular disease. Since that report there have been no studies that would seem to support those conclusions.[7]

Patients with type I diabetes will require insulin to control the blood glucose level. Infection, emotional and physical stress, pregnancy, and surgical procedures will usually disturb the control of the patient's diabetes. This is particularly true in patients who take insulin. Additional control measures must be used during these periods of stress. This often involves increasing the dosage of insulin or administering insulin to patients with type II diabetes for a short period of time.

Insulin shock

It is important that patients treated with insulin follow their diet very closely. If they fail to eat in a normal pattern but continue to take their regular insulin injection, they may experience a hypogly-cemic reaction caused by an excess of insulin (insulin shock). A hypoglycemic reaction can also occur as a result of overdosage of insulin or an oral hypoglycemic agent.

Reactions or shock caused by excessive insulin occurs in three well-defined stages, each more severe and dangerous than the preceding (Table 15-7).

MILD STAGE

The mild stage is the most common and is characterized by hunger, weakness, trembling, tachycardia, pallor, and sweating. It occurs before meals, during exercise, or when food has been omitted or delayed. Paresthesias may be noted on occasion.

MODERATE STAGE

In the moderate stage the patient becomes incoherent, uncooperative, and sometimes belligerent or resistive. Judgment and orientation are defective. The chief danger during this stage is that patients may injure themselves or someone else if they are driving, etc.

SEVERE STAGE

Complete unconsciousness with or without tonic or clonic skeletal movements occurs during the severe stage. Most of these reactions occur during sleep after the first two stages have gone unrecognized. This stage may also occur after exercise or ingestion of alcohol if earlier signs are ignored. Sweating, pallor, rapid thready pulse, hypotension, and hypothermia may be present.

• • •

The reaction to excessive insulin can be corrected by giving the patient sweetened fruit juice or anything with sugar in it. Patients in the severe stage, unconsciousness, are best treated by giving glucose solution IV. Glucagon or epinephrine may be used for transient relief.

DENTAL MANAGEMENT
Medical considerations

Any dental patient who has the cardinal symptoms of diabetes (polydipsia, polyuria, polyphagia, weight loss, and loss of strength) should be

TABLE 15-8. Detection of diabetic patient

I. Known diabetic person
  A. Detection by history
    1. Are you diabetic?
    2. What medications are you taking?
    3. Are you being treated by a physician?
  B. Establishing severity of disease and degree of control
    1. When were you first diagnosed as diabetic?
    2. What was the level of the last measurement of your blood glucose?
    3. What is the usual level of blood glucose for you?
    4. How are you being treated for your diabetes?
    5. How often do you have insulin reactions?
    6. How much insulin do you take with each injection and how often do you receive injections?
    7. Do you test your urine for glucose?
    8. When did you last visit your physician?
    9. Do you have any symptoms of diabetes at present?
II. Undiagnosed diabetic person
  A. History of signs or symptoms of diabetes or its complications
  B. Individuals at high risk for developing diabetes
    1. Parents who are diabetic
    2. Gave birth to one or more large babies
    3. History of spontaneous abortions or stillbirths
    4. Obese
    5. Over 40 years of age
  C. Referral or screening test for diabetes

TABLE 15-9. Screening for diabetes in dental office

I. Selection of patient
II. On each of 3 days before screening, patient's diet should contain 250 to 300 g of carbohydrate
III. Overnight fast day before screening
IV. Have patient come to dental office for 8:30 or 9:00 A.M. appointment day of testing (no breakfast)
  A. Fasting blood glucose test
    1. Make wound on finger pad with sterile blood lancet
    2. Drop blood onto reagent end of Dextrostix
    3. Wash blood off after 1 minute
    4. Using color chart, estimate blood glucose level
  B. 2-hour postprandial blood glucose test
    1. Have patient ingest 75 g of glucose (Glucola)
    2. 2 hours later, obtain blood sample and test as above
V. Refer patient to physician if:
  A. Fasting blood glucose is 140 mg/100 ml or higher
  B. 2-hour postprandial blood glucose is 200 mg/100 ml or higher

referred to a physician for diagnosis and treatment.

Patients with findings that may suggest the possibility of diabetes (headache, dry mouth, marked irritability, repeated skin infection, blurred vision, paresthesias, progressive periodontal disease, multiple periodontal abscesses, or loss of sensation) should be screened by the dentist for hyperglycemia or referred to a clinical laboratory or physician for screening tests (Table 15-8).

Patients who are obese, are over 40 years of age, or have close relatives who are diabetic should be screened once a year for any indication of hyperglycemia that may reveal the onset of diabetes. Women who have given birth to large babies (over 10 pounds) or who have had multiple spontaneous abortions or stillbirths also should be screened once a year for diabetes. These patients are best

screened by their physician if they have one. Patients who do not have a physician can be screened in the dental office or referred to a clinical laboratory or physician for screening.

The dental office screening test for diabetes (hyperglycemia) is simple and inexpensive and, if done with care, is very accurate in detecting patients with moderate to severe elevations of blood glucose. The following procedures are suggested to screen the dental patient for hyperglycemia (see Table 15-9). The patient should be encouraged to eat a normal diet that contains about 250 to 300 g of carbohydrate per day at least 3 days before screening. On the day of screening the patient should eat no breakfast and come into the dental office at about 8:30 to 9:00 A.M. A fasting blood glucose or 2-hour postprandial blood glucose test can be performed. If the 2-hour postprandial blood glucose test is selected, the patient should be given a 75 g glucose load in the form of Glucola, a convenient commercial product.

If the fasting blood glucose test is selected, blood is obtained when the patient comes to the office. In the case of a 2-hour postprandial blood glucose test, blood is obtained 2 hours after inges-

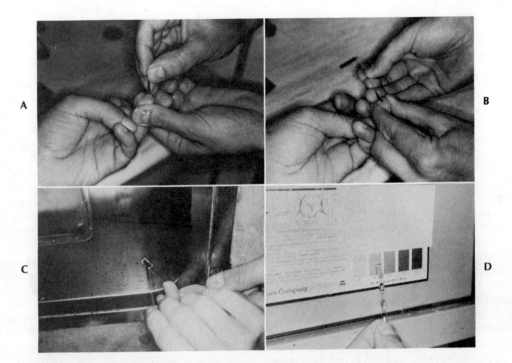

FIG. 15-2. A, Use of sterile lancet to pierce finger pad. B, Collecting blood in capillary tube. C, Transfer of blood from capillary tube to reagent end of Dextrostix. D, Matching activated reagent end of Dextrostix to color chart.

tion of the Glucola. The blood can be obtained from the patient's finger pad using a sterile blood lancet to produce the wound (Fig. 15-2, A). The blood can be collected in a capillary tube (Fig. 15-2, B) and then blown onto the reagent end of a Dextrostix (which contains glucose oxidase and a color-indicating system) (Fig. 15-2, C). After 1 minute the blood is washed from the Dextrostix, and the color of the reagent end is compared to a chart provided by the manufacturer, the Ames Co., to estimate the concentration of glucose (Fig. 15-2, D).

A patient with an estimated fasting blood glucose level of 140 mg/100 ml or higher should be referred to a physician for medical evaluation and treatment if indicated. A patient with a 2-hour postprandial blood glucose level of 200 mg/100 ml or higher should also be referred.

All patients with diagnosed diabetes must be identified by history, and the type of medical treatment they are receiving must be established. The type of diabetes (type I, II, or III) should be determined and the presence of complications noted. Patients being treated with insulin should be asked how much insulin they use and how often they inject themselves each day. The frequency of insulin reactions and when the last one occurred should be determined. The frequency of visits to the physician should be established, as should whether or not the patient checks his urine for glucose. This information will provide the dentist with information concerning the severity and control of the diabetes (see Table 15-8).

Patients with type II diabetes who have no evidence of complications and have their disease under good medical control will require little or no special attention when receiving dental treatment, unless they should develop an acute dental or oral infection. In contrast, patients with complications such as renal disease and cardiovascular disease may need to be managed in special ways. Patients being treated with insulin or who are not under good medical management also will require special attention.

Patients who have not seen their physician for a long time, who have had frequent episodes of insulin shock, or who report signs and symptoms of diabetes may have disease that is out of control. These patients should be referred back to their physician for evaluation, or the physician should be consulted to establish the patient's current status.

Some patients with type I diabetes who are being treated with large doses of insulin will have periods of extreme hyperglycemia and hypoglycemia (brittle diabetes), even with the best of medical management. These patients will require close consultation with their physician before any dental treatment is started.

One of the major problems in the dental management of the diabetic patient who is being treated with insulin is to prevent insulin shock from occurring during the dental appointment. These patients should be told to take their usual insulin dosage and to eat their normal breakfast before the dental appointment, which is usually best scheduled in the morning. When the patient comes for the appointment, the dentist should confirm that the patient has taken his insulin and eaten breakfast. In addition, these patients should be instructed to tell the dentist if at any time during the appointment they feel symptoms of an insulin reaction occurring. A source of sugar, such as orange juice, must be available in the dental office to give to the patient if symptoms of an insulin reaction occur.

Any diabetic patient who is going to receive extensive periodontal or oral surgery procedures other than single simple extractions should have special attention paid to their dietary needs after the surgery. It is important that the total caloric content and the protein to carbohydrate to fat ratio of the diet remain the same so that control of the disease and proper blood glucose balance are maintained. The patient's physician should be consulted concerning the diet recommendation for the postoperative period. One suggestion is to have the patient use a blender to prepare the usual diet so that it can be ingested with minimum discomfort. Special food supplements that are in a liquid form can be used.

Patients who have brittle diabetes or require a high dosage of insulin (type I diabetics) and are going to recieve periodontal or oral surgery procedures may be given prophylactic antibiotics during the postoperative period to avoid infection.

Patients with well-controlled diabetes can be given general anesthesia; however, in the dental office, management with local anesthetics is preferable.

Any diabetic patient with acute dental or oral

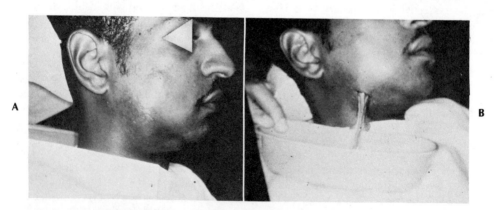

FIG. 15-3. A, Diabetic patient who was treated with insulin. Note swelling in cheek area, which was caused by acute infection of dental origin. This patient required increase in his insulin dosage to control diabetic condition and allow for successful management of oral infection. **B,** Facial abscess was then drained through submandibular incision.

infection presents an immediate problem in management. This problem will be even more difficult for patients who take high insulin dosage and those who have type I diabetes. The infection will often cause loss of control of the diabetic condition; as a result, the infection is not handled by the body's defenses as well as it would be in the nondiabetic patient. Patients with brittle diabetes (difficult to control, high dosage of insulin) may require hospitalization during management of the infection. The patient's physician should be consulted and become a partner in the management of the patient during this period.

The basic aim of treatment is to treat the oral infection and at the same time respond to the need to regain control of the diabetic condition. Patients receiving insulin usually will require additional insulin, which should be prescribed by their physician. Other patients may need more aggressive medical management of their diabetes, which may include insulin during this period. The dentist must treat the infection by drainage, extraction, pulpotomy, warm rinses, and/or antibiotics. Attention also must be paid to the electrolyte balance and the fluid and dietary needs of the patient (Fig. 15-3).

Treatment planning modifications

The diabetic patient who is receiving good medical management without serious complications such as renal disease, hypertension, or coronary atherosclerotic heart disease can receive any indicated dental treatment. Diabetic patients with serious medical complications may need to have an altered plan of dental treatment (see Chapters 5, 7, and 11).

Oral complications

The oral findings in patients with uncontrolled diabetes most likely relate to the excessive loss of fluids by means of urine, the altered response to infection, the microvascular changes, and possibly the increased glucose concentrations in saliva.

The effects of hyperglycemia lead to increased amounts of urine, which depletes the amount of extracellular fluids and reduces the secretion of saliva. The reduced salivary flow results in the complaint of dry mouth. An increase in the rate of dental caries has been reported in young diabetic patients and would appear to be related to reduced salivary flow.

The parotid saliva of persons with uncontrolled diabetes has been reported to contain a slight increase in the amount of glucose.[2] The glucose concentration in parotid saliva from nondiabetic individuals varies from 0.22 to 1.69 mg/100 ml, while the glucose concentration in parotid saliva from persons with uncontrolled diabetes has been reported to range from 0.22 to 6.33 mg/100 ml. The effect of this slight increase in glucose concentration, if any, on the incidence of dental caries and other oral conditions in the diabetic patient remains to be established.

Several studies have reported an increase in the incidence and severity of gingival inflammation, periodontal abscesses, and chronic periodontal disease in diabetic patients[1,39] (Figs. 15-4 and 15-5). On the other hand, a well-controlled study by Shannon et al.[10] failed to demonstrate any difference in the amount or severity of periodontal disease in young diabetic and nondiabetic individuals.

Saadoun[9] reported small blood vessel changes in gingival tissues of diabetic patients. These consisted of flattening of the endothelial cells, accumulation of periodic acid-Schiff–positive material in the basement membrane, and narrowing of the lumen. He also described an increase in the glucose level of the gingival fluids in diabetics. The neutrophils also appear to be affected secondary to the hyperglycemia.They show decreased phagocytosis diapedesis, impaired adherence, and impaired chemotaxis.

Saadoun[9] also reported that adults with uncontrolled diabetes who are prone to periodontal disease will have more severe manifestations of the disease than nondiabetic patients who are prone to peridontal disease. This relationship is not clear in the patient with controlled diabetes. As a group, diabetic patients appear to have more severe periodontal disease than nondiabetic patients, but the differences are not great. Saadoun also concluded that the glucose tolerance test results are not a reliable predictor of the patient's periodontal status. The time relationship between the diabetic state and periodontal disease is yet to be established.

A study performed in Sweden involving children of diabetic mothers showed a much higher frequency of enamel hypoplasia (28%) than in children of nondiabetic mothers (3%).[5] The cause of this difference is not known, but it may be a result of the effects of hyperglycemia on the for-

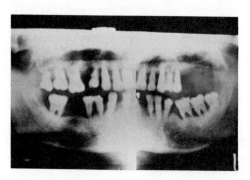

FIG. 15-4. Panoramic radiograph from young adult with very severe, progressive periodontitis. Following positive screening test for diabetes, patient was referred to physician and diagnosis of diabetes mellitus was established. Patient required insulin treatment.

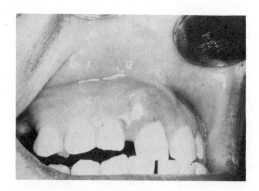

FIG. 15-5. Example of periodontal abscess in patient with multiple abscesses. Patient was evaluated by physician and diagnosis of diabetes mellitus was eventually established.

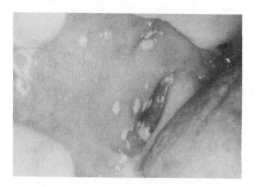

FIG. 15-6. Diabetic patient, who also has end-stage renal disease, with oral candidosis. Note multiple small white lesions on buccal mucosa. These lesions could be scraped off. Cytology and cultures confirmed clinical impression of fungal infection caused by *Candida albicans.*

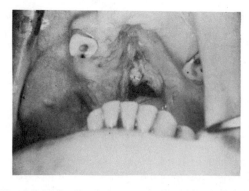

FIG. 15-7. Diabetic patient with lesion involving palate. Cultures established diagnosis of mucormycosis, a serious fungal infection that may occur in patients with systemic diseases such as diabetes or cancer. Treatment usually includes control of diabetes, surgical excision of lesion, and antibiotics and fungicides.

mation and calcification of the enamel matrix.

Oral fungal infections may be found in the uncontrolled diabetic patient. These include moniliasis and the more rare mucormycosis (Figs. 15-6 and 15-7).

There appears to be general agreement that healing is delayed in individuals with uncontrolled diabetes and that they are more prone to various oral infections following surgical procedures.

Several studies have suggested that patients thought to be ''prediabetic'' can have this condition confirmed by gingival biopsy findings of thickened and hyalinized small vessels. However, at present this technique remains to be proved accurate and beneficial.

Emergency dental care

In general, surgical procedures should be avoided in patients with uncontrolled diabetes because of problems with delayed healing and postoperative infection. Acute pulpal problems in the diabetic person can be managed by pulpectomy or analgesics until the diabetes is controlled, after which extraction can be performed if indicated.

The person with controlled diabetes can receive any indicated emergency treatment. However, if acute infection is present the diabetic state may go out of control. If it does, the diabetes must be managed by the physician while at the same time the oral infection is treated by the dentist.

REFERENCES

1. Bartolucci, E.G., et al.: Accelerated periodontal breakdown in uncontrolled diabetes: pathogenesis and treatment, Oral Surg. **52:**387-390, 1981.
2. Campbell, M.J.: Glucose in the saliva of the non-diabetic and the diabetic patient, Arch. Oral Biol. **10:**197-205, 1965.
3. Ellenbergy, M., and Refkin, H.: Diabetes mellitus: theory and practice, New York, 1970, McGraw-Hill Book Co.
4. Goteiner, D.J.: Glycohemoglobin (GHb): a new test for the evaluation of the diabetic patient and its clinical importance, J. Am. Dent. Assoc. **102:**57-58, 1981.
5. Grahnén, H., and Edund, K.: Maternal diabetes and changes in the hand tissues of the primary teeth, Odontol. Rev. **18:**157-162, 1967.
6. Napier, J.A.: Field methods and response rates in Tecumseh community health study, Am. J. Public Health **52:** 208-216, 1962.
7. National Diabetes Data Group: Classification and diagnosis of diabetes mellitus and other categories of glucose intolerance, Diabetes **28:**1039-1057, 1979.
8. Owen, O.E., et al.: Pathogenesis and diagnosis of diabetes mellitus. In Rose, L.F., and Kaye, D., editors: Internal medicine for dentistry, St. Louis, 1983, The C.V. Mosby Co., pp. 1259-1264.
9. Saadoun, A.P.: Diabetes and periodontal disease: a review and update, J. Western Soc. Periodontol. **28:**116-139, 1980.
10. Shannon, I.L., et al.: Glucose tolerance responses in young adults of sharply contrasting periodontal status, SAM-TR-66-9, U.S. Air Force Sch. Aerospace Med., 1-6, Feb. 1966.
11. Williams, R.H., and Porte, D., Jr.: The pancreas. In Williams, R.H., editor: Textbook of endocrinology, ed. 5, Philadelphia, 1974, W.B. Saunders Co., pp. 527-600.

16

ADRENAL INSUFFICIENCY

GENERAL DESCRIPTION
Etiology

Adrenal insufficiency may be either primary or secondary. Primary disease is caused by disorders of either the pituitary gland or of the adrenal glands themselves. Primary adrenal insufficiency occurs infrequently, but when it does it is called Addison disease. Addison disease is characterized by progressive atrophy or destruction of the adrenal glands, classically resulting from chronic granulomatous infectious disease (for example, tuberculosis).[9] There is also an occasional idiopathic form of destruction that is thought to have an autoimmune basis.

Secondary adrenal insufficiency is far more common and is caused by the chronic administration of corticosteroids (steroids), resulting in the suppression of endogenous steroid production. The degree of suppression is related to dosage and length of time of administration; therefore the lower the dose and the shorter the time of administration, the less suppression would be expected. Steroids are used in the treatment of many diseases, including rheumatoid arthritis, asthma, erythema multiforme, erosive lichen planus and various other dermatoses, and systemic lupus erythematosus and other autoimmune disease.[6,8,9]

Though they are not curative, the palliative effects of steroids are extremely useful and serve as powerful adjuncts in the treatment of diseases that are not amenable to curative therapy. It is the principal side effect of secondary adrenal insufficiency that is of interest to the dentist.

Pathophysiology and sequelae

The adrenal glands are located bilaterally at the superior pole of each kidney. They manufacture and secrete at least three hormones, the two principal ones being aldosterone and cortisol. Adrenal function is under the direct control of the pituitary gland, which is regulated by the hypothalamus. When stimulated, the pituitary gland secretes adrenocorticotropic hormone (ACTH), which in turn causes the secretion of cortisol by the adrenal cortex. Aldosterone secretion is mediated by the extracellular fluid volume and sodium.[1,4,6,9]

Aldosterone is a mineralocorticoid, the main function of which is maintaining normal sodium, potassium, and fluid levels by mediating renal tubular function. Aldosterone is regulated by the renin-angiotensin system of the juxtaglomerular apparatus. The system is stimulated by a fall in renal blood pressure resulting from decreased blood volume or electrolyte imbalance, specifically sodium. The result is a release of renin that activates angiotensin, causing vasoconstriction. Aldosterone also is released and causes sodium retention and potassium excretion. Aldosterone production is inhibited through a feedback mechanism that prevents overproduction.[1,4,6,9]

Cortisol is the main glucocorticoid of the body; it has a multitude of functions and effects, some of the more important of which are gluconeogenesis (synthesis of glucose by liver) and antiinflammatory and antiallergic effects.[1] The adrenal glands secrete about 15 to 30 mg of cortisol a day under usual circumstances. The maximum *potential* out-

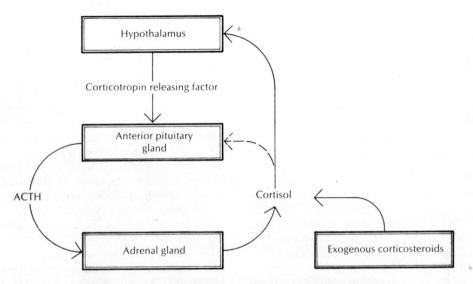

FIG. 16-1. Pituitary-adrenal axis and negative feedback system.

put is around 300 mg for a 24-hour period.[8] The normal pattern of secretion is intimately connected with a person's normal sleep-awake sequence. In the average person who works during daylight hours, the level of serum cortisol is highest on arising in the morning and lowest at bedtime. This pattern is reversed in a person who works nights. This normal variation of serum cortisol levels is called diurnal variation.

The secretion of cortisol is directly dependent on the level of circulating ACTH. As the cortisol level increases and demand is met, the production of ACTH decreases. This drop in ACTH then inhibits the production of cortisol, and the cortisol level begins to drop. When it reaches a certain low point, ACTH is produced and the cycle begins again. With the prolonged administration of high doses of steroids, the feedback system senses the levels of exogenous steroid and inhibits ACTH production, which in turn suppresses the adrenal production of endogenous cortisol (Fig. 16-1). The result is adrenal insufficiency secondary to exogenous steroid administration.[2,5,9] It is generally accepted that significant adrenal suppression will have occurred after 1 month of daily administration of corticosteroid equivalent to 20 mg of hydrocortisone. Topically applied steroids can also

induce adrenal suppression by absorption through the skin or mucous membrane, although this is variable.[3,7] It appears that the amount of topical steroid required to treat small, noninflamed areas usually will not be a cause for concern. On the other hand, the amount required for treatment of an inflamed area for a month or longer should be cause for concern, especially if occlusive dressings are used. In this event one must assume that adrenal suppression may have occurred.

Other than patients with Addison disease or those who have had bilateral adrenalectomy, the potential to regain adrenal function after cessation of steroid therapy is generally retained, each patient requiring variable lengths of time proportional to dosage and duration of therapy. Most people will regain normal function within 9 months, although some patients with severe suppression may take up to a year.

Primary adrenal insufficiency occurs occasionally and is seen as the classical picture of Addison disease. All adrenal cortical hormones may be produced in deficient quantities, and, because the main adrenocortical hormones are aldosterone and cortisol, the disease picture is caused essentially by insufficient quantities of these principal hormones. Lack of aldosterone renders the patient unable to conserve sodium and eliminate potassium and hydrogen ions. The result is an individual who is hypovolemic, hyperkalemic, and acidotic. Cortisol deficiency results in a variety of problems, including impaired glucose metabolism, hypotension, impaired fluid excretion, increased ACTH excretion, excessive pigmentation, and inability to tolerate stress.[1,4,6,9] This disease can be rapidly devastating if left untreated.

CLINICAL PRESENTATION
Signs and symptoms

The signs and symptoms of primary adrenal insufficiency all relate to the deficiency of aldosterone and cortisol. Probably the most common complaints are weakness and fatigue and an abnormal pigmentation of skin and mucous membranes (Fig. 16-2, *A* and *B*). In addition, hypotension, anorexia, and weight loss are common findings.[8] If the patient with Addison disease is challenged by stress, such as infection or surgery, an addisonian crisis may be precipitated, which is a medical emergency. It is manifested by a severe exacerbation of symptoms and includes hypotension, nausea, vomiting, weakness, headache, dehydration, and hyperpyrexia. If not treated rapidly, the patient will die.

Adrenal insufficiency resulting from chronic steroid administration does not usually present any symptoms in the earlier stages unless the patient is stressed and does not have adequate circulating cortisol to cope with the stress. In that event an adrenal crisis may be precipitated. This can usually be prevented by increasing the amount of steroid received to cover the period of stress. It is important to identify patients with diseases that are being treated with steroids to prevent untoward reactions.

More commonly the patient who has been receiving long-term, high-dose steroid therapy may begin to demonstrate signs and symptoms of hyperadrenalism or Cushing syndrome.[2,9] The cushingoid person may complain of weight gain, round or moon-shaped face (Fig. 16-3), "buffalo hump" on back, abdominal striae, and acne. Other findings include hypertension, heart failure, osteoporosis, diabetes mellitus, impaired healing, and mental depression or psychosis.

Laboratory findings

Laboratory confirmation of adrenal insufficiency is accomplished by measuring the response of the adrenal glands to an infusion of ACTH. Cortisol and all of its various metabolites are collectively labeled as 17-hydroxycorticosteroids, and the level of 17-hydroxycorticosteroids is markedly decreased in a person with adrenal insufficiency.

MEDICAL MANAGEMENT

The person with Addison disease is usually treated by replacement of specific hormones that are lacking; most often these are glucocorticoids, mineralocorticoids, and occasionally androgens. The doses will vary from patient to patient. Successfully treated patients usually live normal lives; however, the problem requiring additional steroids to cope with the stress remains.

Acute adrenal crisis requires immediate treat-

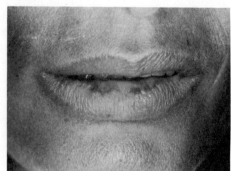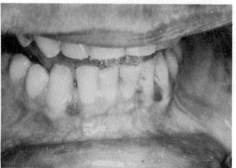

FIG. 16-2. Patient with Addison disease. Note bronzing of skin and pigmentation of lip, **A,** and oral mucosa, **B.**

ment. Therapy is based on fluid and electrolyte replacement, administration of glucocorticoids, and resolving the underlying stress that precipitated the event.

Patients who become cushingoid may require alteration of the steroid dosage to minimize the symptoms.

A variety of glucocorticoids are available, and the dental practitioner may encounter a number of these being taken by patients. Table 16-1 lists the strengths of the various glucocorticoids in common use as compared to hydrocortisone.

Patients with secondary adrenal suppression or

TABLE 16-1. Equivalent dosages of glucocorticoids to hydrocortisone

Compound	Antiinflammatory potency relative to hydrocortisone	Equivalent dosage to hydrocortisone (mg)
Hydrocortisone (cortisol)	1.0	20
Cortisone	0.8	25
Prednisone	4.0	5
Prednisolone	4.0	5
Dexamethasone	25.0	0.75

Adapted from Haynes, R.C., and Murad, F.: Adrenocorticotropic hormone: adrenocortical steroids and their synthetic analogs: inhibitors of adrenocortical steroids biosynthesis. In Gilman, A.G., et al., editors: Goodman and Gilman's the pharmacological basis of therapeutics, ed. 6, New York, 1980, Macmillan Publishing Co., Inc., p. 1482.

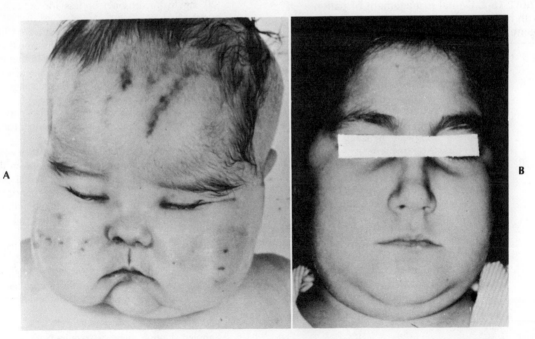

FIG. 16-3. Two patients with Cushing disease demonstrating rounded face and obesity. **A,** Congenital Cushing disease; **B,** acquired Cushing disease. (From Falace, D.A.: Medical considerations. In Wood, N.A., editor: Treatment planning: a pragmatic approach, St. Louis, 1978, The C.V. Mosby Co., p. 56.)

Addison disease do not tolerate stress well; this is the main concern during the delivery of dental treatment. A common treatment modification of steroid therapy is that of alternate-day therapy; that is, steroids are given in the morning of every other day instead of daily, but a double dose is given to maintain the patient's high serum level.[2,8,9] The rationale for this is that the cortisol level normally is high in the morning, thus a dose given at that time does not tend to suppress ACTH abnormally; whereas on the off day the adrenal-pituitary axis is allowed to function normally and produce endogenous steroids. The result is less adrenal suppression than is seen with daily therapy. Unfortunately, this technique is not uniformly successful, and many patients must return to daily therapy.

DENTAL MANAGEMENT
Medical considerations

The following suggestions are to be viewed as general guidelines for managing the dental treatment for individuals who are currently taking steroids or have taken steroids in the past year. *These guidelines are not intended to be definitive and may well need to be modified by the patient's physician.* Consultation and close cooperation with the patient's physician are absolutely essential before initiating treatment for these individuals.

For the purpose of discussion, patients may be divided into two management categories: patients who are currently taking steroids and patients with a past history of steroid use (Table 16-2).

I. Patients currently taking steroids
   When a patient is identified by history as currently taking steroids, inquiry should be made about the disease requiring steroid therapy, the length of time the patient has taken steroids, how often the steroids are taken, the name of the drug, and the dosage. The physician should then be contacted to verify this information and to discuss the patient's status and the proposed management scheme as follows.
   A. Patients taking equivalent of normal daily output (20 mg hydrocortisone) or less for at least a month
      This is an uncertain area, and the patient's adrenal reserve can only be determined by an ACTH challenge; therefore it must be assumed that the patient may have some degree of adrenal suppression. He should be treated as in category B unless the physician directs otherwise.
   B. Patients taking equivalent up to two times normal daily output (20 to 40 mg hydrocortisone) for at least a month
      Routine dental care may be accomplished after doubling the normal daily dose to be taken the morning of the appointment. Major dental procedures such as full-mouth extraction, periodontal surgery, or treatment of traumatic injuries may require hospitalization with parenteral steroids.
   C. Patients taking greater than equivalent of twice normal daily output (40 mg hydrocortisone)
      These patients probably already have adequate coverage with their normal dose of medication and would not usually require additional supplementation.
   D. Patients using topical steroids
      Supplementation may be required if steroids have been applied to large, inflamed areas and occlusive dressings used. The physician should make the determination.

TABLE 16-2. Dental management of patient with history of corticosteroid use (general guidelines)

I. Patients currently taking steroids
   A. Patients taking equivalent of normal daily output (20 mg hydrocortisone) or less for at least a month
      Probably safe to treat but because of variability dentist should assume some suppression and should treat patient as in category B unless physician directs otherwise
   B. Patients taking equivalent of up to two times normal daily output (20 to 40 mg hydrocortisone) for at least a month
      1. Double normal dose day of appointment
      2. Major procedures may require hospitalization
   C. Patients taking greater than equivalent of twice normal daily output (40 mg hydrocortisone)
      No additional medications usually needed
   D. Patients using topical steroids
      Consultation with physician
II. Patients with past history of steroid usage
   A. If no steroids taken in past 12 months, treat normally
   B. If steroids taken in past 12 months, consult physician and treat in appropriate category listed above

---

II. Patients with past history of steroid use

If a patient has not taken any steroids within the past 12 months and is doing well, no steroids are required and the patient may receive normal dental care. If steroids have been taken during the past 12 months, the physician should be consulted for treatment under the appropriate category in I.

Even though precautions are taken and patients are managed with increased steroid levels, the dentist should remain alert to the possibility of an acute adrenal crisis. Signs and symptoms of acute adrenal insufficiency include hypotension, weakness, nausea, vomiting, headache, and frequently fever. Immediate treatment of this problem consists of 100 mg hydrocortisone (Solu-Cortef), IV or IM, and transportation to a medical facility as soon as possible.

As a general rule, when treating patients with a history of present or past steroid usage, it is better to "overtreat" than to risk an acute adrenal crisis. Over short periods, increased amounts of steroids are safe.

Treatment planning modifications

No treatment planning modifications are required.

Oral complications

In primary adrenal insufficiency pigmentation of the oral mucous membranes is a common finding. Patients with secondary adrenal insufficiency may be prone to delayed healing and an increased susceptibility to infection.

Emergency dental care

Should a patient taking less than the equivalent of 40 mg/day of hydrocortisone have an acute dental need (for example, abscess) that will require immediate care (that is, pulpotomy incision and drainage or extraction), he may not be able to wait until his regular medications are available; therefore an acceptable plan is listed in Table 16-3. If the patient is taking the equivalent of more than 40 mg hydrocortisone daily, care should be provided in the normal manner, but the patient should be monitored closely.

TABLE 16-3. Emergency dental care for patient with probable adrenal suppression

100 to 200 mg of hydrocortisone, IM, 1 hour before procedure
Double normal daily dose day after procedure

REFERENCES

1. Dluhy, R.G., Lauler, D.P., and Thorn, G.W.: Pharmacology and chemistry of adrenal glucocorticoids, Med. Clin. North Am. **57:**1155-1165, 1973.
2. Dujovne, C.A., and Azarnoff, D.L.: Clinical complications of corticosteroid therapy, Med. Clin. North Am. **57:**1331-1342, 1973.
3. Gruenberg, J.C., and Mikhail, G.R.: Percutaneous adrenal suppression with topically applied corticosteroids, Arch. Surg. **111:**1165, 1976.
4. Guyton, A.C.: Textbook of medical physiology, ed. 6, Philadelphia, 1981, W.B. Saunders Co., pp. 944-958.
5. Haynes, R.C., and Murad, F.: Adrenocorticotropic hormone: adrenocortical steroids and their synthetic analogs; inhibitors of adrenocortical steroid biosynthesis. In Gilman, A.G., et al., editors: Goodman and Gilman's the pharmacologic basis of therapeutics, ed. 6, New York, 1980, Macmillan Publishing Co., pp. 1466-1496.
6. Liddle, G.W.: The adrenals. In Williams, R.H., editor: Textbook of endocrinology, ed. 6, Philadelphia, 1981, W.B. Saunders Co., pp. 249-292.
7. Maibach, H.I., and Stoughton, R.B.: Topical corticosteroids, Med. Clin. North Am. **57:**1253-1264, 1973.
8. Streeten, D.H.: Corticosteorid therapy. I. Pharmacological properties and principles of corticosteroid use, JAMA **232:**944-947, 1975.
9. Williams, G.H., et al.: Diseases of the adrenal cortex. In Thorn, G.W., et al., editors: Harrison's principles of internal medicine, ed. 9, New York, 1980, McGraw-Hill Book Co., pp. 1711-1736.

17

THYROID DISEASE

The patient with thyroid disease is of concern to the dentist from several aspects. The dentist may detect early signs and symptoms of thyroid disease and refer the patient for medical evaluation and treatment. In some cases this may be lifesaving, whereas in others the quality of life for the patient can be improved and complications of certain thyroid disorders avoided.

Patients with untreated thyrotoxicosis may be in great danger if surgical or operative procedures are performed by the dentist. Although uncommon, dental treatment may precipitate an acute medical emergency (thyrotoxic crisis or thyroid storm). Acute infections and trauma also may precipitate a thyrotoxic crisis in the untreated or inadequately treated patient.[1,2]

In this chapter the emphasis will be placed on disorders involving hyperfunction of the gland (thyrotoxicosis) and hypofunction of the gland (myxedema or cretinism).

GENERAL DESCRIPTION

The thyroid gland develops from the thyroglossal duct and possibly portions of the ultimobranchial body. It is located in the anterior portion of the neck just below and also lateral to the cricoid cartilage. It consists of two lateral lobes connected by an isthmus. In some individuals a superior portion of glandular tissue may be identified, the pyramidal lobe. Thyroid tissue may be found anywhere along the path of the thyroglossal duct from its origin, midline of the posterior portion of the tongue, to the location of the thyroid gland in the neck. However, in most individuals the remnants of the duct atrophy and disappear. Ectopic thyroid tissue may secrete thyroid hormones or become cystic or neoplastic. In a few individuals the only functional thyroid tissue may be in these ectopic locations.

The thyroid secretes three hormones—thyroxine (T_4), triiodothyronine (T_3), and calcitonin. The tissue developing from the ultimobranchial bodies is thought to give rise to the cells that produce calcitonin.

T_4 and T_3 are hormones that affect metabolic processes throughout the body and are involved with oxygen use. The secretion of T_4 and T_3 is controlled by the hypothalamus and pituitary gland by a classic negative feedback mechanism. As the serum level of the hormones decreases, the anterior pituitary gland releases a thyroid-stimulating hormone (TSH) that stimulates the secretion of T_4 and T_3 by the thyroid gland (Fig. 17-1).[1,2]

Iodine must be available for the synthesis of T_4 and T_3. The inorganic form of iodine is used by the gland and comes from the peripheral degradation and deiodination of thyroid hormone and the diet. Iodine is stored in the thyroid gland. It appears to be oxidized to a higher valence by a preoxidase, and then it combines with thyrosyl to form either monoiodotyrosine (MIT) or diiodotyrosine (DIT). These compounds then by an oxidative coupling reaction will form either T_4 or T_3.

In the blood, T_4 and T_3 are almost entirely bound to plasma proteins. The homeostatic regulation of hormone levels in the blood appears to be more directed to the concentration of free rather than bound hormone.[2]

Calcitonin is involved along with parathyroid hormone and vitamin D in regulating serum cal-

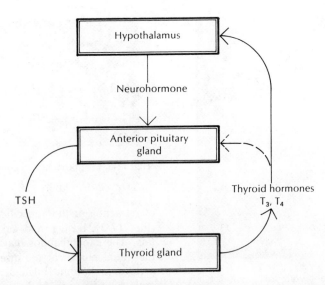

FIG. 17-1. Physiologic control of thyroid hormone secretion. Low levels of T₃ and T₄ will stimulate hypothalamus to release a neurohormone that triggers the anterior pituitary to release TSH, which stimulates thyroid to secrete thyroid hormones. Increased blood levels of T₃ and T₄ then inhibit further release of neurohormone.

cium and phosphorous levels and skeletal remodeling. This hormone and its actions will be considered in greater detail in Chapter 11.

THYROTOXICOSIS (HYPERTHYROIDISM)
Etiology, pathophysiology, and complications

The term *thyrotoxicosis* refers to the excess of T_4 and T_3 in the bloodstream. It may be caused by ectopic thyroid tissue, Graves disease, multinodular goiter, thyroid adenoma, or pituitary disease involving the anterior portion of the gland. In this section the signs and symptoms, laboratory tests, treatment, and dental considerations for the patient with Graves disease will be considered in detail and will serve as the model for other conditions that may result in similar clinical manifestations. It should be emphasized that multinodular goiter, ectopic thyroid tissue, and neoplastic causes of hyperthyroidism are very rare compared to toxic goiter (Graves disease).

Patients with Graves disease often show the presence in the serum of an immunobuin G called long-acting thyroid stimulator (LATS).[2] Tis-

sue culture of lymphocytes from patients with Graves disease stimulated with phytohemagglutinin produce LATS. LATS has been found in the serum of about two thirds of the patients with Graves disease. However, the level of LATS does not correlate with the severity of symptoms of the disease. In addition, infants whose mothers have Graves disease will show a transient period of goiter, ophthalmopathy, and clinical manifestations of the disease. As the clinical disease disappears, the level of serum LATS diminishes.

Recent studies have shown that LATS is a 7S immunoglobulin G produced by B lymphocytes. LATS will stimulate or induce thyroid hyperplasia and iodine accumulation in the thyroid glands, independent of the pituitary gland. A long-acting thyroid stimulator-protector (LATS-P), has been reported that prevents LATS from being neutralized. Graves disease is now considered to be an autoimmune disease.[4,5]

In contrast to the preceding data, a familial tendency has been noted for the transmission of this disorder. An increased incidence has been reported in monozygotic twins as compared to other twins.

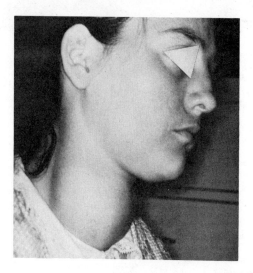

FIG. 17-2. Female patient with toxic goiter (Graves disease).

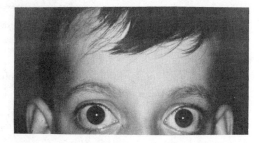

FIG. 17-3. Exophthalmos in child with Graves disease.

In addition, ^{131}I uptake tests have been shown to be increased in about 20% of the immediate relatives of patients with Graves disease, particularly in sisters and daughters.[2]

This disorder is much more common in women (7:1) and may manifest itself at puberty, pregnancy, or menopause (Fig. 17-2). Emotional stress, such as severe fright or separation from loved ones, has been reported to be associated with the onset of the disease. The disease may occur in a cyclic pattern and then "burn itself out" or continue in an active state.

Clinical presentation
SIGNS AND SYMPTOMS

The clinical picture in Graves disease is caused by direct and indirect effects of the excessive thyroid hormones.[1,2]

The patient's skin will be warm and moist. The complexion is rosy, and the patient may blush readily. Palmar erythema may be present. Excessive melanin pigmentation of the skin occurs in many patients. However, pigmentation of the oral mucosa has not been reported. Excessive sweating is common. The patient's hair becomes fine and friable, and the nails become soft and friable.

Most patients will show eye changes that consist of retraction of the upper lid, a bright-eyed stare (Fig. 17-3), lid lag, and jerky movements of the lids. The exophthalmos may be unilateral during the initial phases of the disease but usually progresses to become bilateral. Corneal ulceration, optic neuritis, and ocular muscle weakness may develop as complications in these patients.

The increased metabolic activity caused by excessive hormone secretion increases circulatory demands. An increased stroke volume and rate of the heart often develop. The pulse pressure is widened, and the patient often complains of palpitations. Supraventricular cardiac dysrhythmias develop in many patients. Congestive heart failure may occur and often is somewhat resistant to the effects of digitalis. Patients with thyrotoxicosis are much more sensitive to the actions of pressor amines, and great care must be used if these agents are administered to these patients.

Dyspnea not related to the effects of congestive heart failure may occur in some patients. The respiratory effect is caused by reduction in the vital capacity secondary to weakness of the respiratory muscles.

Weight loss even with an increased appetite is a common finding. The stool is poorly formed, and frequency of bowel movements is increased. Anorexia, nausea, and vomiting are rare, but when they occur may be the forerunners of thyroid storm. Gastric ulcers are rare in patients with thyrotoxicosis. Many of these patients have achlorhydria, and about 3% will develop pernicious anemia.

Thyrotoxic patients are nervous and often will show a great deal of emotional lability. They lose their tempers easily and cry often. Severe psychic reactions may occur. These patients cannot sit still and are always moving. A tremor of the hands, tongue, and lightly closed eyelids is often present. A generalized muscle weakness often occurs, and patients complain of easy fatigability.

The effect of the excessive thyroid hormones on mineral metabolism is complex and not well understood. In addition, the role of calcitonin only complicates the problem. However, thyrotoxic patients have an increased excretion of calcium and phosphorus in the urine and stool. Radiograms demonstrate increased bone loss. Hypercalcemia occurs on occasion, and the serum levels of alkaline phosphatase are usually normal. The bone age of young individuals is advanced (see Chapter 11).

Infection or severe emotional trauma have been suggested to act as a trigger for the onset of clinical manifestations of Graves disease.[2] These relationships are unclear at the present time. The role of oral foci of infection as an etiologic factor in Graves disease is unclear. Some evidence suggests that chronic oral infections may aggravate the symptoms of thyrotoxicosis.

The individual red blood cells in patients with thyrotoxicosis are usually normal. However, the red blood cell mass is increased to carry the additional oxygen needed for the increased metabolic activities. In addition to the increase in total numbers of circulating red blood cells, the bone marrow reveals an erythyroid hyperplasia. The requirements for vitamin B_{12} and folic acid are increased. The white blood cell count may be decreased because of a reduction in the number of neutrophils. The absolute number of eosinophils may be increased. Spleen and lymph node enlargement occurs in some patients. The platelets and clotting mechanism are normal.

The increased metabolic activities associated with thyrotoxicosis lead to increased secretion and breakdown of cortisol, but the serum levels remain within normal limits.

LABORATORY FINDINGS

Thyroid hormone levels in the serum can be measured directly or indirectly. The basal metabolic rate can be used to estimate the amount of free hormone by measuring the rate of oxygen consumption under basal conditions. This test is not used as commonly now because more accurate methods are available to determine hormone levels.

The protein-bound iodine concentration in blood can be measured. Although this test does not measure the concentration of free hormone, the results correlate well with the metabolic status of the patient. The normal level is 4 to 8 μg/100 ml. Values greater than 8 μg/100 ml indicate thyrotoxicosis, whereas reduced levels of free hormone suggest myxedema or cretinism.[1,2]

The uptake of ingested ^{131}I by the thyroid gland can be measured by radioactive scanning procedures. The normal uptake is 15% to 50%. Uptake values greater than 50% suggest hyperthyroidism, whereas values less than 15% suggest hypothyroidism.[1,2]

Other tests are available, such as the thyroid suppression test, thyrotropin stimulation test, hormone binding tests, and serum T_3 and T_4 measurements using various techniques. The reader is referred to a textbook of endocrinology for details concerning these and other thyroid tests.

Medical management

Treatment of patients with thyrotoxicosis may involve antithyroid agents that block hormone synthesis, iodides, radioactive iodine, or subtotal thyroidectomy. The most common antithyroid agents used are propylthiouracil and methimazole. Patients being treated with the antithyroid agents often will be given USP thyroid. The usual length of treatment is 18 to 24 months. The antithyroid agents may cause a mild leukopenia, but drug therapy is not stopped unless the white count is more severely depressed. If exophthalmos is present it follows a course independent of the therapeutic metabolic response to antithyroid treatment modalities. The exophthalmos is usually irreversible.

Management of thyrotoxic crisis

Patients with thyrotoxicosis who are untreated or incompletely treated may develop thyrotoxic crisis.[1,2] This is a very serious complication but fortunately a rare one. It may occur at any age and has an abrupt onset. Precipitating factors are infections, trauma, surgical emergencies, and operations. Early symptoms are extreme restlessness, nausea, vomiting, and abdominal pain. Fever, profuse sweating, marked tachycardia, pulmonary edema, and congestive heart failure soon develop. The patient appears to be in a stupor, and coma may follow. Severe hypotension develops, and death may occur. These reactions appear to be associated at least in part with adrenocortical insufficiency.

Immediate treatment of the patient in thyrotoxic crisis consists of large doses of antithyroid drugs (200 mg of propylthiouracil), potassium iodide, propranolol (to antagonize the adrenergic component), hydrocortisone (100 to 300 mg), IV glucose solution, vitamin B complex, wet packs, fans, and ice packs.[1,2]

HYPOTHYROIDISM

Hypothyroidism is a rare condition. One out of about every 1500 hospital admissions is for this condition. Adult hypothyroidism (myxedema) is five times more common in women and most common between the ages of 30 and 60 years. Childhood hypothyroidism is termed *cretinism*.[1,2]

Hypothyroidism can be congenital or acquired. The acquired form may follow thyroid gland or pituitary gland failure. Radiation of the thyroid gland, surgical removal, and excessive antithyroid drug therapy may cause hypothyroidism. Some cases of the disease appear with no identifiable cause.

Neonatal cretinism is characterized by dwarfism, overweight, broad flat nose, eyes set apart, thick lips, large protruding tongue, poor muscle tone, pale skin, stubby hands, retarded bone age, delayed eruption of teeth, malocclusions, a hoarse cry, umbilical hernia, and mental retardation that can be avoided with early detection and treatment (Fig. 17-4).

Hypothyroidism having its onset in older children and adults is characterized by a dull expression, puffy eyelids, alopecia (hair loss) of the outer third of the eyebrows, palmar yellowing, dry rough skin, dry brittle and coarse hair, increased size of tongue, slowing of physical and mental activity, slurred hoarse speech, anemia, constipation, increased sensitivity to cold, increased capillary fragility, muscle weakness, and deafness.

The accumulation of subcutaneous fluid usually is not as pronounced in patients with pituitary myxedema as in those with primary (thyroid) myxedema. The cholesterol serum levels are

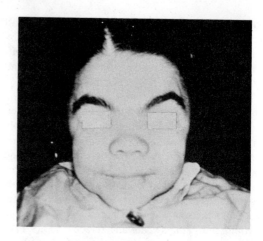

FIG. 17-4. Cretinism.

closer to normal values in the patients with pituitary myxedema. Untreated patients with severe myxedema may develop hypothermic coma that is usually fatal.

Laboratory tests reveal a low basal metabolic rate, increased serum cholesterol levels, a low protein-bound iodine concentration, and a depressed uptake of radioactive iodine.

Patients with untreated hypothyroidism are sensitive to the actions of narcotics, barbiturates, and tranquilizers, and these drugs must be used with care. Stressful situations such as cold, operations, infections, or trauma may precipitate a hypothyroid (myxedema) coma. This condition is treated by parenteral T_3, steroids, and artificial respiration.

Myxedema coma occurs most often in very severe hypothyroid elderly patients.[1,2] It is more common during the winter months and has a high mortality. The condition is characterized by hypothermia, bradycardia, and severe hypotension, and epileptic seizures may occur during the comatose state. Patients with hypothyroidism are treated with either synthetic thyroid hormone or thyroprotein derived from animal thyroid glands.

DENTAL MANAGEMENT
Clinical examination

The clinical examination of the thyroid gland should be part of the head and neck examination performed by the dentist. The anterior neck region

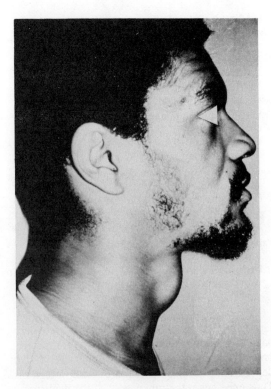

FIG. 17-5. Patient with thyroglossal duct cyst.

TABLE 17-1. Dental management of thyrotoxic patient

Detection of patient
  Symptoms
  Signs
Avoidance in untreated or poorly treated patient
  Surgical or operative procedures
  Acute infection
  Epinephrine and other pressor amines
Recognition and management of initial therapy of crisis
  Wet packs, ice packs
  Hydrocortisone
  IV glucose solution
  Cardiopulmonary resuscitation
  Seeking medical aid
Patient under good medical treatment
  Avoidance of acute oral infections
  Treatment of all chronic oral infections
  Preceeding with normal procedures and management

should be examined for indications of old surgical scars. The posterior dorsal region of the tongue should be examined for a nodule that could represent lingual thyroid tissue. The area just superior and lateral to the cricoid cartilage should be palpated for the presence of a pyramidal lobe. Although difficult to detect, the normal thyroid gland can be palpated in many patients.[2] It feels rubbery to palpation and can more easily be identified by asking the patient to swallow during the examination. As the patient swallows, the thyroid gland will be raised. Lumps found in the neck that may be associated with the thyroid will also rise (move superiorly) with swallowing. An enlarged gland caused by hyperplasia (goiter) will feel softer than the normal gland. Adenomas and carcinomas involving the gland will be firmer to palpation and will usually be seen as isolated swellings in the gland. Patients with Hashimoto disease or Riedel thyroiditis will reveal a gland that is much firmer to palpation than the normal gland.

Nodules found in the midline in the area of the thyroglossal duct will move upward with protraction of the patient's tongue (Fig. 17-5).

If a diffuse enlargement of the thyroid is detected, auscultation should be employed to examine for a systolic or continuous bruit that can be heard over the hyperactive gland of thyrotoxicosis or Graves disease as a result of engorgement of the vascular system in the gland.

Medical considerations (Table 17-1)
THYROTOXICOSIS

The dentist should be aware of the clinical manifestations of thyrotoxicosis so that patients with undiagnosed and poorly treated disease states can be detected and referred for medical evaluation and treatment. By doing this the morbidity and mortality associated with thyrotoxicosis can be reduced.

Palpation and inspection of the thyroid gland should be part of the routine head and neck examination performed by the dentist. If a thyroid enlargement is noted, even if the patient appears euthyroid, the patient should be referred for further evaluation before further dental treatment is rendered. A diffuse enlargement may be simple goiter or subacute thyroiditis. Isolated nodules may turn out to be adenomas or carcinomas.

Patients with untreated or poorly treated thyrotoxicosis are susceptible to developing an acute medical emergency—thyrotoxic crisis. This is another very important reason for detection and referral of these patients for medical management. If surgical procedures are performed on these patients, a crisis can be precipitated. In addition, acute oral infections in these patients may precipitate a crisis. If a crisis should occur, the dentist should be able to recognize what is happening, begin emergency treatment, and seek immediate medical assistance. The dentist can cool the patient with cold towels, administer hydrocortisone (100 to 300 mg), start an IV flow of hypertonic glucose (if equipment is available), and monitor the patient's vital signs and be prepared to initiate cardiopulmonary resuscitation if indicated. Immediate medical assistance should be sought, and when available, other measures such as antithyroid drugs and potassium iodide can be started.

Although the role of chronic infection and thyrotoxicosis is unclear, it is recommended that these foci be treated in these patients as in any other patient. Once the patient has been detected and referred for medical management, the treatment of the oral foci of infection should be accomplished.

Patients with extensive dental caries or periodontal disease or both can be treated after medical management of the thyroid problem has been effected.

The use of epinephrine or other pressor amines must be avoided in the untreated or poorly treated thyrotoxic patient. These patients are very sensitive to the effects of these agents. However, the well-treated thyrotoxic patient presents no problem in this regard and may be given normal concentrations of vasoconstrictors.

Once the thyrotoxic patient is under good medical management, the dental treatment plan will be unaffected. However, if acute oral infection should occur in these patients, consultation with the patient's physician is recommended as part of the management program.

HYPOTHYROIDISM

In general the patient with mild symptoms of hypothyroidism who is untreated is not in danger when receiving dental therapy. However, a few patients with untreated severe symptoms of hypothyroidism may be in danger if dental treatment is

TABLE 17-2. Dental management of hypothyroid patient

Detection of patient
  Symptoms
  Signs

Avoidance in untreated or poorly treated patients
  Surgical or operative procedures
  Oral infections
  Central nervous system depressants—narcotics, barbiturates, etc.

Recognition and management of initial stages of myxedema coma
  Hydrocortisone (100 to 300 mg)
  Artificial respiration
  Seeking immediate medical aid

Patient under good medical management
  Avoidance of acute oral infections
  Proceeding with normal procedures and management

---

rendered. This is particularly true of the elderly patients with myxedema. A myxedema coma can be precipitated by the use of central nervous system depressants, surgical procedures, and infections. Thus once again the major goal of the dentist is to detect these patients and refer them for medical management before any dental treatment is rendered (Table 17-2).

Patients with less severe forms of hypothyroidism also should be identified when possible, because the quality of their life can be greatly improved with medical treatment, and in very young individuals permanent mental retardation can be avoided with early medical management. In addition, oral complications of delayed eruption of teeth, malocclusion, enlargement of the tongue, and skeletal retardation can be prevented with early detection and medical treatment.

Once the hypothyroid patient is under good medical care, no special problems are presented in terms of dental management except for dealing with the malocclusion and enlarged tongue if present.

Treatment planning modifications

No treatment planning modifications are required as long as the medical problems are well controlled.

Oral complications

THYROTOXICOSIS

Osteoporosis may be found involving the alveolar bone. Dental caries and periodontal disease appear to develop more rapidly in these patients. The teeth and jaws develop more rapidly, and premature loss of the deciduous teeth with early eruption of the permanent teeth is common. Euthyroid (normal thyroid function) infants of hyperthyroid mothers have been reported to have erupted teeth at birth. A few patients with thyrotoxicosis have been found to have lingual "thyroid" consisting of thyroid tissue below the area of the foramen caecum.[3]

If the dentist detects a lingual tumor in a euthyroid patient, the patient should be evaluated by a physician for the presence of a normal thyroid gland before the mass is surgically removed. This is usually done with radioactive iodine scanning.

HYPOTHYROIDISM

Infants with cretinism may demonstrate thick lips, enlarged tongue, delayed eruption of teeth, and resulting malocclusion.[3] The only specific oral change manifested by adults with acquired hypothyroidism is an enlarged tongue.

Emergency dental care

In a patient with untreated thyroid disease (hyperthyroid or hypothyroid), emergency treatment should consist of:
1. Pain control with analgesics (nonnarcotic)
2. Infection control with antibiotics
3. Immediate referral to a physician

In patients with treated and controlled thyroid disease, any treatment that is necessary should be rendered.

REFERENCES

1. Barnes, H.V.: The thyroid gland. In Harvey, A., editor: Osler's the principles and practice of medicine, ed. 19, New York, 1976, Appleton-Century-Crofts, pp. 1072-1108.
2. Ingbar, S.H., and Woeber, K.A.: The thyroid gland. In Williams, R.H., editor: Textbook of endocrinology, ed. 5, Philadelphia, 1974, W.B. Saunders Co., pp. 95-227.
3. Miller, M.F.: Diseases of the endocrine organs. In Lynch, M.A., editor: Burket's oral medicine, diagnosis and treatment, ed. 7, Philadelphia, 1977, J.B. Lippincott Co., pp. 443-470.
4. Ingbar, S.H., and Woeber, K.A.: Diseases of the thyroid. In Petersdorf, R.G., et al., editors: Harrisons principles of internal medicine, ed. 10, New York, 1983, McGraw-Hill Book Co., pp. 614-634.
5. Nikolai, T.F.: The thyroid gland. In Rose, L.F., and Kaye, D.: Internal medicine for dentistry, St. Louis, 1983, The C.V. Mosby Co., pp. 1126-1153.

18

PREGNANCY AND BREAST-FEEDING

The pregnant patient, though not "medically compromised," poses a unique set of management problems for the dentist. Therapeutic dental care must be rendered to the mother without adversely affecting the fetus. Although providing routine dental care to pregnant patients is generally safe, it must be recognized that the delivery of dental care involves some potentially harmful elements, including ionizing radiation, drug administration, pain, and stress. Thus the prudent practitioner minimizes exposure to potentially harmful procedures or avoids them altogether.

Additional considerations arise during the postpartum period if the mother elects to breast-feed her infant. Most drugs are transmitted from the maternal serum to the breast milk, so the infant is exposed to these compounds. Obviously, the dentist should avoid any drug known to be harmful to the infant.

GENERAL DESCRIPTION

To define rational management guidelines, it is first necessary to review the normal occurrences of pregnancy and fetal development.

Endocrine changes are the most significant basic changes that occur with pregnancy, and they result in most of the systemic alterations with which we will be concerned. An increase occurs in the production of maternal hormones, and placental hormones begin to be produced.

Common neurologic findings in the first trimester include fatigue and hyperemesis (nausea and vomiting). There is also a tendency for syncope and postural hypotension. During the second trimester, the patient may demonstrate a sense of well-being and have relatively few symptoms. During the third trimester, increasing fatigue and mild depression may be seen.[12]

Cardiovascular changes are varied. There is commonly a slight decrease in blood pressure. Blood volume increases approximately 45% to 50%, and cardiac output increases 20% to 30%. Corresponding to these volume changes are tachycardia and functional heart murmurs. There may also be dyspnea at rest that is aggravated by a supine position.[11-13]

During late pregnancy, a phenomenon known as supine hypotensive syndrome or vena cava syndrome may occur in about 10% of patients. This syndrome is manifested by an abrupt fall in blood pressure and a sudden loss of consciousness that occur when the patient is in a supine position. It is caused by impairment of venous return to the heart by the compression of the inferior vena cava by the gravid uterus. The impairment results in decreased blood pressure, decreased cardiac output, and loss of consciousness. The remedy for the problem is to roll the patient over to her side to lift the uterus off the vena cava. The patient should rapidly regain consciousness (Fig. 18-1).

Hematologic changes in pregnancy include a decreased hematocrit and anemia.[11-13] Because of the increased blood volume, there is a marked need for additional iron; it is not surprising that 20% of

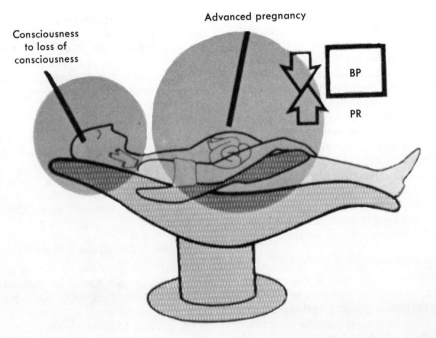

FIG. 18-1. Supine hypotensive syndrome of late pregnancy. (From Falace, D.A.: Medical considerations. In Wood, N.A., editor: Treatment planning: a pragmatic approach, St. Louis, 1978, The C.V. Mosby Co., p. 61.)

pregnant women have some degree of iron deficiency.[12] These problems are exaggerated after significant blood loss.

Pregnancy sometimes predisposes to increased appetite and an appetite for unusual foods. As a result the diet may not be nutritious or balanced and may be high in sugars.

The general pattern of fetal development should also be understood when formulating dental management principles. Briefly, normal pregnancy lasts approximately 40 weeks. During the first trimester, formation of organs and systems occurs; thus the fetus is most susceptible to malformation during this period. After the first trimester, formation has been completed, and the remainder of fetal development is devoted to growth and maturation. Thus the chances of malformation are markedly diminished after the first trimester. A notable exception to this is dental staining caused by administration of tetracycline during pregnancy.

Another consideration relating to fetal growth is spontaneous abortion (miscarriage). Spontaneous abortion—the natural termination of pregnancy before the twentieth week of gestation—occurs in approximately 10% to 20% of all pregnancies.[6] Even though it is unlikely that a dental procedure could induce spontaneous abortion, it is wise to avoid any procedure during the first trimester and thus avoid any questionable relationship if spontaneous abortion occurs. Factors to be avoided include radiographs, drugs, chemicals, and stress. Additionally, it is known that febrile illnesses and sepsis can precipitate miscarriage; therefore prompt treatment of infection is advised.

Finally, it must be kept in mind that the fetus has a limited ability to metabolize drugs because of its immature liver and immature enzymatic system.

DENTAL MANAGEMENT
Medical considerations

Management recommendations during pregnancy should be viewed as general guidelines and not as hard-and-fast rules. If at all possible the first step in dental management should be to contact the patient's obstetrician or physician to discuss the patient's medical status, her dental needs, and the dentist's proposed plan of treatment. This is not only beneficial from the standpoint of planning treatment, but it also demonstrates to the patient your caring and concern about her and her baby from a total-health point of view.

Pregnancy is a very special event in a person's life and as such is emotionally charged. Therefore establishment of a good patient-dentist relationship that encourages openness, honesty, and trust is an integral part of successful patient management. This kind of relationship greatly decreases stress and anxiety for both patient and dentist.

PREVENTIVE PROGRAM

The most important objective in planning dental treatment for the pregnant patient is to establish a healthy oral environment and an optimum oral hygiene level. This essentially consists of a plaque control program, which will minimize the exaggerated inflammatory response of gingival tissues to local irritants that commonly accompanies the hormonal changes of pregnancy. The relationship of plaque and other local irritants, hormonal alterations, and periodontal disease is well known and should be clearly explained to the patient. Acceptable oral hygiene techniques should be taught, reinforced, and monitored throughout pregnancy. Coronal scaling and polishing or root curettage may be performed whenever necessary. All of these control measures should be stressed throughout pregnancy, including the first trimester.

The question of the benefits of prenatal fluoride frequently arises, and until recently no good evidence existed to support its use. However, in one excellent study of 492 children by Glenn et al.[7] it was shown that when a daily 2.2 mg tablet of sodium fluoride was administered to mothers during the second and third trimesters in combination with fluoridated water, the offspring were virtually free of caries for up to 10 years. In addition to the elimination of caries, the prematurity rate was significantly reduced, there were slight increases in height and birth weight. There was no evidence of medical or dental defects (including fluorosis) in any of the children. Therefore it was concluded that fluoride tablet supplementation from the third through the ninth month of pregnancy is safe and effective.[5]

TREATMENT TIMING (Table 18-1)

Other than a good plaque control program, no elective dental care should be undertaken during the first trimester because of the vulnerability of the fetus.

The second trimester is the safest period in which to provide routine dental care. Even though this is a relatively safe period, it is advisable to limit care to routine treatment, such as simple operative procedures. Emphasis should be placed on controlling active disease and eliminating potential problems that could occur late in pregnancy or immediately after, because dental care during these periods is difficult. Extensive reconstructive procedures or significant surgical procedures should be postponed if possible until after delivery. It should be borne in mind that there is no rush, because prenancy is a temporary condition.

The early part of the third trimester is still a relatively good time to provide routine dental care, but after the middle of the third trimester, no elec-

TABLE 18-1. Treatment timing during pregnancy

First trimester	Second trimester	Third trimester
Plaque control	Plaque control	Plaque control
Oral hygiene instruction	Oral hygiene instruction	Oral hygiene instruction
Scaling/polishing/curettage	Scaling/polishing/curettage	Scaling/polishing/curettage
Emergency care only ------------------------------Routine dental care --------------------------------Emergency care only		
No elective treatment		

tive dental care is advisable. This is because of the increasing feeling of discomfort of the mother. Prolonged chair time should be avoided to prevent the complication of supine hypotensive syndrome. This can be done by scheduling short appointments, allowing the patient to assume a semireclining position, and encouraging frequent changes of position.

DENTAL RADIOGRAPHS

Dental radiography is one of the more controversial areas in the management of the pregnant patient. It is most desirable not to have any irradiation during pregnancy, especially during the first trimester, because the developing fetus is particularly susceptible to radiation damage. However, should dental treatment become necessary, radiographs will generally be needed to provide an accurate diagnosis and to plan proper treatment. Therefore the dentist must be aware of how to proceed safely in this situation.

The safety of dental radiography has been well established, provided features such as high-speed film, filtration, collimation, and lead apron are used. Of all aids the most important in the case of the pregnant patient is the protective lead apron, because studies have shown that when it is used during dental radiography, gonadal radiation is virtually unmeasurable.[2,14]

The dentist should keep in perspective the scope of this problem. Brent[4] has stated that an absorbed dose of 10 rads is the threshold dose for radiation-induced genetic damage. Accepting this figure as the ultimate danger point, some comparisons are revealing. Table 18-2 compares the amount of radiation received from various medical and dental x-ray examinations to the cosmic radiation one receives from living on the face of the earth for 1 day. From these figures, it is evident that with use of the lead apron, one or two intraoral films are truly of no significance in terms of radiation to the fetus.

Even in light of the obvious safety of these procedures, the dentist should not be cavalier in the approach to x-ray examinations during pregnancy (or any other time for that matter). X-rays should be used selectively and only when appropriate to aid in diagnosis and treatment. Therefore when modern x-ray techniques including the lead apron

are used, the dentist can safely make the examinations that he or she considers absolutely necessary to render proper dental care during pregnancy. In most instances the type of dental care recommended can be accomplished using only bitewings, a panoramic film, or selected periapical films.

Drug administration
DURING PREGNANCY

Another controversial area in treating pregnant dental patients is drug administration. The principal concern is that a given drug may cross the placenta and be toxic to the fetus or be teratogenic. Also, any drug that is a respiratory depressant can cause maternal hypoxia, resulting in fetal hypoxia, injury, or death. Thus it is critical to avoid periods of hypoxia in the mother.

It is best that no drugs be administered during pregnancy, especially in the first trimester; however, it is sometimes impossible to adhere to this rule. It is therefore fortunate that most of the commonly used drugs in dental practice can be used with relative safety, with a few notable exceptions. Table 18-3 is a suggested approach to drug use for pregnant patients.

As an additional aid to the dentist who wishes to prescribe or administer a drug to a pregnant patient, the Food and Drug Administration[10] has

TABLE 18-2. Comparative radiation exposures to gonadal or genetic tissues

Source of radiation	Exposure
Chest x-ray film	.001 to .010 rad; .070 to 2.0 rad with fluoroscopy
Lower gastrointestinal series	.350 to 6.00 rad; higher with fluoroscopy
Intravenous pyelogram	.400 to 2.0 rad
Daily background radiation	.0004 rad
Full-mouth dental x-ray examination (18 intraoral films); D film, *lead apron*	.00001 rad

Adapted from Bean, L.R., Jr., and Devore, W.D.: The effects of protective aprons in dental roentgenography, Oral Med. **28:** 505, 1969.

TABLE 18-3. Dental drug administration in pregnancy

Drug	First trimester	Second and third trimester
Local anesthetics		
Lidocaine	Yes	Yes
Mepivacaine	Yes	Yes
Analgesics		
Aspirin	Yes	Yes, but avoid in late third trimester
Acetaminophen	Yes	Yes
Codeine	Yes	Yes
Phenacetin	No	No
Antibiotics		
Penicillin	Yes	Yes
Erythromycin	Yes	Yes
Tetracycline	No	No
Streptomycin	No	No
Sedatives/hypnotics		
Nitrous oxide with 50% oxygen	No	Yes
Diazepam	No	No
Barbiturates	No	No

adopted a format of categorizing prescription drugs for pregnant patients based on their risk of causing fetal injury. This format will be required on prescription drug information by November, 1984.

Briefly, the format is as follows:

A = Controlled studies in humans fail to demonstrate a risk to the fetus, and the possibility of fetal harm appears remote.

B = Animal studies do not indicate fetal risk and there are no human studies, *or* animal studies show a risk but controlled human studies do not.

C = Animal studies have shown a risk but there are no controlled human studies, *or* no studies are available in humans or animals.

D = Positive evidence of human fetal risk exists, but in certain situations the drug may be used despite its risk.

X = Positive evidence of human fetal risk exists, and the risk outweighs any possible benefit of use.

Obviously, drugs in category A or B would be preferable for prescribing.

It should be recognized that individual physicians may advise against the use of some of the preferred drugs or, conversely, may suggest the use of a contraindicated drug. The listed guidelines are general ones. An example of the occasional use of a contraindicated drug would be IV sedation with diazepam or a narcotic for a frightened patient or a patient in severe pain.

Although it is unlikely that a single administration of nitrous oxide would be teratogenic, the drug is not recommended during the first trimester. This recommendation is based on findings in animal studies relating chronic nitrous oxide administration and birth defects. Although these results cannot be extrapolated to humans, it seems prudent to avoid nitrous oxide use during organogenesis.[5] If nitrous oxide is used in the second or third trimester, at least 50% oxygen should be delivered to ensure adequate oxygenation at all times. Special precautions should also be taken to avoid diffusion hypoxia at the termination of nitrous oxide administration. An additional consideration is for the female dentist or dental auxiliary who is pregnant. It is advisable that she not be exposed to persistent trace levels of nitrous oxide in the operatory, because this may be associated with increased incidence of spontaneous abortion.[5]

DURING BREAST-FEEDING

A perplexing problem for the dentist arises when a nursing mother requires the administration of a drug in the course of dental treatment. The concern is that the administered drug will find its way into breast milk and be transferred to the nursing infant, in whom exposure may result in adverse effects.

Unfortunately, the data on which to draw definite conclusions about drug dosage and effects via breast milk are sparse; however, retrospective clinical studies and empiric observations coupled with known pharmacologic pathways allow recommendations to be made. A significant known fact is that the amount of drug excreted in breast milk is usually not more than 1% to 2% of the maternal dose; therefore it is highly unlikely that most drugs are of any pharmacologic significance to the infant.[5]

Agreement seems to exist that a few drugs, or categories of drugs, are definitely contraindicated

TABLE 18-4. Dental drug administration during breast-feeding

Drug	Compatible with breast-feeding
Local anesthetics	
Lidocaine	Yes
Mepivacaine	Yes
Analgesics	
Aspirin	Yes, but in occasional therapeutic doses
Acetaminophen	Yes
Codeine	Yes
Antibiotics	
Penicillin	Yes; however, development of sensitivity should be considered; may affect gastrointestinal flora
Erythromycin	Yes; however, development of sensitivity should be considered; may affect gastrointestinal flora
Tetracycline	No; may cause dental discoloration; may affect gastrointestinal flora
Streptomycin	No; may cause deafness
Cephalosporins	Yes; however, development of sensitivity should be considered; may affect gastrointestinal flora
Sedatives	
Nitrous oxide	Yes
Diazepam	Yes, but in small, occasional doses
Barbiturates	Yes

Adapted from Platzker, A.C.D., et al.: Drug "administration" via breast milk, Hosp. Pract. 15:111-117, 1980.

for nursing mothers. These include lithium, anticancer drugs, radioactive pharmaceuticals, phenindione, chloramphenicol, and isoniazid[1,3,9,15] Table 18-4 is a compilation of recommendations regarding administration of commonly used dental drugs during breast-feeding. As with drug use in pregnancy, individual physicians may wish to modify these recommendations. As such the recommendations shown in Table 18-4 should be viewed as general guidelines for treatment.

In addition to careful drug selection for the nursing mother, it is desirable for the mother to take the drug just after breast-feeding and then to avoid nursing for 4 hours or more if possible. This will markedly decrease the drug concentration in the breast milk.[3]

Treatment planning modifications

There are no technical modifications required for the pregnant patient. However, reconstructive procedures, crown and bridge procedures, and significant surgical procedures are best delayed until after pregnancy.

Oral complications

The most common oral complication of pregnancy (found in essentially 100% of patients) is a marked increase in gingival inflammation, which represents an exaggerated inflammatory response to local irritants as a result of hormonal influence. This is frequently labeled "pregnancy gingivitis" (Fig. 18-2). On occasion a pyogenic granuloma may result as an exaggerated localized inflammatory hyperplastic tissue response; this is called a "pregnancy tumor" (Fig. 18-3). Gingival changes become apparent around the second month and continue until the eighth month, at which time the gingival tissues rapidly return to normal.[8] It should be stressed that pregnancy does not cause periodontal disease but modifies and worsens that which is already present.

The relationship between dental caries and pregnancy is not well defined; however, evidence suggests that pregnancy does not directly contribute to the carious process. More than likely, an increase in caries activity can be attributed to poor oral hygiene, which is commonly the result of sore, inflamed gingival tissues.

Many people are convinced that pregnancy causes tooth loss ("a tooth for every pregnancy") or that calcium is withdrawn from the maternal dentition to supply fetal requirements ("soft teeth"). Calcium is present in the teeth in a stable crystalline form and as such is not available to the systemic circulation to supply a calcium demand. On the other hand, calcium is readily mobilized from bone to supply these demands. Therefore calcium supplementation for the purpose of preventing tooth loss or "soft teeth" is unwarranted; however, the physician may prescribe calcium for general nutritional requirements of mother and infant.

A final dental finding is tooth mobility, which may be generalized. This sign is probably related

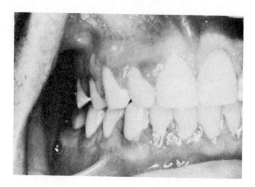

FIG. 18-2. Generalized gingivitis in woman in sixth month of pregnancy—"pregnancy gingivitis."

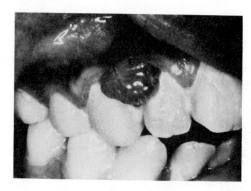

FIG. 18-3. Pyogenic granuloma occurring during pregnancy—"pregnancy tumor."

to the degree of gingival disease and disturbance of the attachment apparatus as well as some mineral changes of the lamina dura. The condition is reversible after delivery.

Emergency dental care

Should it become necessary to provide acute or nonelective care at any time during pregnancy, the practitioner should not hesitate to render whatever is necessary. As stated earlier, it is unlikely that dental procedures would cause any significant problem for the mother or fetus; however, the stress and effects of pain or infection could be detrimental and thus should be effectively treated. In essence, this means doing what must be done to remedy the dental problem while adhering to management guidelines as much as possible. The physician should be consulted before treatment is begun.

REFERENCES

1. American Academy of Pediatrics Committee on Drugs: Psychotropic drugs in pregnancy and lactation, Pediatrics **69:**241-244, 1982.
2. Bean, L.R., Jr., and Devore, W.D.: The effects of protective aprons in dental roentgenography, Oral Med. **28:**505-508, 1969.
3. Berlin, C.M.: Pharmacologic considerations of drug use in the lactating mother, Obstet. Gynecol. **58**(suppl.):1755-2355, 1981.
4. Brent, R.L.: Environmental factors: radiation. In Brent, R.L., and Harris, M.I., editors: Prevention of embryonic, fetal and perinatal disease, Fogarty International Center series on preventive medicine, vol. 3, DHEW Pub. No. 76-853, pp. 179-197, 1976.
5. Bussard, D.A.: Congenital anomalies and inhalation anesthetics, J. Am. Dent. Assoc. **93:**606-609, 1976.
6. Cavanagh, D., and Comes, M.R.: Spontaneous abortion. In Danforth, D.N., editor: Obstetrics and gynecology, ed. 4, Hagerstown, Md., 1982, Harper & Row, Publishers, Inc., pp. 378-392.
7. Glenn, F.B., et al.: Fluoride tablet supplementation during pregnancy for caries immunity: a study of the offspring produced, Am. J. Obstet. Gynecol. **143:**560-564, 1982.
8. Loe, H.: Periodontal changes in pregnancy, J. Periodontol. **36:**209-217, 1965.
9. Platzker, A.C.D., et al.: Drug "administration" via breast milk, Hosp. Pract. **15:**111-117, 1980.
10. Pregnancy categories for prescription drugs, FDA Drug Bull. **12**(3):26, 1982.
11. Pritchard, J.A., and MacDonald, P.C.: Williams obstetrics, ed. 16, New York, 1980, Appleton-Century-Crofts., pp. 221-260.
12. Quilligan, E.J.: Maternal physiology. In Danforth, D.N., editor: Obstetrics and gynecology, ed. 3, Hagerstown, Md., 1977, Harper & Row, Publishers, Inc.
13. Sexton, J., et al.: Surgery in a gravid patient, J. Oral Surg. **36:**878-886, 1978.
14. Warheit, A.: Dental roentgenology in the obstetric patient, Clin. Obstet. Gynecol. **9:**71-74, 1966.
15. Wilson, J.T., et al.: Drug excretion in human breast milk: principles, pharmacokinetics, and projected consequences, Clin. Pharmokinet. **5:**1-66, 1980.

19

ALLERGY

There are primarily three reasons why it is important for the dentist to know about allergy. First, oral soft-tissue changes may be caused by an allergic reaction. Second, acute medical emergencies may occur in the dental office because of an allergic reaction. Third, patients who have severe alterations of their immune system because of radiation or drug therapy may need dental care. The dentist must be able to identify and manage each of these problems and thus must have a basic understanding of allergy.

GENERAL DESCRIPTION
Incidence and etiology

Two types of lymphocytes are involved in the immune system, thymic-mediated lymphocytes (T cells) with the cellular component, and lymphocytes not "processed" by the thymus (B cells) with the humoral portion.

T cells can be differentiated from B cells by various laboratory techniques (Table 19-1). Based on these methods it has been estimated that about 60% to 80% of the circulating lymphocytes in blood are T cells. When certain foreign materials (antigens) are introduced into the body, unsensitized B cells may be transformed into lymphoblasts under the influence of macrophages and T cells that act as helper cells (Table 19-2). The lymphoblasts then divide into a plasma cell and a sensitized B cell or memory cell. The plasma cell then produces antibodies that are specific for the involved antigen. These antibodies are released into the bloodstream and circulate or become fixed to mast cells in various locations in the body. The memory B cells can differentiate into plasma cells on future contact with the antigen and produce specific antibodies.

Other types of foreign material such as certain bacteria will, when introduced into the body, affect unsensitized T cells to become lymphoblasts. These will divide into an effector cell and a sensitized T cell or memory cell (Table 19-3). Future contact with the antigen will transform the sensitized T cell into an immunoblast that will release various lymphokines (Table 19-4). Over 20 different lymphokines have been identified. These include a transfer factor that can sensitize nonsensitized T cells, a lymphotoxin that can cause local tissue injury, interferon that acts as a nonspecific antiviral agent, and a migration-inhibition factor that localizes and activates macrophages.

Under some circumstances the repeated contact or exposure to an antigen may cause an inappropriate response, allergy, that can be harmful or destructive to the host's tissues. Allergic reactions

TABLE 19-1. Classification of T and B lymphocytes

	T cells	B cells
Surface membrane		
Immunoglobulins	0	+
Complement receptors	0	+
E rosettes*	+	0
Response to mitogens		
Phytohemagglutinin	+	0
Concanavalin A	+	0

*Of all blood lymphocytes, 60% to 80% are T cells.

233

TABLE 19-2. Lymphocyte response—B cells

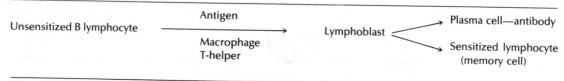

| Unsensitized B lymphocyte | $\xrightarrow{\text{Antigen}}$ Macrophage T-helper | Lymphoblast | $\nearrow$ Plasma cell—antibody $\searrow$ Sensitized lymphocyte (memory cell) |

TABLE 19-3. Lymphocyte response—T cells

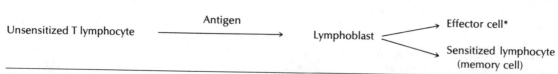

| Unsensitized T lymphocyte | $\xrightarrow{\text{Antigen}}$ | Lymphoblast | $\nearrow$ Effector cell* $\searrow$ Sensitized lymphocyte (memory cell) |

*Serves as helper cell or releases lymphokines.

TABLE 19-4. Lymphocyte response—T cells

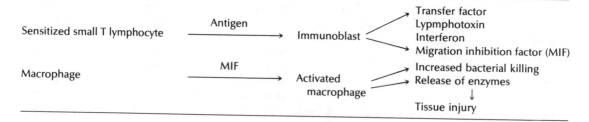

| Sensitized small T lymphocyte | $\xrightarrow{\text{Antigen}}$ | Immunoblast | Transfer factor Lypmphotoxin Interferon Migration inhibition factor (MIF) |
| Macrophage | $\xrightarrow{\text{MIF}}$ | Activated macrophage | Increased bacterial killing Release of enzymes ↓ Tissue injury |

can thus involve the cellular or humoral component of the immune system.

Reactions that involve the humoral system most often occur soon after the contact with the antigen. Four types of allergic responses related to the humoral immune system will be discussed here: (1) anaphylaxis, (2) atopy, (3) immune-complex injury, and (4) cytotoxic immune reaction.[2]

Allergic reactions that involve the cellular immune system often are delayed in onset. There are four types of delayed allergic reactions associated with the cellular immune system. These are: (1) infectious, (2) contact, (3) graft rejection, and (4) graft-vs.-host reaction.[2]

In summary, allergy may be defined as an immunologic response, cellular or humoral, to an exogenous antigen that is inappropriate or damaging and is not shown by all members of the species.[2]

Pathophysiology and complications
HUMORAL IMMUNE SYSTEM

Allergic responses related to the humoral immune system usually occur soon after the second contact with the antigen. However, it is common to find individuals who have repeated contacts with a drug or material before finally becoming allergic to it (Fig. 19-1). *Anaphylaxis* is an acute reaction involving the smooth muscle of the bronchi, where the antigen-antibody complex is formed and where it causes histamine release from surrounding mast cells. The smooth muscle contracts, and this may lead to acute respiratory distress or failure. *Atopy* (hayfever, asthma, and urticaria) occurs when an antigen reacts with its antibody, which usually is fixed to a target tissue; the antigen-antibody complex causes the release of histamine from mast cells. This histamine causes an increase in permeability of adjacent vascular structures, which

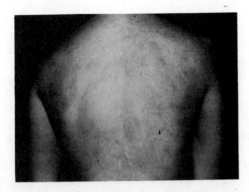

FIG. 19-1. This patient had taken penicillin a number of times without any problem. However, patient developed this generalized urticarial reaction following injection of penicillin for treatment of acute oral infection.

results in the loss of intravascular fluid into the surrounding tissue spaces. This reaction accounts for the swelling and urticaria (angioneurotic edema) and the secretions associated with hayfever. The antibodies involved in anaphylaxis and atopy are immunoglobulin E (IgE) antibodies. These humoral antibodies are fixed to and sensitize mast cells, so that when they encounter the antigen, they release histamine. IgE-related allergies are usually treated with antihistamines, vasopressors such as epinephrine, oxygen, and in some cases steroids.[2,3,14]

Immune-complex injury involves circulating immunoglobulin or immunoglobulin antibodies, which are produced by plasma cells. The antigen-antibody reaction occurs *within* the vascular system; a vasculitis with thrombosis occurs, and necrosis of adjacent tissue may follow. This is not a histamine-mediated reaction, so antihistamines are not effective in its treatment. Diseases caused by immune-complex reaction are usually treated with corticosteroids. The pathogenesis of lupus erythematosus and acute glomerulonephritis is thought to involve an immune-complex reaction.[2,3,14]

A fourth group of antibodies, immunoglobulin A antibodies, is associated with secretory cells. These antibodies are thought to protect mucosal cells from certain infectious agents. No specific disease has yet been demonstrated to be related to this group of antibodies.[2]

Cytotoxic immune reaction involves circulating cells whose surfaces serve as the antigen that reacts with circulating antibodies. The antigen-antibody complex results in the destruction of the cell. This is *not* a histamine-mediated reaction. Erythroblastosis fetalis, transfusion reactions, and some cases of thrombocytopenia are examples of diseases caused by cytotoxic allergic reaction. Diseases produced by cytoxic reaction are usually treated with corticosteroids.

CELLULAR IMMUNE SYSTEM

The cellular immune system allergic reactions are usually delayed and will appear about 48 to 72 hours after contact with the antigen.

The *infectious* allergic reaction is seen in the tuberculin skin test. In this test, a person who has been previously exposed to *Mycobacterium tuberculosis* will, with the second exposure in the form of an intradermal injection of an altered form of the bacterium, develop a delayed response, usually within 48 to 72 hours. The response is characterized by redness, swelling, and sometimes ulceration at the site of injection. *Contact* allergy occurs when a substance of low molecular weight that is not antigenic by itself comes in contact with a tissue component (primarily a protein) and forms an antigenic complex. This small molecule is called a hapten, or one half of an antigen. The complex will cause sensitization of lymphocytes. Poison ivy is an example of a contact allergy. The reaction is delayed, with response occurring 48 to 72 hours after contact with the antigen. The *graft rejection* phenomenon occurs when organs or tissues from one body are transplanted into another body. There is a cellular rejection of the transplanted tissue unless the donor and recipient are genetically identical or the host's immune response has been suppressed. *Graft-vs.-host reaction* is an unusual phenomenon that is primarily produced in experimental animals. If the animal receiving a graft has been rendered immune deficient with whole-body radiation, lymphocytes transferred to the host will "destroy" the animal in a few days.[2] This type of reaction is now being seen to some extent in patients who receive bone marrow transplants for cancer treatment.

MEDICAL MANAGEMENT

Patients with atopy may receive injections to desensitize them so that they are no longer allergic to the antigen. Some individuals with severe asthma may be forced to move to areas of the country that do not contain the antigen in the case of allergy to pollen. Patients with asthma, immune-complex injury, and cytotoxic immune reactions may be treated with steroids.

Patients who have received organ transplants often will be taking steroids and immunosuppressive drugs. A variety of treatments have been used for patients with contact dermatitis, including topical steroids. From a dental standpoint, a patient being treated for an allergic problem will have an increased chance of being allergic to another substance, and if a patient is taking steroids, his reaction to stress may be impaired. Additionally, if a patient has received an organ transplant he may be susceptible to infection.

DENTAL MANAGEMENT
Medical considerations

A dentist will be faced with several clinical problems caused by allergic reactions. When the dentist is obtaining a history from a patient, the patient may say that he is "allergic" to a local anesthetic. The dentist should question the patient further to determine if the classical signs of allergy occurred (Table 19-5). Patients who fail to associate these symptoms are usually describing toxic, vasoconstrictor, or fainting reactions that had nothing to do with a true allergy to the local anesthetic (Table 19-6).

The most common reaction associated with local anesthetics is a toxic reaction, resulting usually from the IV injection of the anesthetic or being a reaction to the vasoconstrictor used with the anesthetic. This reaction consists of nausea, seizurelike activity, tachycardia, apprehension, sweating, and hyperactivity. Another common reaction to "local anesthetics" involves the anxious patient who, be-

cause of his concern about receiving a "shot," will experience tachycardia, sweating, paleness, and syncope. True allergic reactions to the local anesthetics now used in dentistry are rare.

If the patient's history supports a toxic or vasoconstrictor reaction, the dentist should explain the nature of the previous reaction and avoid injecting the local anesthetic solution into the vascular system by aspirating before injecting. If the patient's history supports an interpretation of fainting and not an allergic reaction, the dentist's primary task will be to work with the patient to reduce anxiety during dental visits. If the history supports a true allergic reaction to a local anesthetic, the dentist should try to identify the type of anesthetic that was used. Once this has been done, a new anesthetic that has a different basic chemical structure can be used. There are two main groups of local anesthetics available for use in dentistry: (1) esters (procaine [Novocain], tetracaine [Pontocaine], and propoxycaine [Ravocaine]); and (2) amides (lidocaine [Xylocaine], mepivacaine [Carbocaine], and prilocaine [Citanest]).[1]

Procaine is the local anesthetic used in dentistry that has the highest incidence of allergic reactions associated with its use. The antigenic component appears to be PABA, which is one of the metabolic breakdown products of procaine. Cross-reactivity has been reported between lidocaine and procaine. This has been traced to a germicide, methylparaben, that is used in small amounts as a preservative in local anesthetics. Methylparaben is chemically very similar to PABA. Thus a patient who is allergic to procaine may react to lidocaine if it contains methylparaben. Lidocaine that does not contain methylparaben can now be obtained, and it should be used when dealing with a patient with history of allergy to procaine.[8,11,15]

Patients who have a history of being "allergic"

TABLE 19-5. Signs and symptoms suggestive of allergic reaction

Urticaria
Swelling
Skin rash
Chest tightness
Dyspnea, shortness of breath
Rhinitis

TABLE 19-6. Adverse reaction to local anesthetics

Toxic reactions
   Central nervous system stimulation
   Central nervous system depression

Vasoconstrictor reaction
Anxiety reaction
Allergic reaction

to local anesthetics but are unable to identify the specific agent used present a real problem to the dentist. The nature of the reaction must be established. If it is consistent with an allergic reaction, the next step should be to attempt to identify the anesthetic agent that was used. When the patient is unable to provide this information, the dentist can attempt to contact the previous dentist involved.

If this fails, the dentist has two options: (1) use of an antihistamine, diphenhydramine (Benadryl), as a local anesthetic, or (2) referral of the patient to an allergist for a provocative dose testing (PDT). Under most circumstances, the use of diphenhydramine is the most practical. A 1% solution of diphenhydramine that contains a 1:100,000 concentration of epinephrine can be made up. This solution has a average duration of anesthesia of about 30 minutes. It can be used for infiltration or block anesthesia. When it is used for a mandibular block, 1 to 4 ml of solution is needed. Some patients have reported a burning sensation, swelling, and/or erythema after a mandibular block using 1% diphenhydramine. These effects were not serious and cleared within 1 to 2 days. No more than 50 mg of diphenhydramine should be used during any given appointment. Diphenhydramine can also be used as a local anesthetic for the patient who gives a history of being allergic to local anesthetics from both of the major groups—esters and amides.[12]

The dentist may elect to refer to an allergist the patient who has a history of an allergic reaction to a local anesthetic that cannot be identified or who gives a history of being allergic to agents from

both of the major groups of local anesthetics. Most investigators agree that skin testing for allergy to local anesthetics is of no real benefit. However, the allergist may perform a PDT procedure.[10] The allergist would review the patient's allergic history. The concept of PDT would be discussed with the patient, and then the test would be performed (Table 19-7).

Based on the patient's history, the allergist would select a local anesthetic that would be least likely to cause an allergic reaction for testing. At 15-minute intervals, 0.1 ml of test solution would be injected subcutaneously with concentrations increasing from a dilution of 1:10,000 to 1:1,000, 1:100, 1:10, and then undiluted; then 0.5 ml of undiluted test solution; and finally 1.0 cc of undiluted solution. During the PDT the allergist would be prepared to deal with any adverse reaction that might occur. The allergist would report back to the dentist on the drug selected, the final dose given, and the absence of any adverse reaction. Under these conditions a local anesthetic thus tested (with no reaction) could be used in the tested patient. The risk of an allergic reaction would be no greater than in the general population.[10]

When administering an alternative anesthetic to a patient with a history of a local anesthetic allergy the dentist should follow these steps: (1) inject slowly, aspirating first to make sure that a vessel is not being injected; (2) put 1 drop of the solution to be injected into the tissues; and (3) withdraw the needle and wait 5 minutes to see what reaction, if any, occurs. If no allergic reaction occurs, as much anesthetic as needed for the procedure should be deposited. Be sure to aspirate before making the second injection (Table 19-8).

The use of penicillin has been increasing tremendously throughout the world, particularly in the United States, during the last 30 years. Approximately 2.5 million people in the United States are allergic to penicillin. Allergic reactions occur in 5% to 10% of the people who receive penicillin and related drugs. About 0.004% to 0.04% of the patients treated with penicillin develop an anaphylactic reaction, and about 10% of these individuals die. This accounts for about 100 to 300 deaths per year. Another way of looking at these data is that about 1 to 10 deaths occur per 10,000,000 injections of penicillin.[9]

The possibility of sensitizing a patient to penicil-

TABLE 19-7. Referral of patient with history of anesthetic allergy to allergist for evaluation of best local anesthetic to use

---

1. Patient identified by history to have had reaction consistent with allergic reaction
   a. Allergic to anesthetic that is identified
   b. Allergic to anesthetic that cannot be identified
   c. Allergic to several anesthetics involving both groups of local anesthetics
2. Skin testing not indicated because of variable results
3. Provocative dose testing (PDT)
4. Selection and recommendation of alternative local anesthetic based on results of PDT

TABLE 19-8. Dental management of local anesthetic allergy

I. Establish history of previous reaction following use of local anesthetic

II. Establish nature of previous reaction and type of anesthetic used
    A. Syncopal
    B. Allergic
        1. Soft-tissue swelling
        2. Skin rash
        3. Rhinitis
        4. Difficulty breathing

III. If reaction is consistent with allergic reaction
    A. Select anesthetic from different chemical group
        1. Ester—procaine
        2. Amide—lidocaine, mepivacaine
    B. Aspirate, inject 1 drop of alternate anesthetic, and wait 5 minutes; if no reaction occurs, inject (after aspiration) rest of anesthetic needed (be prepared to deal with allergic reaction if one should occur)
    C. In cases of allergic reaction to several local anesthetic agents or if anesthetic used previously cannot be identified, diphenhydramine may be used as local anesthetic

IV. If history of multiple allergies is present or if type of local anesthetic that was used cannot be identified, patient may be referred to allergist for PDT

---

lin increases according to the route of administration as follows: oral administration results in sensitization of only about 0.1% of patients; IM injection, 1% to 2%; and topical application, 5% to 12%.[1,17] Based on these data, it is obvious that the use of penicillin in a topical ointment is contraindicated. Also, if the dentist has a choice, the oral route should be selected for penicillin administration whenever possible. Antibodies produced against penicillin will cross-react with the semisynthetic penicillins and can cause severe reactions in patients allergic to penicillin. However, the synthetic penicillins do seem to have a reduced rate of causing new sensitizations in patients who are not allergic to penicillin at the time of administration.[9] Patients with a history of penicillin allergy should be given erythromycin for the treatment of oral infections or for prophylaxis against infective endocarditis.

Skin testing for allergy to penicillin is much more reliable than skin testing for allergy to a local anesthetic. There is, however, some risk involved, and the allergist must be prepared for adverse reactions. When skin testing for penicillin sensitivity is performed both of the metabolic breakdown products of penicillin must be tested. These are the major derivative, penicilloyl polylysine (PP), and the minor derivative mixture (MDM). If skin tests are negative to both breakdown products the patient is considered not to be allergic to penicillin. If positive tests are obtained for one or both of the breakdown products the patient is considered to be allergic to penicillin, and the drug should not be used.[9] Patients with a positive skin test to MDM have a higher incidence of anaphylactic reactions than patients with positive skin tests to PP.[9]

Penicillin reactions can be prevented by not using penicillin in patients who have a history of penicillin allergy. Drugs that may cross-react should also be avoided in these patients. These drugs include ampicillin, carbenicillin, methicillin, cephalosporins, and others.[9]

Patients with a negative history of allergy to penicillin can be treated with the drug when indicated. It should be given by the oral route whenever possible. The patient should be observed for 30 minutes after the first dose if possible and should be informed to seek immediate care if any of the signs or symptoms of an allergic reaction occur after he has left the dental office.

Allergic patients being treated with steroids should be managed as described in Chapter 16. Patients with transplanted organs should be protected against postoperative infection by antibiotics if surgical procedures are performed.

The dental management of the patient with asthma is primarily concerned with preventing severe asthmatic attacks from occurring in the dental office and dealing with an attack if one happens. In addition, certain important drug considerations must be needed for these patients.

Routine dental care should be planned for the asthmatic patient during the time of year when the attacks are less frequent and severe. Emotional stress may precipitate an attack; thus every effort must be made to make the dental visit as free of anxiety as possible. This would include showing interest and concern in the patient, scheduling relatively short appointments in the morning, giving

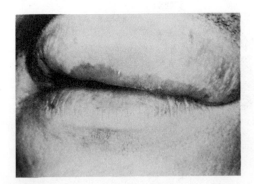

FIG. 19-2. Patient with angioneurotic edema of upper lip, which occurred soon after injection of a local anesthetic.

TABLE 19-9. Oral atopic reactions

I. Urticarial swelling (angioneurotic edema)
   A. Reaction occurs soon after contact with antigen
   B. Reaction consists of painless swelling
   C. Itching and burning may occur
   D. Lesion may remain for 1 to 3 days

II. Treatment
   A. Reaction not involving tongue, pharynx, or larynx; no respiratory distress—50 mg diphenhydramine four times a day until swelling diminishes
   B. Reaction involving tongue, pharynx, or larynx; respiratory distress
      1. 0.5 ml of epinephrine 1:1000, IM or subcutaneously
      2. Oxygen
      3. Once immediate danger is over, 50 mg diphenhydramine four times a day until swelling diminishes

premedication with 5 to 10 mg of diazepam (Valium), and terminating the appointment if the patient becomes overstressed.

If an acute asthmatic attack occurs in the dental office, the patient should be treated with an aerosol preparation of 0.25% isoproterenol.[2] Patients who have been given this drug by their physician should be told to bring it for each dental visit. A subcutaneous injection of 0.1 ml of epinephrine 1:1000 may be used in severe attacks. Oxygen may be used for the acute attack. If the attack continues, the patient's physician must be called and arrangements made to hospitalize the patient.

Patients with a history of severe asthma should not be given a general anesthetic or nitrous oxide in the dental office. Bilateral mandibular blocks should not be given, and a rubber dam should not be used. Central nervous system depressant drugs such as morphine are contraindicated in these patients (see Chapter 9).

About 0.5% of all individuals with asthma are allergic to aspirin.[3] Thus this drug should be used with caution in these patients. The middle-aged female patient with asthma and nasal polyps has the greatest incidence of allergic reactions to aspirin. Antihistamines should be avoided in patients with asthma, because excessive drying of secretions may occur. Patients with asthma may be treated with steroids, additional steroids may be needed to avoid averse reactions to the stress of certain dental procedures (see Chapter 16).

Treatment planning modifications

Most allergic patients can receive any indicated dental treatment as long as the antigen is avoided and special preparations are made for patients receiving steroids.

Oral complications

Oral lesions may be produced by humoral allergic reactions. *Atopic reactions* to various foods, drugs, or anesthetic agents may occur within the oral cavity. This reaction is usually characterized by urticarial swelling (angioneurotic edema) (Fig. 19-2). The reaction is usually very rapid, with a lesion developing within a short time after contact with the antigen. The lesion is a painless, soft-tissue swelling produced by a transudate from surrounding vessels. It may lead to itching and burning. These lesions will usually be present for 1 to 3 days and then begin to resolve spontaneously. Because they are histamine-mediated reactions, antihistamines are often effective in treating the lesions. Epinephrine is of value in the more severe reactions (Table 19-9).

Stomatitis medicamentosa is a condition that may be found following contact with various foods, drugs, or agents that are placed within the oral cavity[8] (Fig. 19-3). The reaction occurs rather quickly, usually within a 24-hour period after con-

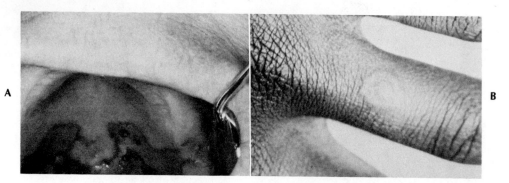

FIG. 19-3. Patient with erythema multiforme that developed following oral administration of drug to treat oral infection. **A,** Ulceration of palatal mucosa. **B,** Target lesion on finger.

TABLE 19-10. Stomatitis medicamentosa

1. Usually occurs within 24 hours after contact with antigen
2. Consists of
   a. Erythema
   b. Rash
   c. Ulceration
3. Treatment
   a. Topical steroids
   b. In severe cases, systemic steroids
   c. Identification of antigen
   d. Avoidance of any future contact with antigen if possible

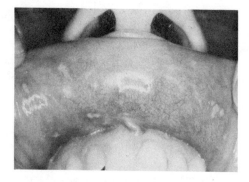

FIG. 19-4. Patient with aphthous stomatitis who was found to be allergic to toothpaste he was using.

tact with the offending antigen. The tissue reaction is characterized by erythema, rash, and/or ulceration. The exact allergic mechanism involved in stomatitis medicamentosa has not been established, but it would seem to fit the immune-complex type of injury, partly because antihistamines have not been found to be of any value in treating these types of reactions. Some cases of aphthous stomatitis and erythema multiforme may represent an immune-complex type allergic reaction. Topical steroids have been found to be useful in controlling symptoms, and in some cases they speed the healing of the lesion. In severe reactions systemic steroids are useful (Table 19-10).

Contact stomatitis may occur following the placement of various alloys, denture material, toothpaste, or cosmetics (lipstick, face creams, and powder) into the mouth.[8] Alloys used in the construction of partial dentures may cause contact stomatitis in the following manner: (1) corrosion of the metal releases metal ions that penetrate the oral mucosa; (2) these ions then combine with a tissue protein to form an antigen complex; (3) the antigen complex is carried to lymphoid tissue, where it sensitizes lymphocytes; and (4) the sensitized lymphocytes are released into circulation. When these lymphocytes reach the oral mucosa, they may react with new antigens, causing tissue destruction by means of rash, vesicles, or ulceration. Some cases of aphthous stomatitis (Fig. 19-4) are

TABLE 19-11. Contact stomatitis

Basis for reaction
  Contact with antigen
  Thymic-mediated lymphocytes become sensitized when first contact with antigen occurs
  Next contact with antigen results in release of lymphokines by sensitized lymphocytes—lymphokines result in tissue destruction
  Clinical evidence of reaction is delayed—48 to 72 hours
  Reaction usually leads to ulceration of oral mucosa

Management of reaction
  Identification of antigen
  Avoidance of future contact with antigen
  Topical steroids

TABLE 19-12. Substances that may cause allergic stomatitis

Agents	Common examples
Topical medications	Antibiotic troches, benzocaine
Systemic medications	Antibiotics, sulfa drugs
Metals	Nickel, gold
Mouth rinses and dentifrices	Phenolic compounds such as oils and parapens; antiseptics and astringents; flavoring agents
Detergents	Hand soap used by dentists and dental auxiliaries
Dental materials	Impression compounds, acrylic monomer, latex
Foods	Shellfish, berries, chewing gum

From Eversole, L.R.: Allergic stomatitides, J. Oral Med. 34:93-102, 1979.

thought to be caused by contact allergy to foods, dental products, or cosmetics (Table 19-11).

Oral epimucous testing for contact stomatitis consists of placing the suspected antigen in contact with the oral mucosa and observing over a period of time for any reaction (erythema, sloughing, or ulceration) that might indicate an allergy to the test material. In most cases a reaction would not be expected to develop for at least 48 to 72 hours. Various techniques have been used for epimucous testing for suspected allergens. One of these is to place the suspected allergen in a rubber suction cup, place the cup on the buccal mucosa, and observe at intervals for erythema or ulceration under the cup. Another technique is to place a sample of the suspected antigen in a depression on the palatal aspect of an overlay denture. The denture is put into place, and it holds the allergen in contact with the palatal mucosa. Another technique consists of incorporating the allergen into Orabase and applying the Orabase in the mucobuccal fold and periodically observing for reaction. Alternately, the antigen can be incorporated into an oral adhesive spray. Skin testing and oral epimucous testing for potential antigens are not foolproof by any means. These techniques are reliable in their responses in certain patients. The tissue response in some cases may be caused by trauma, and in others in which no tissue reaction occurs, the patient may in fact still be allergic to the substance.

In patients who have recurrent aphthous stomati-

tis of a possible allergic cause, it is necessary to identify by history the types of materials, including foods, cosmetics, toothpaste, etc., that the patient has been using and then to use substitutes, one by one, or eliminate the use of these substances to see if the lesions go away. Once the lesions clear, the indicated agent can be used again to see if it will precipitate the lesions. If it does, the diagnosis is established, and the substance should no longer be used by the patient (Table 19-12).

Management of allergic reactions

The dentist should obtain a history of any previous allergic reactions from each of his or her patients. If any patient has a history of allergy to drugs or materials that may be used in dentistry, a clear entry should be made in the dental record, and any further contact or use of the antigen(s) must be avoided in that patient (Fig. 19-5).

Even when the dentist has followed these precautions, allergic reactions may occur in patients. Most of these will be mild and of a nonemergency nature; however, some may be severe and life threatening. The dentist must be ready to deal with either type of reaction. When dealing with a mild, nonemergency allergic reaction, the dentist should first attempt to identify and eliminate any further

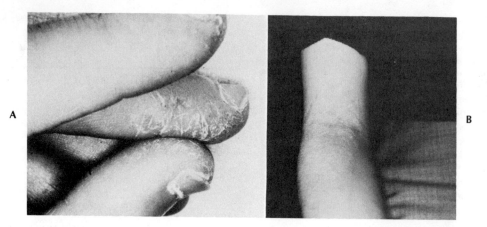

FIG. 19-5. Examples of contact dermatitis. **A,** Fingers of dentist who developed allergy to procaine. **B,** Patient who developed allergy to a soap.

TABLE 19-13. Symptomatic treatment of patients with multiple oral ulcerations

Action	Purpose
1. Rinse with bland mouthwash—1 teaspoon baking soda in 8-ounce glass of warm water.	To remove materials from surface of ulcers.
2. Rinse with and then swallow elixir of diphenhydramine (Benadryl). One teaspoon of elixir—hold in mouth for 1 to 2 minutes and then swallow. Each 5 ml contains 12.5 mg of diphenhydramine.	Diphenhydramine is very good topical anesthetic and will provide relief from pain.
3. Apply Orabase to lesions in areas such as floor of mouth and mucobuccal fold.	To protect surface of ulcer(s) from irritation.
4. Prescribe bland diet.	To protect surface of ulcer(s) from irritation.
5. Repeat procedure four times a day.	

contact by the patient with the specific antigen. At the same time, the dentist may need to initiate antiallergic therapy to deal with the lesions resulting from the allergic reaction.

The management of most common types of mild, nonemergency allergic reactions can be grouped under the headings described here.

STOMATITIS MEDICAMENTOSA

Stomatitis medicamentosa reactions are thought to be related to the humoral immune system and may represent an immune-complex type of allergic reaction. Erythema multiforme may represent this type of etiology. About one half of the patients with erythema multiforme are found to have a predisposing factor, such as a drug or herpes simplex infection, involved in the onset of their diseases.[6,16] Sulfa antibiotics are the most common drugs associated with the onset of erythema multiforme. Sulfonylurea hypoglycemic agents used to treat some diabetics have been found to be associated with the onset of erythema multiforme. Many patients with erythema multiforme can be managed by symptomatic therapy including a bland mouthwash (sodium bicarbonate in warm water), syrup of diphenhydramine, and/or triamcinolone acetonide (Kenalog) in Orabase (Table 19-13). A few patients with more severe involvement may require systemic steroids.

If a drug appears to be associated with the onset of the disease, any further contact with the drug should be avoided.

CONTACT STOMATITIS

Contact stomatitis is a delayed allergic reaction associated with the cellular immune response in most cases. Because of the delayed nature of the reaction following contact with the allergen in cases of contact stomatitis, the dentist must inquire about contacts with materials that may have occurred 2 to 3 days before the lesions appeared.[6] The antigen may be found in dental materials, toothpaste, mouthwashes, lipsticks, face powders, etc. In many cases no further treatment is necessary once the source of the antigen has been identified and removed from further contact with the patient. However, if the tissue reaction is severe or persistent, topical corticosteroids should be used. A good preparation to use topically is triamcinolone acetonide in Orabase.

Various dental materials have been reported to cause allergic reactions in patients. Impression materials containing an aromatic sulfonate catalyst, Scutan and Impregum, have been reported to cause a delayed allergic reaction in postmenopausal women. The reaction consisted of tissue ulceration and necrosis that got progressively worse with each exposure.[45]

On rare occasions, dental composite materials have been reported to cause allergic reactions.[13] The acrylic monomer used in denture construction has been reported to cause allergic reactions[7]; however, the vast majority of tissue changes under dentures are caused by trauma and secondary infection with bacteria or fungi.[7]

LICHENOID DRUG ERUPTION

Some patients with skin and/or oral lesions identical to those of lichen planus have been found to have taken certain drugs before the onset of the lesions. If these drugs are withdrawn, the lesions clear within several days in most patients or within a few weeks in others. The agents most commonly found to be associated with the onset of the lichenoid lesions are almeyda, Levantine, and the quinidine drugs. Other agents found to be associated in some cases are the thiazide drugs and photographic dyes such as paraphenylenediamine. Biopsy of the lichenoid lesions shows a microscopic picture the same as that found in lichen planus with the additional finding of eosinophils in the subepithelial infiltrate.[6] It would appear that these lesions are related to the cellular immune system and therefore could be placed under the heading of contact stomatitis. However, the true nature of the reaction is not clear at this time.

URTICARIA

Urticarial reactions usually occur faster than contact reactions and are related to the humoral immune response. The antigens are usually drugs, but many other agents or materials may serve as antigens. If the reaction is mild and of a non-emergency nature, oral antihistamines should be given. Diphenhydramine, 50 mg every 4 hours, orally, is the recommended treatment.[2] Once again, the source of the antigen should be identified and the patient informed that he should have no further contact with the antigen.

• • •

In both contact and urticarial types of reactions listed previously, the patient should be referred to an allergist if the problem becomes more severe or is prolonged.

In some patients the allergic reaction may be more severe. In dealing with the emergency type of reaction the dentist should take the following initial steps[2]:

1. Place the patient in a head-down or supine position.
2. Make certain that the patient has a patent airway.
3. Administer oxygen.
4. Be prepared to send for help and to support respiration and circulation. The rate and depth of respiration should be noted as should the patient's vital signs.

Most reactions in dental patients will consist of simple fainting, which will be managed well by the preceding actions. In addition, the dentist may administer aromatic spirits of ammonia by inhalation, because this will encourage breathing through reflex stimulation.

If the initial steps have not solved the emergency

TABLE 19-14. Anaphylaxis

Basis of reaction
  First contact with antigen results in formation of antibodies by plasma cells
  IgE antibodies circulate in blood stream
  Antibodies attach to target tissues (mast cells near smooth muscle of bronchi)
  Next contact with antigen may result in combination of antigen and antibody
  Antigen-antibody complex causes destruction of mast cell(s) with release of histamine
  Smooth muscle contracts, and vessels lose fluids, etc.
  Acute respiratory distress and cardiovascular collapse may occur within minutes
Management of reaction
  Call for medical help
  Place patient in supine position
  Check for open airway
  Administer oxygen
  Check pulse, blood pressure, and respirations
    If depressed or absent, inject 0.5 of epinephrine IM or subcutaneously
  Provide cardiopulmonary resuscitation if indicated
  Repeat injection of 0.5 ml of epinephrine if no response

problem and it is indeed of allergic cause, the dentist is faced with either an edematous-type reaction or an anaphylactic reaction.

If the immediate-type allergic reaction (humoral) has resulted in edema of the tongue, pharyngeal tissues, or larynx, the dentist will have to take additional emergency steps to prevent death from respiratory failure. At this point, if the patient has not responded to the initial procedure and is having acute respiratory distress, the dentist should do the following:[2]

1. Inject 0.5 ml of 1:1000 epinephrine IM or subcutaneously.
2. Support respiration, if indicated, by mouth-to-mouth breathing or bag and mask; be sure the chest moves when either of these methods are used.
3. Check the patient's carotid or femoral pulse; if a pulse cannot be detected, closed chest cardiac massage should be initiated.
4. By this time someone in the office should have called a nearby physician or hospital.

ANAPHYLAXIS

An anaphylactic reaction usually takes place in a very short period of time—minutes. In contrast to the severe edematous reaction, in which respiratory distress occurs first, both respiratory and circulatory depression occur early in the anaphylactic reaction. Anaphylactic reaction is often fatal unless vigorous, immediate action is taken. Because this reaction occurs within minutes after contact with the antigen, the dentist should take the following steps[2] (Table 19-14):

1. Have someone in the office call for medical aid, nearby physician, or hospital.
2. Place the patient in a supine position.
3. Make certain the airway is patent.
4. Administer oxygen.
5. Check carotid or femoral pulse and respiration; if no pulse is present and respiration is depressed:
   a. Inject 0.5 ml 1:1000 epinephrine IM or subcutaneously.
   b. Inject 0.5 ml 1:1000 epinephrine slowly IV.
   c. Support circulation by closed chest cardiac massage
   d. Support respiration by mouth-to-mouth breathing.

Emergency dental care

Patients with a history of allergy can receive any emergency dental treatment indicated as long as the antigen or antigens are avoided. Special preparations must be made for patients who are receiving steroids. Patients with an altered immune response should be given an antibiotic.

REFERENCES

1. American Dental Association: Accepted dental therapeutics, Chicago, 1975, The Association.
2. Bickley, H.C.: Practical concepts in human disease, Baltimore, 1974, The Williams & Wilkins Co., pp. 60-79.
3. Criep, L.H.: Allergy and clinical immunology, New York, 1976, Grune & Stratton, Inc., pp. 507-529.
4. Dahl, B.L.: Tissue hypersensitivity to dental materials, J. Oral Rehabil. **5**:117-120, 1978.
5. Duxbury, A.J., Turner, E.P., and Watts, D.C.: Hypersensitivity to epimine containing dental materials, Br. Dent J. **147**:331-333, 1979.
6. Eversole, L.R.: Allergic stomatitides, J. Oral Med. **34**:93-102, 1979.
7. Fernstrom, A.I.: Location of the allergenic monomer in

warm-polymerized acrylic dentures. Part I, Swed. Dent. J. **4:**253-260, 1980.

8. Giovannitti, J.A.: Assessment of allergy to local anesthetics, J. Am. Dent. Assoc. **98:**701-706, 1979.

9. Holroyd, S.V., and Wynn, R.L.: Clinical pharmacology in dental practice, ed. 3, St. Louis, 1983, The C.V. Mosby Co., pp. 245-278.

10. Incando, G., et al.: Administration of local anesthetics to patients with a history of prior adverse reaction, J. Allergy Clin. Immunol. **61:**339-345, 1978.

11. Larson, C.E.: Methylparaben, an overlooked cause of local anesthetic hypersensitivity, Anesth. Prog. **24:**72-74, 1977.

12. Malamed, S.F.: Diphenhydramine hydrochloride, its use as a local anesthetic in dentistry, Anesth. Prog. **20:**76-82, 1973.

13. Nathanson, D.: Delayed extra-oral hypersensitivity to dental composite materials, Oral Surg. **47:**329-333, 1979.

14. Norman, P.S., and Lichtenstein, L.M.: Immune responses in man. In Harvey, A., editor: Osler's the principles and practice of medicine, ed. 19, New York, 1976, Appleton-Century-Crofts, pp. 1317-1324.

15. Reuben, B.M.: A current practical review of local anesthesia, Dent. Surv. **56:**38-43, 1980.

16. Shafer, W.G., Hine, M.K., and Levy, B.M.: A textbook of oral pathology, ed. 3, Philadelphia, 1974, W.B. Saunders Co., pp. 531-537.

17. Weinstein, L.: Chemotherapy of microbial diseases. In Goodman, L.S., and Gilman, A., editors: The pharmacological basis of therapeutics, ed. 5, New York, 1975, Macmillan Publishing Co., Inc., pp. 1090-1224.

20

BLEEDING DISORDERS

A number of procedures that are performed in dentistry may cause bleeding. Under normal circumstances these procedures can be performed with very little risk to the patient. However, the patient whose ability to control bleeding has been altered by drugs or disease may be in grave danger unless the dentist identifies the problem before performing any dental procedure. In most cases, once the patient with a bleeding problem has been identified, steps can be taken to greatly reduce the risks associated with dental procedures.

This chapter is designed to provide the dentist with an understanding of the mechanisms involved in the normal control of bleeding, to describe the common causes of bleeding problems, to present an approach for the dentist to use in identifying patients with possible bleeding abnormalities, and to describe in general terms the management of these patients once they have been identified.

GENERAL DESCRIPTION
Incidence

Most bleeding disorders are iatrogenic, or produced by a physician. Each of the many patients who receive coumarin drugs to prevent recurrent thrombosis has a potential bleeding problem. Most of these patients are receiving anticoagulant medication because they have had a recent myocardial infarction, a cerebrovascular accident, or thrombophlebitis. Patients who have had open heart surgery to correct congenital defects, to replace diseased arteries, or to replace damaged heart valves also may be receiving long-term anticoagulation therapy. In addition, some individuals treated with aspirin for chronic illnesses such as rheumatoid arthritis have potential bleeding problems.

True hemophilia, factor VIII deficiency, is the most common of the inherited coagulation disorders. The overall prevalence of hemophilia in the United States is about 1 case for every 20,000 people. However, because of its genetic mode of transfer, certain areas of the United States are found to contain many more persons with hemophilia than other areas. About 80% of all cases of genetic coagulation disorders are true hemophilia, 13% are Christmas disease (factor IX deficiency), and 6% are factor XI deficiency.[7,8]

Patients with acute or chronic leukemia may have clinical bleeding tendencies because of thrombocytopenia, which may result from overgrowth of malignant cells in the bone marrow that leaves no room for red blood cells or platelet precursors. In addition, leukemic patients may develop thrombocytopenia from the toxic effects of the various chemotherapeutic agents used to treat the disease.

The incidence of acute leukemia in the United States for all ages is about 3 to 4 cases per 100,000 persons. Chronic lymphocytic leukemia is rare in children but increases in incidence to about 10 cases per 100,000 persons over the age of 75 years. Chronic granulocytic leukemia is rare in those under the age of 30 years and over the age of 70 years.[4,7,8]

The incidence of acute leukemia does not vary much among races. In contrast, chronic leukemia is rare in eastern countries, less common in blacks, and more common in northern countries.[7,8]

It is difficult to obtain accurate information about the incidence of other systemic conditions that may render the patient susceptible to prolonged bleeding following injury or surgery. However, when considering the prevalence of the drug-influenced or disease-produced defects in the normal control of blood loss, it is clear that a busy dental practice will contain a large number of patients who may be "bleeders."

Etiology

A pathologic alteration of a blood vessel wall, a significant reduction in the number of platelets, defective platelets, a deficiency of one or more of the coagulation factors, anticoagulant drugs, and the inability to destroy free plasmin may result in significant clinical bleeding. This bleeding may occur even following minor injuries and could lead to death in some patients if immediate action is not taken.

The classification given in Table 20-1 is based on bleeding problems in patients with normal numbers of platelets (nonthrombocytopenic purpuras) and decreased numbers of platelets (thrombocytopenic purpuras) and in patients with disorders of coagulation.

Infections, chemicals, or certain types of allergy may alter the structure and function of the vascular wall to the point at which the patient may have a clinical bleeding problem.

A patient may have normal numbers of platelets, but the platelets may be defective or unable to perform their proper function in the control of blood loss from damaged tissues.

If the total number of circulating plates is reduced below 60,000 to 80,000/mm^3 of blood, the patient may be a "bleeder."[4,7] In some cases the total platelet count is reduced by unknown mechanisms—this is called primary thrombocytopenia. Chemicals, radiation, and various systemic diseases such as leukemia may have a direct effect on the bone marrow and result in secondary thrombocytopenia.

Patients may be born with a deficiency of one of the factors needed for blood coagulation, for example, factor VIII deficiency (hemophilia) or factor IX deficiency (Christmas disease).

Acquired coagulation disorders are the most common cause of prolonged bleeding and may become apparent in patients only after trauma or surgical procedures.

The liver produces all of the coagulation factors except factor VIII and possibly factor XIII; thus

TABLE 20-1. Classification of bleeding disorders

I. Nonthrombocytopenic purpuras
  A. Vascular wall alteration
    1. Scurvy
    2. Infections
    3. Chemicals
    4. Allergy
  B. Disorders of platelet function
    1. Genetic defects
    2. Drugs—aspirin
    3. Allergy
    4. Autoimmune disease

II. Thrombocytopenic purpuras
  A. Primary
  B. Secondary
    1. Chemicals
    2. Physical agents—radiation
    3. Systemic disease—leukemia

III. Disorders of coagulation
  A. Inherited
    1. Hemophilia—deficiency of factor VIII
    2. Christmas disease—deficiency of factor IX
    3. Others
  B. Acquired
    1. Liver disease
    2. Vitamin deficiency
      Biliary tract obstruction
      Malabsorption
      Excessive use of broad-spectrum antibiotics
    3. Anticoagulation drugs
      Heparin
      Coumarin drugs
    4. Other

any patient with significant liver disease may have a bleeding problem. In addition to a possible disorder in coagulation, the patient with liver disease who develops portal hypertension with hypersplenism may be thrombocytopenic as a result of the overactivity of the spleen, which may destroy circulating platelets.

Any condition that disrupts the intestinal flora so that vitamin K is not produced in sufficient amounts will result in a decreased plasma level of prothrombin, because vitamin K is needed by the liver to produce prothrombin (factor II) and factors VII, IX, and X. Biliary tract obstruction, malabsorption syndrome, and excessive use of broad-spectrum antibiotics also may lead to low levels of prothrombin on this basis.

Other drugs such as heparin, coumarin derivatives, and aspirin may cause a bleeding disorder because of disruption of the coagulation process. Aspirin also may interfere with platelet function.

Pathophysiology

Under normal conditions any spontaneous bleeding is abnormal, with the exception of menstruation. Also, under normal conditions even large injuries will result in little blood loss; but when the body's ability to control bleeding has been altered, even a very slight injury may result in massive blood loss. For hemostasis to be maintained, the blood vessels must be normal, an adequate number of functional platelets must be present, and the coagulation mechanisms must be intact. Thus the control of bleeding can be described as involving three phases: vascular, platelet, and coagulation[7] (Table 20-2).

The vascular phase begins immediately following injury and involves vasoconstriction of arteries and arterioles in the area of injury, retraction of arteries that have been cut, and buildup of extravascular pressure by blood loss from cut vessels. This pressure aids in collapsing the adjacent capillaries and veins in the area of injury.

The platelet phase begins only seconds following injury and consists first of the platelets becoming "sticky," which allows them to adhere to the endothelium of damaged vessels and the collagen in the surrounding injured tissue. Soon the platelets begin to stick to each other. This adhesion and aggregation of platelets produces "plugs" that seal off the openings of cut vessels. This process is helped by the slowing of blood flow, which occurs soon after injury. The adhesion and aggregation of platelets is influenced by the plasma factor adenosine diphosphate (ADP), which is released from the injured tissue, the red blood cells, and the platelets themselves. Platelet prostaglandin activity will stimulate the aggregation of platelets. Cyclo-oxygense and thromboxane are the prostaglandins that are involved.[1] Thus the role of platelets in hemostasis is both mechanical and biochemical. The plug of platelets seals the damaged vessel mechanically, and various substances within platelets play an important biochemical role in the coagulation phase.

In the past, coagulation of blood was described

TABLE 20-2. Normal control of bleeding

1. Vascular phase
   a. Vasoconstriction in area of injury
   b. Occurs soon after injury
2. Platelet phase
   a. Platelets and vessel wall become "sticky"
   b. Mechanical plug of platelets seals off openings of cut vessels
   c. Occurs soon after injury
3. Coagulation phase
   a. Blood lost into surrounding area coagulates by extrinsic and common pathways
   b. Blood in vessels in area of injury coagulates through intrinsic and common pathways
   c. Takes place more slowly than other phases

TABLE 20-3. Blood coagulation factors

Factor	Name
I	Fibrinogen
II	Prothrombin
III	Thromboplastin
IV	Calcium
V	Labile factor, proaccelerin, accelerator (Ac-) globulin
(VI)	Not assigned
VII	Proconvertin, serum prothrombin conversion accelerator (SPCA), cothromboplastin, autoprothrombin I
VIII	Antihemophilic factor (AHF), antihemophilic globulin (AHG)
IX	Plasma thromboplastin component (PTC) (Christmas factor)
X	Stuart-Prower factor
XI	Plasma thromboplastin antecedent (PTA)
XII	Hageman factor
XIII	Laki-Larand factor (LLF); fibrin stabilizing factor

as taking place in four stages. Stage I was said to involve the formation of thromboplastin, stage II to deal with the formation of thrombin from thromboplastin, stage III to consist of the conversion of fibrinogen to fibrin in the presence of thrombin, and stage IV to involve the lysis of the fibrin clot. Other coagulation factors were thought to be involved, but their roles were not well understood, and thus they were not assigned a definite function in this scheme.

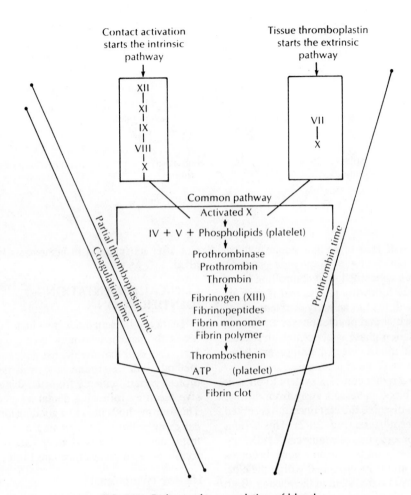

FIG. 20-1. Pathways for coagulation of blood.

Because of recent advances in hematology, the coagulation process can now be described better in regard to the role of the 12 known coagulation factors (Table 20-3). Each factor is commonly referred to by its Roman numeral, with the exceptions of prothrombin and fibrinogen.

The coagulation factors are thought to be proenzymes that are normally inert but that are transformed into proteolytic enzymes when activated The activation of the coagulation factors is by contact and takes place in a "waterfall" manner; that is, one factor becomes activated and it in turn activates another and so on in an ordered sequence.[7]

Blood coagulation is now described as being ini-

tiated by two separate mechanisms, extrinsic (activated outside the blood vessels) and intrinsic (activated within the blood vessels), and then proceeding to completion along a common pathway[7] (Fig. 20-1). Coagulation may be initiated either by contact activation of factor XII (intrinsic pathway) or by tissue thromboplastin (extrinsic pathway) and is then completed along a common pathway that involves the transformation of prothrombin to thrombin and then fibrinogen to fibrin. The intrinsic pathway is much slower than the extrinsic pathway. Both systems are necessary for normal coagulation to occur.

A significant disorder in either the vascular or

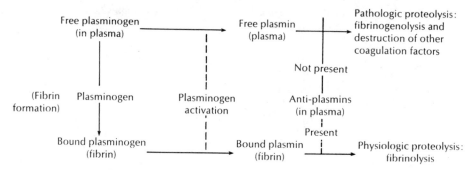

FIG. 20-2. Plasminogen system.

platelet phase will lead to an immediate clinical bleeding problem following injury or surgery. These phases are concerned with controlling blood loss immediately following injury, and if they are defective this will lead to an early problem. However, if the vascular and platelet phases are normal and the coagulation phase is abnormal, the bleeding problem will not be detected until several hours after the injury or surgical procedure.

There is also a rather complex system to prevent coagulation of blood in vessels away from the site of injury and to dissolve the clot once it has served its function in hemostasis (Fig. 20-2). This system involves the proenzyme plasminogen.[7,8] During fibrin formation some plasminogen becomes bound to fibrin and is incorporated within the clot. The rest remains in a free state in the plasma. Both bound and free plasminogen may be converted to the active enzyme form plasmin, which causes fibrinolysis. Plasminogen can be activated by extracts of vascular endothelium, bacterial enzymes, factor XII, thrombin, and various forms of stress, such as emotional stress, hypoglycemia, and vigorous exercise.

Various antiplasmin factors also are present in circulating blood, and these rapidly destroy free plasmin but are relatively ineffective against plasmin that is bound to fibrin. Thus under normal conditions, once an injury has occurred, coagulation will proceed to the formation of fibrin. At the same time, both bound and free plasminogen become activated to plasmin. The free plasmin is rapidly destroyed; thus it does not interfere with the formation of the clot. The bound plasmin is not inactivated, and it is free to dispose of the fibrin

clot after its function in hemostasis has been fulfilled.

CLINICAL PRESENTATION—IDENTIFICATION

There are four methods by which the dentist can detect the patient who may have a bleeding problem. The skill that the dentist develops with these methods will determine how well he or she can protect certain patients from the danger of excessive bleeding following dental surgical treatment. The four methods are (1) a good history, (2) physical examination, (3) screening clinical laboratory tests, and (4) observation of excessive bleeding following a surgical procedure (Table 20-4).

History (symptoms)

A good history is the best single screening procedure to identify the patient with a possible disorder. The history should include questions concerning the following six topics:
1. Presence of bleeding problems in relatives
2. Excessive bleeding following operations
3. Excessive bleeding following trauma
4. Use of drugs for prevention of coagulation or chronic pain
5. Past and present illnesses
6. Occurrence of spontaneous bleeding

BLEEDING PROBLEMS IN RELATIVES

Hemophilia and Christmas disease, the two most common inherited coagulation disorders, will be discussed here to show how a history of bleeding in a patient's relatives may give a clue to the presence of a congenital bleeding problem. These

TABLE 20-4. Detection of the patient who is a "bleeder"

I. History
   A. Bleeding problems in relatives
   B. Bleeding problems following operations and tooth extractions
   C. Bleeding problems following trauma—cuts, etc.
   D. Medications that may cause bleeding problems
      1. Aspirin
      2. Anticoagulants
      3. Long-term antibiotic therapy
   E. Presence of illnesses that may have associated bleeding problems
      1. Leukemia
      2. Liver disease
      3. Hemophilia
      4. Congenital heart disease
   F. Spontaneous bleeding from nose, mouth, ears, etc.

II. Examination findings
   A. Jaundice, pallor
   B. Spider angiomas
   C. Ecchymoses
   D. Petechiae
   E. Oral ulcers
   F. Hyperplastic gingival tissues
   G. Hemarthrosis

III. Screening laboratory tests
   A. Prothrombin time.
   B. Partial thromboplastin time
   C. Tournique test
   D. Bleeding time
   E. Platelet count

IV. Surgical procedure—excessive bleeding following surgery may be first clue to underlying bleeding problem

coagulation disorders are transmitted by a sex-linked recessive mode of inheritance. The X chromosome contains the altered gene for these diseases. In most cases the female serves as the carrier and the diseases manifest themselves only in the male.[7] To demonstrate the various possibilities of inheritance of these diseases, the following symbols will be used:

xx	Normal female
xy	Normal male
x*	Abnormal recessive gene for the disease
x*y	Affected male
xx*	Female carrier
x*x*	Affected female

An affected male will not transmit the disease to any of his sons. However, all of his daughters will be carriers.

	x*	y
x	xx*	xy
x	xx*	xy

One half of the sons of a female carrier married to a normal male will be affected by the disorder, and one half of her daughters will be carriers.

	x	y
x	xx	xy
x*	x*x	x*y

One combination is possible that would produce a daughter with one of these coagulation disorders.[7] This occurs when a female carrier marries an affected male. One half of the daughters would have the disorder, one half of the daughters would be carriers, one half of the sons would be affected, and one half of the sons would be normal. The probabilities for this type of union are very small, and this explains why so very few females are affected with these diseases.

	x*	y
x*	x*x*	x*y
x	xx*	xy

About 25% of the patients who have been proved to have a hereditary coagulation disorder have a negative family history.[7] The reason for this is the relatively high rate of mutation producing new cases. Therefore a negative family history in itself does not always preclude a genetic coagulation disorder.

BLEEDING PROBLEMS FOLLOWING OPERATIONS AND TOOTH EXTRACTIONS

Each new patient should be questioned concerning excessive bleeding following major or minor operations. The number of individuals who have had appendectomies, tonsillectomies, or tooth extractions is very large. Persons who have had such a procedure without a bleeding problem do not have a significant inherited coagulation disorder. They also did not have a significant acquired bleeding problem at the time the operative procedure was performed. However, this does not mean that the patient is free of a bleeding problem that could have been acquired since the last surgical procedure.

BLEEDING PROBLEMS FOLLOWING TRAUMA

All new patients should be asked if they have experienced any recent trauma, and if so whether it was followed by excessive bleeding. The more severe the trauma, the more likely that it would reveal the presence of an underlying bleeding disorder. Small cuts in patients with coagulation disorders may not cause excessive bleeding, because the vascular and platelet phases may be sufficient to control blood loss even if there is a defect in coagulation. However, small cuts in patients with platelet or vascular deficiencies usually will result in excessive bleeding.

When excessive bleeding does occur following trauma in patients with coagulation disorders, it is usually delayed. This is because the immediate control of blood loss by vasoconstriction, extravascular pressure, and platelet plugging proceeds normally. However, when these effects begin to lessen, they are not replaced by the formation of a good clot of fibrin as happens in normal coagulation. This is when the bleeding begins in the patient who has a coagulation defect.

MEDICATIONS THAT MAY CAUSE BLEEDING PROBLEMS

All new patients should be asked if they are taking an anticoagulant drug such as heparin or a coumarin derivative. If the patient is receiving one of these drugs, the dentist should contact the patient's physician and determine what degree of anticoagulation is being maintained and why the drug is being used. All patients should be asked if they have been taking aspirin or drugs that contain aspirin and in what dosage and over what length of time. They should also be asked if they have had recent treatment with broad-spectrum antibiotics.

PRESENCE OF ILLNESSES WITH ASSOCIATED BLEEDING PROBLEMS

The past and current medical status of patients should be reviewed. They should be questioned concerning a history of liver disease, biliary tract obstruction, malabsorption problems, infectious diseases, genetic coagulation disorders, chronic in-

flammatory diseases, and leukemia or other types of cancer and whether they have received radiation therapy or have been exposed to large amounts of radiation.

SPONTANEOUS BLEEDING

Each patient should be asked about a history of spontaneous bleeding. This would include gingival, nasal, urinary, rectal, gastrointestinal, oral, pulmonary, and vaginal sources of bleeding. If spontaneous bleeding has occurred, the frequency, amount of blood loss, appearance of blood, and steps that were taken to stop the bleeding should be determined.

Physical examination (signs)

It is important that the exposed skin and oral mucosa be examined for objective signs that may indicate the presence of a bleeding disorder. Jaundice, spider angioma, and ecchymosis may be seen in the person with liver disease. A fine tremor of the hands when they are held out also may be observed in these patients. In about 50% of persons with liver disease there is a reduction of platelets secondary to hypersplenism that results from the effects of portal hypertension. These individuals may show petechiae on the skin and mucosa.[7,8]

The most common objective findings in patients

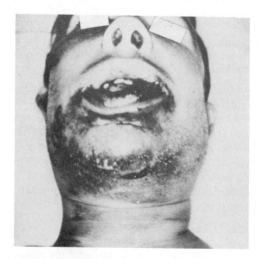

FIG. 20-3. Patient with hemophilia who has massive areas of ecchymosis secondary to trauma.

with genetic coagulation disorders are ecchymoses, hemarthrosis, and dissecting hematomas (Fig. 20-3). The signs seen most commonly in patients with abnormal platelets or thrombocytopenia are petechiae and ecchymoses (Fig. 20-4).

Patients with acute or chronic leukemia may reveal one or more of the following signs: ulceration of the oral mucosa, hyperplasia of the gingiva, petechiae of the skin or mucous membranes, ecchymoses of skin or mucous membranes, and lymphadenopathy (Figs. 20-5 and 20-6).

A number of patients with bleeding disorders may show no objective signs that suggest their underlying problem.

Screening laboratory tests

Five clinical laboratory tests can be used to screen patients for bleeding disorders. These tests are the platelet count, Ivy bleeding time, tourniquet test, partial thromboplastin time (PTT), and prothrombin time (PT) (Table 20-5).

From a functional viewpoint the platelet count does not have to be ordered to screen a patient, because the bleeding time will reflect problems with both the number and the quality of platelets. However, by obtaining a platelet count better insight can be gained as to the nature of the problem in patients with a prolonged bleeding time. For example, if the bleeding time was prolonged and

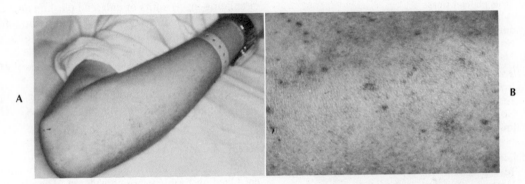

FIG. 20-4. **A,** Patient with thrombocytopenia who has numerous petechiae on arm. **B,** Close-up view of petechiae on arm.

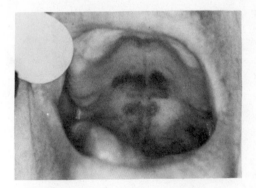

FIG. 20-5. Patient with chronic lymphocytic leukemia who has several areas of ecchymoses on mucosa of hard and soft palate.

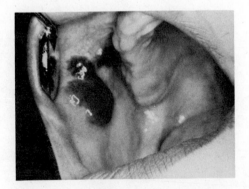

FIG. 20-6. Patient with cheek lesion that could appear to be area of ecchymosis; however, lesion blanched with pressure and was capillary hemangioma.

TABLE 20-5. Laboratory tests for detection of a potential "bleeder"

1. Prothrombin time
   a. Tests extrinsic and common pathways
   b. Control should be run
   c. Normal—11 to 14 seconds (depends on laboratory)
   d. Control must be in normal range
2. Partial thromboplastin time
   a. Tests intrinsic and common pathways
   b. Control should be run
   c. Normal—25 to 40 seconds (depends on laboratory)
   d. Control must be in normal range
3. Ivy bleeding time
   a. Tests platelet phase
   b. Normal if adequate number of platelets of good quality present
   c. Normal—1 to 6 minutes
   d. Also may test vascular phase, but tourniquet test is better
4. Tourniquet test
   a. Tests vascular phase
   b. Normal if just a few petechiae found on arm below blood pressure cuff
   c. Also may test platelet phase
5. Platelet count
   a. Tests platelet phase
   b. Normal—200,000 to 300,000/mm³
   c. Clinical bleeding problem if less than 80,000/mm³

the platelet count was within normal limits, a problem in platelet function would be indicated.

The Ivy bleeding time is the best test to measure for the presence of adequate platelet function (Fig. 20-7).

The tourniquet test, although it may be positive in patients who are thrombocytopenic, is the best test to measure the status of the vascular phase. Increased numbers of petechiae will be found on the arm as the severity of vascular wall defects increase.

The PTT test is used to measure the status of the intrinsic and common pathways of coagulation. This test reflects the ability of blood still contained within vessels in the area of injury to coagulate. Both the PTT and the PT will be prolonged if the circulating inactivators of unbound plasmin are defective or if a significant deficiency of one or more of the common pathway coagulation factors is present.

The PT will be prolonged in cases of factor VII deficiency. The PTT will be prolonged in cases of a deficiency of one or more of the intrinsic pathway coagulation factors—factors VIII, IX, XI, and XII.

MEDICAL MANAGEMENT

In this chapter conditions that may cause a clinical bleeding problem are considered. The emphasis is on the detection of patients with a potential bleeding problem and the management of these patients if surgical procedures are needed. The

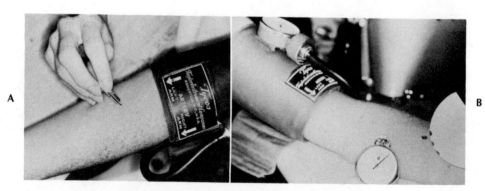

FIG. 20-7. A, Blood pressure cuff in place and stab wound just being made for Ivy bleeding time. **B,** Ivy bleeding time midway to completion; blood can still be blotted onto filter paper.

medical treament of the specific disorders will not be covered. The reader is referred to one of the textbooks listed at the end of this chapter for this information.

DENTAL MANAGEMENT
Medical considerations

No surgical procedures should be performed on a patient suspected to have a bleeding problem based on history and examination findings. Such a patient should be screened with the appropriate clinical laboratory tests and, if indicated, referred to a hematologist for diagnosis and treatment. Patients under medical management who may have bleeding problems should receive no dental treatment until consultation with the patient's physician has taken place and appropriate preparations have been taken to avoid excessive bleeding following dental procedures.

Nine different clinical situations often present the dentist with the problem of whether or not a given patient has a bleeding problem. Each of these situations will be discussed in detail (see Table 20-6).

NO CLINICAL OR HISTORICAL CLUES TO BLEEDING PROBLEM

A person with a potential bleeding problem may have no subjective or objective findings that suggest an underlying bleeding problem. The first indication may be prolonged bleeding following a surgical dental procedure. Local measures should be taken to control the bleeding, and if these fail a hematologist may have to be consulted. Once the problem is under control, the patient should be screened with the appropriate laboratory tests—PT, PTT, bleeding time, and tourniquet test—because there are no clues to the cause of the problem.

HISTORY OR CLINICAL FINDINGS OR BOTH SUGGEST POSSIBLE BLEEDING PROBLEM BUT NO CLUES TO CAUSE

When there are no clues concerning the cause of a potential bleeding problem in a patient, all five screening laboratory tests should be performed. The patient's physician can order these tests, or the dentist can order them from a clinical laboratory facility (Table 20-7).

TABLE 20-6. Selection of screening laboratory tests for detecting patient with potential bleeding problem based on history and examination findings

No clinical or historical clues to bleeding problem—problem develops following surgical procedure

History or clinical findings or both suggest possible bleeding problem but no clues to cause
  Prothrombin time
  Partial thromboplastin time
  Bleeding time
  Tourniquet test
  Platelet count

Aspirin therapy
  Bleeding time
  Partial thromboplastin time

Coumarin therapy
  Prothrombin time

Possible liver disease
  Bleeding time
  Prothrombin time

Chronic leukemia
  Bleeding time

Malabsorption syndrome or long-term antibiotic therapy
  Prothrombin time

Renal dialysis (heparin)
  Partial thromboplastin time

Vascular wall alteration
  Tourniquet test

ASPIRIN THERAPY

Patients receiving aspirin therapy may have a bleeding problem based on the drug's effect on platelets. Usually these patients have been receiving high doses (20 grains or more) of aspirin each day for a long time (more than a week). Not all patients taking aspirin as described will have a bleeding problem, but all of them should be screened to make certain of this. One test should be ordered to screen this type of patient: a bleeding time to screen the platelet function (aspirin can affect the platelet phase). If this test is abnormal, the patient's physician should be consulted before any dental surgical procedures are performed.

TABLE 20-7. Results of screening tests*

Condition	Screening tests				
	Platelet count	Bleeding time	PTT	PT	Tourniquet test
Thrombocytopenia	+ +	+ +	−	−	+
Dicumarol therapy	−	−	+ +	+ +	−
Liver disease	+	+	+ +	+ +	+
Vascular wall defect	−	+	−	−	+ +
Hemophilia	−	−	+ +	−	−
Aspirin therapy	+	+	+	+	+
Leukemia	+	+	−	−	+
Malabsorption syndrome or long-term antibiotic therapy	−	−	+ +	+ +	−
Factor VII deficiency	−	−	−	+ +	−
Renal dialysis (heparin)	+	+	+ +	−	+

*−, Normal; +, may be abnormal; + +, abnormal.

COUMARIN THERAPY

If the history establishes that a patient is receiving one of the coumarin drugs, the dentist should consult the patient's physician concerning the reason the patient is taking the drug, the level of anticoagulation (reported in terms of the PT—most patients are held at about 2 to 3½ times the normal PT of 11 to 14 seconds), and the current medical status of the patient. Most physicians are aware of the recommendations of the American Medical Association and the American Dental Association suggesting that the patient be brought down to at least a level of anticoagulation of about 1½ to 2 times the normal PT before the surgical procedure is attempted. If bleeding occurs, local measures can be used to control it.[4] If the physician agrees to this approach, he or she will reduce the dosage of anticoagulant. Some physicians may have the patient discontinue anticoagulant therapy before surgery. In either case, it will take at least 2 to 3 days for the effect of the reduced dosage to be reflected in a decrease in the PT.[7] On the day of surgery, the physician or dentist should order a PT to be certain that the desired degree of anticoagulation reduction has occurred. If PT is still greater than twice normal, the dosage of anticoagulant should be reduced again by the physician and the surgery should be postponed for 2 or 3 more days. Then the PT should be repeated.

If infection is present no surgery should be done until the patient has been treated with antibiotics. When the patient is free from acute infection and the PT is in the acceptable range (1½ to 2 times normal), surgery can be performed. The procedure should be done with as little trauma as possible, and the patient should be administered antibiotics to prevent postoperative infection. If excessive postoperative bleeding occurs, Gelfoam with thrombin can be used to control it. In some patients it may be helpful to construct a splint before surgery to cover the surgical area. This will protect the clot, and Gelfoam with thrombin can be packed beneath the splint. Primary closure over sockets is desirable.

Oxycel or Surgicel may be used in place of the Gelfoam. However, thrombin should not be used with these agents, because it is inactivated as a result of pH factors, thus representing additional cost with no real benefits (Table 20-8).

POSSIBLE LIVER DISEASE

A patient with a history of jaundice or heavy alcohol use may have significant liver disease. Most of the coagulation factors are produced in the liver; therefore, if enough liver damage has occurred, the patient could have a serious bleeding problem because of a defect in the coagulation phase. In addition, about 50% of patients with sig-

TABLE 20-8. Dental management of the patient taking dicumarol

I. Detection by history

II. Consultation with physician
  A. Status of underlying problem
  B. Level of anticoagulation expressed in PT
    1. If greater than 2 times normal, request that dicumarol dosage be reduced
    2. The effects of the reduction in dicumarol dosage will take 2 or 3 days
    3. On day of procedure, check to see if PT is 2 times normal or less

III. If scaling or surgical procedures are planned, patient should be free of active infection

IV. Prophylactic antibiotics are suggested following surgery to prevent postoperative infection, which may complicate the control of bleeding problem

V. If excessive bleeding should occur following surgery it can be controlled by local measures
  A. Splints
  B. Gelfoam with thrombin
  C. Oxycel, Surgicel
  D. Pressure packs

VI. Have patient return in 4 to 5 days, and if healing is normal call physician and have patient returned to usual dosage of anticoagulant

nificant liver disease will have a defect in the platelet phase as a result of platelet destruction by the spleen. The PT test can be used to screen for a defect in the coagulation phase in patients with a history that indicates liver disease. A bleeding time also should be obtained to see if the platelet phase has been affected. It is possible that the amount of liver damage would not be great enough to affect the coagulation phase, but the effect on the platelet phase could be severe enough to lead to a serious bleeding problem. If both the PT and bleeding time are normal, surgery can be performed on these patients with little risk of a postoperative bleeding problem.

CHRONIC LEUKEMIA

Patients with chronic leukemia should have their platelet status checked before they undergo dental surgery. A bleeding time should be performed on the day of surgery. If abnormal results are ob-

tained, surgery should be postponed if possible. If the surgery must be done, platelet replacement will have to be considered before the procedure. The patient's physician must be involved with this evaluation and preparation.

MALABSORPTION SYNDROME OR LONG-TERM ANTIBIOTIC THERAPY

In patients with malabsorption syndrome or patients receiving long-term antibiotic therapy, the bacteria in the intestine that produce vitamin K may be adversely affected. Vitamin K is needed by the liver for the production of prothrombin. The PT test can be ordered to screen for a possible bleeding problem. If the PT is normal, surgery can be performed on these patients without risk of a bleeding problem. The patient's physician should be consulted regarding the patient's health status before surgery, because there may be complicating factors, in addition to the possible bleeding problem, that would contraindicate surgery.

RENAL DIALYSIS (HEPARIN)

During hemodialysis the patient is usually given heparin, a short-acting anticoagulant. Heparin has a half-life of 4 hours; therefore effects may be variable for up to 24 hours after administration. If such a patient reports for dental care the day of hemodialysis treatment, the appointment should be postponed if possible until the following day to be certain that the effect of heparin has worn off.

VASCULAR WALL ALTERATION

Some patients with autoimmune disease may have alterations of the vessel wall that may result in excessive bleeding following surgical procedures. The tourniquet test can be used to identify the presence of significant vascular wall changes in these patients.

Management of patient with serious bleeding problem

Patients found to be thrombocytopenic or to have a severe coagulation disorder will most often require hospitalization and special preparation for surgery. A hematologist should be involved with the diagnosis, presurgical evaluation, preparation, and postsurgical management of these patients.

The patient with hemophilia (factor VIII deficiency) can be used to illustrate some of the management problems involved in dealing with a patient who has a serious bleeding problem. Consultation with a hematologist is necessary. The hematologist first establishes the diagnosis and determines the degree of factor VIII deficiency and whether any factor VIII inhibitors are present. He or she then selects the type of replacement material to be used, such as a cryoprecipitate of fresh plasma, and determines the dosage of the replacement material. A 7- to 10-day replacement period is usually planned so that healing is well underway before replacement is stopped.[2,3,5]

If factor VIII inhibitors are found, the hematologist may use epsilon-aminocaproic acid (EACA) therapy to help maintain the fibrin clot that does form. Cortisone also may be used to interfere with the action of the inhibitors.[4,7,8]

Splints should be made by the dentist before surgery so that mechanical displacement of the clot by the patient's tongue can be prevented.

The patient should be hospitalized for the surgery. The dentist and hematologist must observe the patient for any signs of an allergic reaction to the replacement therapy and be prepared to take appropriate action (Table 20-9).

TABLE 20-9. Dental management of hemophilia

1. Detection and referral
2. Consultation with hematologist
   a. Diagnosis
   b. Level of factor VIII deficiency
   c. Presence of factor VIII inhibitors
   d. Selection of replacement factor
   e. Dosage of replacement factor
   f. Need for EACA for clot maintenance
   g. Need for steroids to interfere with action of inhibitors
   h. Hospitalization of patient for surgical procedures
3. Construction of splints if multiple extractions or flap procedures are planned
4. Patient should be free of active infection
5. Use of good surgical techniques and sutures for closure whenever possible (at extraction site)
6. Prophylactic antibiotics to prevent postoperative infection

It may soon be possible for the dentist to treat some hemophilic patients in the dental office without factor VIII replacement therapy. Hemophilic patients are now being given EACA and microfibrillar collagen hemostat on an experimental basis, after which surgical procedures such as extractions and scaling procedures are performed. The EACA prevents the clot from breaking down, and the microfibrillar collagen hemostat used locally aids in formation of a clot.

Treatment planning modifications

With proper preparation, most indicated dental treatment can be provided for patients with various bleeding problems. Patients with congenital coagulation defects must be encouraged to improve and maintain good oral health, because most dental treatment for these patients at present is complicated by the need for replacement of the missing factor. Dental treatment often requires hospitalization. Patients with bleeding problems secondary to diseases that may be in the terminal phase should in general only be offered conservative dental treatment. Aspirin should not be used for pain relief in patients who have known bleeding disorders or who are receiving anticoagulant medication.

Oral complications

Patients with bleeding disorders may complain of spontaneous gingival bleeding. Oral tissues may show petechiae, ecchymoses, jaundice, pallor, and ulcers. Patients with leukemia may reveal a generalized hyperplasia of the gingiva. Patients with neoplastic disease may show osseous lesions on radiographs. These patients may show drifting and loose teeth. They may complain of paresthesias, such as burning of the tongue or numbness of the lip.[4,6]

Emergency dental care

The patient with a dental emergency who is identified as having a possible bleeding disorder by history or examination or both should not undergo surgery under any condition. Conservative means should be used to control any pain and infection.

After the patient has been diagnosed and treated for the medical problem, the dentist can begin to make plans for the extraction, pulpotomy, etc. If replacement of missing coagulation factors or platelets is indicated, it will be necessary for the dentist to work closely with the patient's physician before and after surgery.

REFERENCES

1. Catalamo, P.M.: Platelet and vascular disorders. In Rose, L.F., and Kaye, D., editors: Internal medicine for dentistry, St. Louis, 1983, The C.V. Mosby Co., pp. 400-408.
2. Cohen, S.G.: Hemophilia. In Rose, L.F., and Kaye, D., editors: Internal medicine for dentistry, St. Louis, 1983, The C.V. Mosby Co., pp. 427-428.
3. Lucas, D.N., and Albert, T.W.: Epsilon Amino Caproic Acid in hemophiliacs: a concise review, Oral Surg. **51:**115-120, 1981.
4. Lynch, M.A.: Hematologic diseases and related problems. In Lynch, M.A., editor: Burket's oral medicine, diagnosis and treatment, ed. 7, Philadelphia, 1977, J.B. Lippincott Co., pp. 409-443.
5. Nossel, H.L.: Bleeding. In Petersdorf, R.G., et al., editors: Harrison's principles of internal medicine, ed. 10, New York, 1983, McGraw-Hill Book Co., pp. 292-299.
6. Shafer, W.G., Hine, M.K., and Levy, B.M.: A textbook of oral pathology, ed. 4. Philadelphia, 1983, W.B. Saunders Co., pp. 726-736.
7. Wintrobe, M.M.: Clinical hematology, ed. 8, Philadelphia, 1981, Lea & Febiger, pp. 354-436.
8. Zieve, P.D.: Bleeding disorders. In Harvey, A., editor: Osler's the principles and practice of medicine, ed. 19, New York, 1976, Appleton-Century-Crofts, pp. 653-669.

21

BLOOD DYSCRASIAS

The purpose of this chapter is to present the most common disorders of the white and red blood cells that may influence dental treatment (see Table 21-1). The dentist should be able to detect patients with these diseases by history, clinical examination, and screening laboratory tests. Patients with disorders of the white or red blood cells may be susceptible to abnormal bleeding, delayed healing, infection, or mucosal ulceration. In addition, some of these diseases can be fatal. Thus they must be detected and the patient who has one referred to a physician for diagnosis and treatment before any dental procedure is performed. Patients with known disorders who are under medical care should have no dental care until consultation with the physician is obtained.

Anemia

GENERAL DESCRIPTION

Anemia is defined as a reduction in the oxygen-carrying capacity of the blood. It is usually related to a decrease in the number of circulating red blood cells or to an abnormality in the hemoglobin contained within the red blood cells. Anemia is not a disease but rather a symptom complex. Anemia may result from iron deficiency, decreased production of red blood cells, or increased rate of destruction of circulating red blood cells.

Excessive blood loss from menses or bleeding from the gastrointestinal tract can lead to iron deficiency anemia. Individuals with gastrectomy or malabsorption syndrome may have reduced absorption of iron from the gastrointestinal tract,

TABLE 21-1. Classification of blood dyscrasias

I. Red blood cell disorders
  A. Anemia
  B. Polycythemia

II. White blood cell disorders
  A. Leukopenia
  B. Leukocytosis
  C. Myeloproliferative disorders
    1. Acute leukemia
    2. Chronic leukemia
    3. Others
  D. Lymphoproliferative disorders
    1. Acute leukemia
    2. Chronic leukemia
    3. Multiple myeloma
    4. Lymphomas

which can result in anemia. Children and pregnant women may have an inadequate dietary intake of iron, which may also lead to anemia.

Factors that reduce the capacity of the bone marrow to produce red blood cells will cause anemia. Patients with gastric changes that result in the failure to produce the intrinsic factor needed for absorption of vitamin B_{12} will be unable to produce adequate numbers of red blood cells and will become anemic. Leukemia and metastatic tumors to bone will lead to replacement of the red blood cell precursors in the bone marrow and result in decreased production of red blood cells. The bone marrow cells may be destroyed by radiation or by the effects of drugs or chemicals, resulting in decreased production of red blood cells as well as white blood cells and platelets.

The bone marrow may be functioning normally, but the red blood cells may be destroyed at an increased rate once in circulation because of the effects of toxins, transfusion reactions, hyperactivity of the spleen, or defects in the construction of the red blood cells. The increased rate of destruction of red blood cells can lead to anemia.

All the various causes of anemia will not be covered in detail in this chapter. Examples have been selected to demonstrate the clinical problems involved in the management of patients with anemia.

Menses and pregnancy

It is very common for women who are menstruating or are pregnant to develop a mild iron deficiency anemia. The repeated blood loss associated with menses can lead to depletion of iron and result in a mild state of anemia. When taking a history from a woman patient it may be necessary for the dentist to ask if she is having periods, when the periods first started, if they have been regular, the number of days involved, and the number of pads used. Patients with a history of regular periods but with heavy flow may be anemic and should receive medical advice and treatment. A patient with a change in pattern, onset, length, or rate of flow of her periods should be encouraged to seek medical evaluation. A patient who has stopped having periods long before expected should be referred for medical evaluating. The patient who has had bleeding in between her regular periods should also be referred for medical evaluation.

During pregnancy there is an increased demand on the expectant mother for additional iron and vitamins to support the growth of the fetus. Unless sufficient amounts of these nutrients have been provided in some form, the mother may become anemic. In obtaining the health history the dentist should establish if the patient has other children and when they were born. The closer together the pregnancies were, the greater the chances for the patient to have developed iron deficiency anemia. Once the baby has been born, the mother may lose additional iron if she breast-feeds the baby.

In contrast to women, mild anemia in men usually indicates the presence of a serious underlying medical problem. Under normal conditions men lose very little iron, and iron deficiency anemia on a physiologic basis is very rare. Therefore, any man found to be anemic *must* be referred for medical evaluation.

Pernicious anemia

Vitamin B_{12} and folic acid are needed for the maturation of the red blood cell in the bone marrow. A deficiency in the daily intake or absorption of these vitamins can result in anemia. Pernicious anemia results from a deficiency of the intrinsic factor, a substance secreted by the parietal cells of the stomach. Intrinsic factor is necessary for the absorption of vitamin B_{12}, which is needed for maturation of the red blood cell. Pernicious anemia is a disease of late adult life. Early symptoms include tingling of the fingers and toes, numbness, uncoordination, and muscular weakness. Early detection is important so that treatment can be begun before neurologic symptoms have progressed so far that they cannot be corrected. Treatment involves vitamin B_{12} injections. Folic acid will correct the anemia but will not stop the progression of the neurologic symptoms. The vitamin B_{12} deficiency would still exist but could be undetected. This is why Federal regulations have stated that vitamin preparations sold over the counter cannot contain a significant amount of folic acid.

Glucose 6-phosphate dehydrogenase deficiency

Glucose 6-phosphate dehydrogenase deficiency is an intracorpuscular defect found most commonly in black Americans. The defect is transmitted on the X chromosome and may occur in both males and females. About 10% to 15% of the black population may be affected. The life span of the red blood cell is reduced to about two-thirds of normal. Infection, diabetes, and certain drugs may cause an acute acceleration of hemolysis of the red cells.[4,7]

Sickle cell anemia

A defect in the beta chain of hemoglobin can cause the red blood cell to become sickle shaped when placed in the presence of either lowered blood oxygen tension or increased blood pH. Sickle cell anemia is a hereditary disorder found in blacks.

The disease may manifest itself as either sickle

cell trait or sickle cell disease. About 9% of the black population is thought to have sickle cell trait.[4,7] These individuals have no symptoms unless they are placed in situations in which abnormally low concentrations of oxygen are present, such as in an unpressurized airplane or in injudicious administration of general anesthesia.

Patients with sickle cell disease usually show marked clinical manifestations and often die before the age of 40 years. About 0.15% of the black population has sickle cell anemia.[4,7] Clinical signs and symptoms include jaundice, pallor, cardiac failure, leg ulcers, stroke, and attacks of abdominal and bone pain. Aplastic crises, in which the patient becomes acutely ill, red cell production stops, and severe anemia develops, may develop from infection or hypersensitivity reactions. Folic acid deficiency may play a part in the cause of the crises, and for this reason folic acid dietary supplements are given to most patients with sickle cell anemia. Once a crisis develops, high doses of folic acid and blood transfusions are used to treat the patient.

Renal disease

The kidney produces the hormone erythropoietin, which stimulates red blood cell production by the bone marrow. If there is significant renal damage, the lack of production of this hormone will result in anemia.

CLINICAL PRESENTATION
Signs and symptoms

Symptoms of anemia include fatigue, shortness of breath, abdominal pain, bone pain, tingling of fingers and toes, and muscular weakness. Signs of anemia may include jaundice, pallor, spooning, cracking, and splitting of the fingernails, increased size of liver and spleen, lymphadenopathy, and blood in the stool. Patients with anemia may complain of sore, painful tongue, smooth tongue, or redness of the tongue. Some patients may complain of a loss of taste sensation.

Screening laboratory tests

If the dentist identifies a patient with signs or symptoms that suggest anemia, the patient should be sent to a commercial laboratory for screening tests or referred to a physician for evaluation. The hemoglobin level and hematocrit are the tests used to screen the patient. In addition to these tests, a total white blood cell count and platelet count should be obtained.

Black patients can be screened for the sickle cell trait by use of the *Sickledex Test* distributed by Johnson & Johnson. This is a simple test that uses a small amount of blood, and it can be performed in the dental office.

White blood cell disorders

GENERAL DESCRIPTION

Three groups of white blood cells are found in the peripheral circulation—granulocytes, lymphocytes, and monocytes. There are three types of granulocytes—polymorphonuclear leukocytes, or "polys," eosinophils, and basophils. Circulating lymphocytes are of two types—thymus-mediated lymphocytes and those that originate from lymphoid tissue found in association with the gastrointestinal tract. The granulocytes and monocytes are produced by cells of the bone marrow.

The prime function of the polymorphonuclear leukocytes is to defend the body against certain infectious agents by phagocytosis and enzymatic destruction of the invaders. Eosinophils and basophils are involved in inflammatory allergic reactions. The thymus-mediated lymphocytes are involved with the delayed, or cellular, immune reaction. The other lymphocytes play an important role in the immediate, or normal, immune system. The monocytes serve as phagocytes and appear to be involved in some way with the immune response (see Chapter 19).

The majority of white blood cells are produced primarily in the bone marrow (granulocytes and monocytes), and there are several "pools" of these cells in the marrow. The first is the mitotic pool, which consists of immature precursor cells. The second is a maturing pool that consists of cells that are undergoing maturation. Finally, there is a storage pool of functional cells that can be released as needed.

The white blood cells released by the bone marrow that are found circulating in the peripheral blood form two pools of cells, a marginal one and a circulating one. Cells in the marginal pool adhere to vessel walls and are readily available when needed. When infection threatens the body, the storage and marginal pools can be called on to help fight the invading infectious agents.

Leukocytosis and leukopenia

The number of circulating white blood cells is expressed as the number of cells found in a cubic millimeter of blood. This count normally ranges from 5000 to 10,0000/mm³ in the adult.[7] The differential white cell count is an estimation of the percentage of each cell type per cubic millimeter of blood. A normal differential count would be as follows: polymorphonuclear leukocytes, 50% to 60%; eosinophils, 3%; basophils, less than 1%; lymphocytes, 20% to 30%; and monocytes, 3% to 7%. The term *leukocytosis* is defined as an increase in the number of circulating white blood cells to more than 10,000/mm³. The term *leukopenia* is defined as a reduction in the number of circulating white blood cells, usually to less than 5000/mm³.[7]

There are many causes of leukocytosis. Exercise, pregnancy, and emotional stress can lead to increased numbers of white blood cells in the peripheral circulation. Leukocytosis resulting from these causes is called physiologic leukocytosis. Pathologic leukocytosis can be caused by infections, neoplasia, and necrosis. Pyogenic infections cause a type of leukocytosis characterized by an increased number of polymorphonuclear leukocytes. If a number of immature polymorphonuclear leukocytes (stab cells) are released into circulation in response to a bacterial infection, a shift to the left is said to have occurred. Viral infections often produce a type of leukocytosis characterized by an increased number of lymphocytes. Tuberculosis and syphilis also primarily cause a lymphocytosis. Protozoan infections often produce a type of leukocytosis that appears as an increase in numbers of monocytes. Allergies and infections caused by certain helminths (worms) usually result in a type of leukocytosis caused primarily by an increase in the number of circulating eosinophils. Necrosis (cell death) will result in a type of leukocytosis brought about by increased numbers of circulating neutrophils. Leukemia, cancer of the white blood cells, usually is characterized by a great increase in the numbers of circulating white blood cells. Carcinomas of glandular tissues may cause an increase

in the number of circulating neutrophils. Acute bleeding also can result in a leukocytosis, because blood loss serves not only as a stimulus for red blood cell production but also can lead to leukopenia. An important form of leukopenia involves the depression of the circulating polymorphonuclear leukocytes. This disorder is called cyclic neutropenia. Patients with this disorder have a cyclic decrease in the number of neutrophils that occurs about every 28 days. During the period in which few circulating polymorphonuclear leukocytes are present, the patient is very susceptible to infection.[4,6] These patients often show very progressive forms of periodontal disease and may develop oral ulcers. A patient with severe leukopenia is very susceptible to infection.

Infectious mononucleosis

Infectious mononucleosis is a viral infection that results in a marked lymphocytic response. It is caused by Epstein-Barr virus, which is a lymphotropic herpesvirus. Infectious mononucleosis is usually asymptomatic when found in children. When young adults are affected, about 50% will be symptomatic. The virus is transmitted via the oropharyngeal route during close personal contact. The incubation time is about 30 to 50 days. A prodromal period of 3 to 5 days precedes the clinical phase, which lasts for 7 to 20 days. About 10% to 20% of asymptomatic, seropositive adults (antibodies to Epstein-Barr virus) carry the virus in the oropharyngeal region.

The prodromal period lasts about 3 to 5 days, and the patient may complain of headache, malaise, myalgia, and fatigue. The clinical phase consists of fever, sore throat, and cervical lymphadenopathy. About one third of the patients will develop palatal petechiae during the first week of the illness, and about 10% will develop a generalized skin rash. Laboratory studies will reveal a lymphocytosis, heterophil antibodies, and antibodies to the Epstein-Barr virus. Many of these clinical findings can be confused with the symptoms of leukemia, hence the importance of the laboratory tests.

Treatment of infectious mononucleosis is symptomatic and consists of bed rest, salicylates for pain control, and gargling and irrigation with saline solution to provide symptomatic relief of pharyngitis and stomatitis. In some patients with severe toxic exudative pharyngotonsillitis and pharyngeal edema, a short course of prednisone may be given. About 20% of the patients with symptomatic infectious mononucleosis will have concurrent beta-hemolytic streptococcal pharyngotonsillitis and should be treated with 250 mg of penicillin V four times a day for 10 days if they are not allergic to penicillin. Ampicillin should be avoided because of the high incidence of skin rash in patients with infectious mononucleosis treated with this drug.[5]

Acute leukemia

Acute leukemia has a sudden onset and will lead to death in 1 to 2 months if untreated. It consists of increased numbers of immature white blood cells in the peripheral circulation. There are two types of acute leukemia, acute lymphoblastic leukemia (ALL) and acute nonlymphoblastic leukemia (ANLL).

Cases of ALL can be placed into one of three groups: L-1, which consists of small cells; L-2, which consists of large cells; and L-3 (Burkitt type), which consists of large homogenous B-marker cells. ANLL can be grouped into six types; M-1, M-2, and M-3, which show different forms of granulocytic differentiation; M-4, which consists of granulocytes and monocytes; M-5, which consists of monocytes; and M-6, which reveals 50% or more erythroblasts.

The incidence of leukemia has remained stable in the United States since about 1956. The mortality also has remained stable at about 6.8 deaths per 100,000 population per year for all types of leukemia. About 50% to 60% of the deaths are caused by acute leukemia. All types of leukemia are a little more common in males than females. The male-to-female ratio in acute leukemia is about 3:2, and in chronic leukemia about 2:1.

Acute leukemia accounts for about 50% of all neoplasms found in children. ALL is found most often in 2- to 4-year old children. Fewer than 20% of cases of ANLL occur in patients under the age of 15 years. Hence ALL is a disease mostly of children, and ANLL is a disease of older adults.

Marked advances have been made in the treatment of leukemia, particularly ALL, during the last 10 to 15 years. About 90% of children with

ALL gain complete remission, and 85% of adults with ALL gain complete remission using current treatment regimens. As stated previously, untreated patients with ALL will be dead within 1 to 2 months following the onset of the disease. The first phase of treatment of ALL consists of prednisone and vincristine. These are followed by other antileukemic agents. It is important that the first attempt at treatment be as effective as possible, because prolonged remission is difficult to obtain after ineffective initial treatment attempts.

ANLL does not respond to treatment as well as ALL. It is more difficult to obtain remission of the disease, and when remission occurs it does not last as long.

Only about 60% to 80% of patients with ANLL who receive the best treatment available will go into remission. When remission is obtained, it only lasts for about 1 year, and only about 10% to 15% of the patients stay in remission for 5 years or longer. Because of this poor response to chemotherapy, patients with ANLL are candidates for bone marrow transplants. Patients who have received bone marrow transplants may develop graft-vs.-host disease, in which the transplanted cells "attack" the host tissues.

Symptoms of acute leukemia include fever; bleeding; pallor; weakness; recurrent infection; enlargement of tonsils, lymph nodes, spleen, and gingiva; oral ulcerations; and small hemorrhages of the skin and mucous membranes. Patients with acute leukemia are very susceptible to excessive bleeding, poor healing, and infection following dental surgical procedures.[3]

Chronic leukemia

There are two types of chronic leukemia, chronic granulocytic leukemia (CGL) and chronic lymphocytic leukemia (CLL). Chronic leukemia has a slower onset of symptoms, a better prognosis, and more mature white blood cells than acute leukemia.

The majority of patients with CGL are 30 to 50 years of age at the onset of the disease. The white blood cell count is usually around 200,000/mm^3 at the time of diagnosis. The symptoms associated with CGL include enlarged and painful spleen, pallor, weight loss, fever, bleeding problems and increased serum vitamin B$_{12}$ levels. Lymphadenopathy is rare in the early phase of CGL. The alkylating agent busulfan is the most common agent used to treat CGL. Busulfan can cause skin pigmentation, dryness of skin and mucosa, and pulmonary fibrosis as side effects. When the vitamin B_{12} serum levels fall back to normal levels, the patient is usually in a state of remission. If more immature cells are formed in the peripheral blood, the patient is said to be in blastic phase of CGL. This phase is very resistant to therapy, and death often occurs in 2 to 3 months. A few patients in this phase (about 20%) will respond to prednisone and vincristine.

Patients with CLL are older than those with CGL; the median age is 60 years. The white blood cell count is usually lower than that found in patients with CGL. Patients with CLL often have associated anemia and thrombocytopenia. They also have enlarged spleens and lymphadenopathy. Patients who have CLL with anemia and thrombocytopenia will live for about 24 months, in contrast to those who have lymphocytosis and lymphadenopathy only, who live for about 8 to 10 years. Treatment of CLL may include radiation of isolated lymph nodes and the use of an alkylating agent such as chlorambucil or cyclophosphamide.

In general, patients with chronic leukemia have anemia and bleeding problems associated with thrombocytopenia. These can be caused by leukemia itself and the effects of the chemotherapy used to treat the disease. Infection is less of a problem in patients with chronic leukemia than in those with acute leukemia. This is because the cells are more mature and functional in chronic leukemia. However, in the later stages of both CGL and CLL, infection becomes a serious complication.[2]

Lymphoproliferative disorders

Lymphoproliferative disorders other than ALL and CLL that are of importance to the dentist include lymphomas and multiple myeloma (Figs. 21-1 to 21-3). Patients with these disorders may have difficulties with infection, wound healing, and bleeding. The problem with infection results from an alteration of the patient's immune response and a secondary neutropenia. Poor healing is a result of a combination of factors, including anemia, neutropenia, and altered immune response. The bleeding problem is associated with a thrombocytopenia

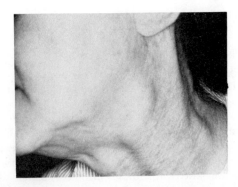

FIG. 21-1. Patient with lymphadenopathy involving cervical lymph nodes. This patient had a form of lymphoma, Hodgkin's disease.

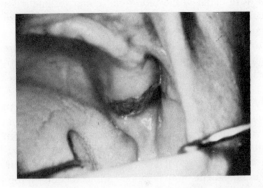

FIG. 21-2. Patient who complained of loose maxillary denture. This patient had a form of lymphoma, reticulum cell sarcoma.

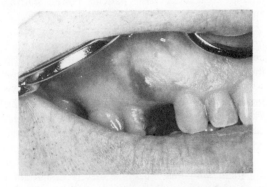

FIG. 21-3. Lesion on alveolar ridge was found on radiographs to involve underlying alveolar bone. This patient had a form of lymphoma, lymphosarcoma.

caused by the decreased production of platelets in the bone marrow.

DENTAL MANAGEMENT
Medical considerations

The dentist should search for signs and symptoms of anemia or white blood cell disorders in patients who are seen for dental treatment. A patient with classical signs or symptoms of anemia or leukemia, for example, should be referred directly to a physician. Patients with signs and symptoms less suggestive of these disorders should be screened by appropriate laboratory tests. These can be obtained by sending the patient to a commercial clinical laboratory or to a physician. Screening tests should include a total white blood cell count, a differential white blood cell count, a smear for cell morphology, a hemoglobin or hematocrit count, and a platelet count. If the screening tests are ordered by the dentist and one or more are abnormal, the patient should be referred for medical evaluation and treatment.

Patients with anemia may have a serious underlying disease, such as peptic ulcer or carcinoma, in which early detection may be lifesaving. Patients with sickle cell anemia may be in grave danger in the dental office if the disease is not detected before dental treatment is started. Undetected leukemic patients may develop serious bleeding problems following any surgical procedure. They may also have problems with healing of surgical wounds, and they are very prone to postsurgical infections. Thus it is important for the dentist to attempt to identify these patients before starting any dental treatment.

Patients under medical treatment for leukemia must be identified by their health history and their current status established by consultation with their physician. With special considerations, the patient who is in a state of remission can receive most indicated dental treatment (see Table 21-2). Patients with acute signs or symptoms of the disease in general should receive only conservative emergency dental care.

If scaling or surgical procedures are planned for a patient who has leukemia that is under good medical control, a bleeding time should be obtained on the day of the procedure. This is done to establish that an adequate number of functional

TABLE 21-2. Dental management of the leukemic patient

I. Detection
  A. History
  B. Examination
  C. Screening laboratory tests
      1. White blood cell count
      2. Differential white blood cell count
      3. Smear for cell morphology
      4. Hemoglobin or hematocrit level
      5. Platelet count

II. Referral
  A. Medical diagnosis
  B. Treatment

III. Consultation before any dental care is rendered
  A. Current status
  B. Review of dental treatment needs
  C. Dental management plan

IV. Routine dental care
  A. None for patient with acute symptoms
  B. Once disease is under control, patient may receive indicated dental care
  C. Scaling and surgical procedures
      1. Bleeding time day of procedures; if normal, proceed; if prolonged, delay or obtain platelet replacement
      2. Prophylactic antibiotic therapy to prevent postoperative infection

V. Emergency dental care
  A. Symptomatic treatment of oral ulcers
      1. Antibiotics
      2. Bland mouth rinse—sodium bicarbonate
      3. Syrup of promethazine (Phenergan)
      4. Orabase
  B. Oral moniliasis—treat with suspension of nystatin (100,000 units/ml)
  C. Conservative management of pain and infection
      1. Antibiotic sensitivity testing
      2. Antibiotics, heat for infection
      3. Strong analgesics for pain

platelets are present. Platelets can be depressed in numbers in these patients, either by the leukemic process or by the agents used to treat the leukemia. If the bleeding time is abnormal, the procedure should be cancelled and the patient's physician consulted. In patients whose disease is under good control but who are still thrombocytopenic, platelet replacement by the physician can be considered if the dental procedures must be done. In general, we would suggest prophylactic antibiotic therapy for leukemic patients who receive surgical treatment to prevent postoperative infection.

Patients with glucose 6-phosphate dehydrogenase deficiency have an increased incidence of drug sensitivity, with sulfonamides, aspirin, and chloramphenicol being the prime offenders.[1,4] Dental infection and drugs that contain phenacetin may accelerate the rate of hemolysis of the red blood cells in patients with this type of anemia; [1,4] thus dental infections should be avoided and, when they do occur, must be dealt with effectively. Drugs containing phenacetin should not be used in these patients.

Patients with sickle cell trait or disease may develop a serious crisis if they are exposed to reduced levels of oxygen.[4,6] Therefore general anesthesia in the dental office is contraindicated for these patients. Nitrous oxide analgesia should not be used in patients with sickle cell anemia, and the patient's physician should be consulted before it is used in patients with sickle cell trait. Whenever possible, patients at high risk for these disorders (blacks) should be screened by clinical laboratory tests before dental treatment is started. Patients with sickle cell anemia may heal slowly; thus extensive elective surgery is not indicated in these patients. Infections also may precipitate an aplastic crisis in patients with sickle cell anemia. Patients with this disorder should be encouraged to maintain healthy dentition. If infections do develop, they must be managed effectively and with speed.

Treatment planning modifications

Patients with acute leukemia should receive only conservative treatment for emergency dental problems. Routine dental treatment is not indicated for these patients. Special attention should be given to oral hygiene procedures for patients who have leukemia to avoid dental caries and gingival inflammation and infection. Leukemic patients whose disease is in a state of remission or control can receive any indicated dental treatment, as long as the preceding special considerations are followed.

Patients with acute infections should not receive routine dental care until the infection has been treated and the patient has returned to a normal state.

Elective surgical procedures are best avoided in

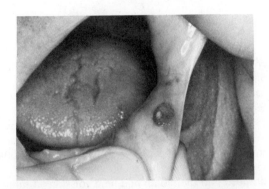

FIG. 21-4. Patient who had multiple intraoral ulcers; one is shown that involved labial mucosa of lower lip. This patient had chronic lymphocytic leukemia.

patients with sickle cell anemia. Routine dental care can be rendered for patients with sickle cell trait and disease. Special emphasis should be placed on oral hygiene procedures to avoid dental caries and gingival inflammation and infection.

Oral complications

Patients with leukemia may develop multiple oral ulcers that can be very painful and are prone to secondary infection (Fig. 21-4). These patients should be administered antibiotics and should receive symptomatic treatment for the ulcers. A bland mouth rinse of 1 teaspoon of sodium bicarbonate in a glass of warm water can be used to clean the surface of the ulcers. Commercial mouth rinses are not recommended because they tend to irritate ulcerated tissues. Following the bland mouth rinse, the patient should be instructed to place a teaspoon of promethazine hydrochloride syrup (6.25 mg/5 ml) into the mouth, hold it there for several minutes, and move it from side to side with the tongue. The syrup then can be swallowed. Promethazine has local anesthetic properties that will provide relief from the pain. Lesions in the mucobuccal fold or under the tongue can then be coated with a thin layer of Orabase, which will protect the surface of the ulcer from irritation. This sequence can be repeated four to six times a day.

Patients with leukemia are usually very prone to infection because of the immature nature of the malignant white blood cells. When oral infection develops in a leukemic patient, a specimen of exudate should be sent for antibiotic sensitivity testing and penicillin therapy should be begun (if the patient is not allergic to penicillin). If the clinical course shows little or no improvement in several days, the antibiotic sensitivity testing data may be used to select an antibiotic that may be more effective.

Leukemic patients are prone to oral moniliasis. When this complication occurs the patient can be treated with a suspension of nystatin (100,000 units/ml). One milliliter of the suspension is dropped into the mouth and held for several minutes before being swallowed. This should be repeated four to six times a day. The medication should be continued for at least 48 hours after the disappearance of clinical signs of the disease.[1]

Small or large areas of submucosal hemorrhage may be found in the leukemic patient (Fig. 21-5). These lesions result from minor trauma and relate to the thrombocytopenia. Leukemic patients also may complain of spontaneous gingival hemorrhage. Some patients may complain of paresthesias resulting from leukemic infiltration of peripheral nerves.

Leukemic patients with poor oral hygiene are prone to develop localized or generalized gingival inflammation (Figs. 21-6 and 21-7). This finding is most common in patients who have monocytic leukemia.

The oral findings in patients with anemia usually relate to the underlying cause of the anemia. The oral mucosa will often appear pale. Patients with nutritional causes of anemia, such as vitamin B_{12}

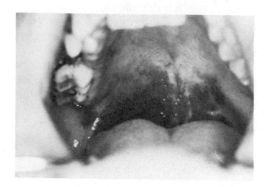

FIG. 21-5. Ecchymoses involving palate of leukemic patient.

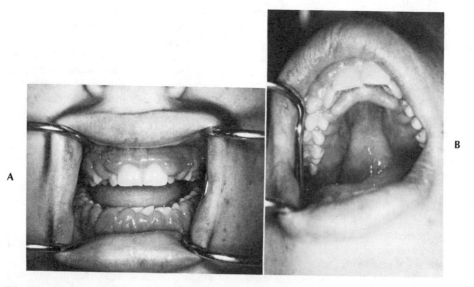

FIG. 21-6. A, Patient with monocytic leukemia who has developed severe generalized gingival hyperplasia. Gingival biopsy revealed numerous immature white blood cells in tissues. B, Palatal view of gingival hyperplasia in leukemic patient.

or iron deficiency, may show loss of papillae from the tongue and atrophic changes of the oral mucosa (Fig. 21-8). An angular cheilitis may be found in some patients. These patients also may complain of burning or sore tongue. Some patients with iron deficiency anemia may have Plummer-Vinson syndrome. This syndrome consists of sore mouth, dysphagia (resulting from muscular degeneration in the esophagus and stenosis of the esophageal mucosa), and an increased frequency of carcinoma

of the oral cavity and pharynx. Patients with this syndrome should be followed up closely for any oral or pharyngeal tissue changes that may be early indicators of carcinoma.[4,6]

In addition to pallor, patients with hemolytic anemia may show oral evidence of jaundice caused by hyperbilirubinemia secondary to excessive erythrocyte destruction. The trabecular pattern of the bone on dental radiographs may be affected because of hyperplasia of marrow elements in response to increased destruction of red blood cells. The bone will appear more radiolucent with very prominent lamellar striations.[4,6]

Patients with sickle cell anemia also may show evidence of jaundice in the oral tissues as well as pallor. Erythropoietic activity is increased, and dental radiographic findings associated with the bone marrow hyperplasia may be found. The trabeculae between teeth may appear as horizontal rows (Fig. 21-9). The lamina dura may appear

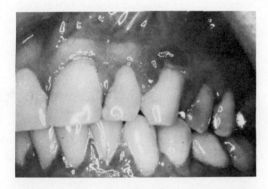

FIG. 21-7. Localized area of gingival inflammation in patient with moderate oral hygiene. Lesion would not clear up following removal of local irritants. Biopsy revealed immature white blood cells compatible with leukemic infiltrate. Patient was referred, and diagnosis of acute monocytic leukemia was established.

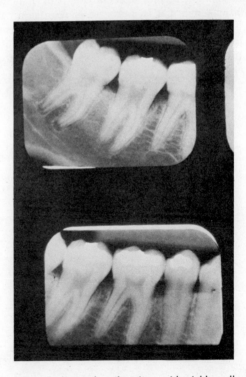

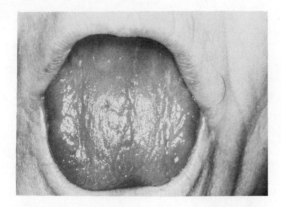

FIG. 21-8. Patient with smooth red tongue. This patient was found to have pernicious anemia (vitamin B_{12} deficiency caused by lack of intrinsic factor).

FIG. 21-9. Radiographs of patient with sickle cell anemia. Note prominent horizontal trabeculations and dense lamina dura.

more dense and distinct. Areas of sclerosis have been reported. Patients with sickle cell anemia may show delayed eruption of teeth, and hypoplasia of teeth may occur.[4,6]

Emergency dental care

Patients who have anemia without thrombocytopenia and leukopenia can usually receive any indicated emergency dental care. Extra caution must be taken in patients who have sickle cell trait and sickle cell anemia to avoid precipitating a crisis. Infections in these patients and patients with other forms of hemolytic anemia must be treated at once. Antibiotics, drainage, heat, etc. are indicated. If thrombocytopenia is present, surgical procedures must be avoided.

Patients with acute signs and symptoms of leukemia should receive no surgical treatment for emergency dental problems. Conservative treatment consisting of antibiotics and strong analgesics is indicated for infection and pain. Patients with leukemia that is in a state of remission can receive any indicated emergency dental treatment, as long as the bleeding time is normal and prophylactic antibiotics are used to prevent infection following surgery.

REFERENCES

1. American Dental Association: Accepted dental therapeutics, ed 39, Chicago, 1982, The Association.
2. Canellos, G.P.: The chronic leukemias. In Petersdorf, R.G., et al., editors: Harrison's principles of internal medicine, ed. 10, New York, 1983, McGraw-Hill Book Co., pp. 808-811.
3. Clarkson, B.: The acute leukemias. In Petersdorf, et al., editors: Harrison's principles of internal medicine, ed. 10, New York, 1983, McGraw-Hill Book Co., pp. 778-808.
4. Lynch, M.A.: Hematologic diseases and related problems. In Lynch, M.A., editor: Burket's oral medicine, diagnosis and treatment, ed. 7, Philadelphia, 1977, J.B. Lippincott Co., pp. 409-443.
5. Niederssam, J.C.: Epstein-Barr infection, including infectious mononucleosis. In Petersdorf, R.G., et al., editors: Harrison's principles of internal medicine, ed. 10, New York, 1983, McGraw-Hill Book Co., pp. 1170-1175.
6. Shafer, W.G., Hine, M.K., and Levy, B.M.: A textbook of oral pathology, ed. 4, Philadelphia, 1983, W.B. Saunders Co., pp. 726-734.
7. Wintrobe, M.M., et al.: Clinical hematology, Philadelphia, 1974, Lea & Febiger, pp. 35-126.

22

ORAL CANCER

The effective management of the patient with oral cancer often requires a team approach that involves dental, medical, surgical, radiotherapeutic, chemotherapeutic, reconstructive, and psychiatric considerations. The management of the patient with oral cancer presents many of the same types of problems to the dentist as the management of a patient with a systemic medical condition such as diabetes mellitus. However, the emphasis on the various roles of the dentist is different with the cancer patient. For example, the dentist assumes a more primary role for the detection of the cancerous lesion. The dentist also carries a more active part in the pretreatment and posttreatment phases for the cancer patient who needs reconstruction following surgery and/or radiation therapy.

All patients who have lesions involving the oral cavity require a diagnosis of the problem. Often a final or definitive diagnosis can be made by the dentist based on history and clinical findings. This is most often true with conditions such as geographic tongue, lichen planus, and aphthous stomatitis. In cases in which the dentist is unable to make a final diagnosis based on clinical findings, additional steps must be taken. These steps may include biopsy or referral to an individual more qualified to deal with the diagnostic problem, i.e., an oral surgeon or oral pathologist.

If the initial clinical impression of the lesion is cancer, it is best under most circumstances to refer the patient directly to a cancer treatment center for diagnosis and therapy. There are two reasons for this recommendation (Fig. 22-1). First, it minimizes the time from the finding of the lesion to the initiation of therapy. Second, it allows the individuals who will make decisions concerning the selection of treatment the opportunity to see the lesion before it has been altered by the biopsy procedure. In some cases, this is very important in determining the stage of the tumor, on which the selection of therapy may be used. In general, if any patient has a lesion for which the suspicion of cancer is low, the lesion should be biopsied by the dentist or the patient referred to an oral surgeon for biopsy to establish a definitive diagnosis (Fig. 22-2). In cases in which a diagnosis of cancer is established by the biopsy, the patient can then be referred for appropriate therapy.

GENERAL DESCRIPTION
Incidence

During 1978* about 660,000 cases of cancer were identified (excluding superficial skin cancers).[3] 67,000 of these cases involved the head and neck region. Excluding cancers of the central nervous system, eyes, and thyroid gland and sarcomas, lymphomas, and cutaneous melanomas, all of which accounted for about 30,000 cases, there were about 37,000 new cases of squamous cell carcinoma involving the head and neck (5.5% of all cancers). 17,400 of these cases were oral carcinomas, which accounted for about 2.6% of all new cancers for the year (see Table 22-1). Other studies have estimated the incidence of all types of oral cancer at about 5% of all new cancers per year. Again, the vast majority of these lesions were squamous cell carcinomas.[4]

The most common location for oral cancer reported by the 1979* Public Health Service report[3]

---

*More recent reports are less complete but continue to support these data.

271

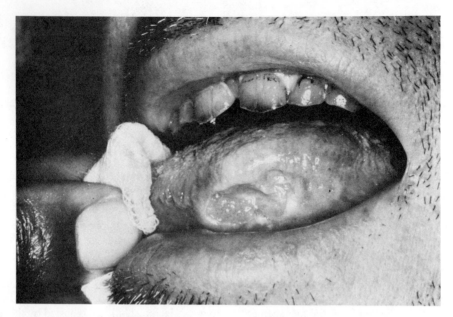

FIG. 22-1. This tongue lesion has very high chance of being cancer based on its clinical appearance. Direct referral to cancer treatment center for diagnosis and therapy is indicated. Diagnosis: squamous cell carcinoma.

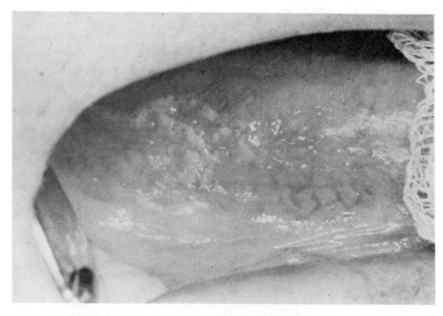

FIG. 22-2. No clinical causes for this tongue lesion could be identified. Its clinical appearance is not highly suggestive of cancer. It would be appropriate for dentist to biopsy this lesion to establish diagnosis. Diagnosis: early squamous cell carcinoma.

TABLE 22-1. Location and incidence of head and neck cancer*

Location	Incidence	Percentage of head and neck cancers	Percentage of all cancers
Oral (including salivary)	17,400	48	2.6
Nasopharynx	1,300	4	0.2
Oropharynx	3,500	10	0.5
Hypopharynx	1,800	5	0.5
Larynx	9,200	25	1.4
Nose and paranasal sinuses	1,500	4	0.2
Maxillary sinus	1,100	3	0.2
Other	400	1.3	0.1
Esophagus (cervical)	800	2	0.1
Trachea (cervical)	100	1	0.1
Ear	300	1	0.1
Unknown Primary	800	2	0.1
TOTALS	36,700	100%	5.5%

From Public Health Service: Management guidelines for head and neck cancer, U.S. Department of Health, Public Health Service, National Institute of Health, pub. no. 80-2037, 1979.
*Does not include thyroid, central nervous system, eye, soft tissue and bone, melanoma, and lymphoma, which account for another 30,600 cases, or 4.6% of all cancers.

TABLE 22-2. Location and frequency of oral cancer

Location	Incidence	Percentage of oral cancer
Lip	4200	24
Tongue	4600	26
Floor of mouth	2200	13
Buccal	1500	9
Gingival	1500	9
Palate	900	5
Salivary gland	2400	14

From Public Health Service: Management guidelines for head and neck cancer, U.S. Department of Health, Public Health Service, National Institute of Health, pub. no. 80-2037, 1979.

was the tongue (4600 cases), followed by the lip (4200 cases). The location with the lowest incidence was the palate (see Table 22-2). The male to female incidence ratio was over 3:1 for head and neck cancer. The male to female ratio for lip cancer was 2.2:1 and for the other oral locations was 11:1.[3] The vast majority of head and neck cancer, including oral cancer, is found in patients over the age of 50. The incidence increases with each decade over age 40 for both males and females.[3]

Etiology

The cause of oral cancer is not known at present. Several factors have been found to be associated with the development of oral cancer (Table 22-3). In the case of lip cancer, exposure to the sun and smoking have been found to have a very strong association in the development of cancer. Tobacco use, smoking, and/or excessive alcohol intake have been found to be associated with most cases of intraoral squamous cell carcinoma. Other factors have been suggested to have a minor role in the etiology of oral cancer. These include tertiary syphilis, arsenic compounds used in the treatment of syphilis, nutritional deficiencies, and heavy exposure to materials such as fumes from wood and metal dusts.[3,4]

The factors that come the closest to a cause and effect relationship in the etiology of oral cancer are smoking and actinic radiation. However, a direct cause and effect relationship has yet to be established.

Pathophysiology and complications

The vast majority of oral cancers are of epithelial origin, with most of these developing from the lining tissues of the oral cavity (Table 22-4).

Hence about 90% of oral cancers are squamous cell carcinomas. The remaining lesions are glandular carcinomas arising from salivary gland tissues and lesions of other tissue types, such as sarcomas and lymphomas.[3] The remainder of this chapter will deal primarily with squamous cell carcinoma, although many of the management recommendations may apply to patients with other types of primary oral cancer.

Squamous cell carcinoma may develop in normal-appearing tissue or, as is more often the case, in preexisting benign white or red lesions involving the oral mucosa (Fig. 22-3). Various studies have shown that white lesions that cannot be scraped off and that are nonspecific clinically (leukoplakia) may be benign, premalignant, or malignant at the time of initial biopsy. About 19% of these white epithelial lesions show evidence of dyskeratosis at the time of initial biopsy, and about 4% are squamous cell carcinoma. Patients with

TABLE 22-3. Predisposing factors in oral cancer development

Major

Smoking
Tobacco use
Excessive alcohol intake
Actinic radiation
Nutritional deficiencies

Minor

Tertiary syphilis
Arsenic compounds used to treat syphilis
Chronic physical and thermal trauma

TABLE 22-4. Classification of oral carcinomas

Squamous cell carcinoma
    Carcinoma in situ
    Well differentiated
    Moderately well differentiated
    Poorly differentiated
    Undifferentiated

Verrucous carcinoma

Glandular epithelial tumor

Unclassified carcinoma

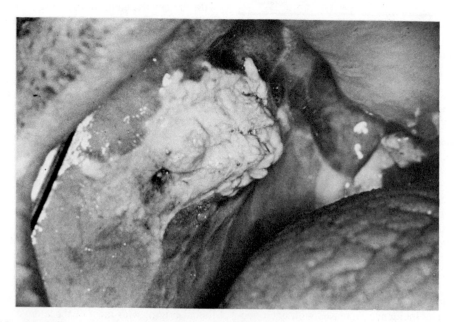

FIG. 22-3. Diffuse white lesion involving buccal mucosa. Biopsy revealed one area of squamous cell carcinoma.

white epithelial lesions that were not cancerous when first biopsied will have about a 6% chance of the lesion developing into cancer when followed up over time.[4] Thus the incidence of squamous cell carcinoma in nonspecific white epithelial lesions found in the oral cavity is about 10%. Nonspecific red lesions involving the oral mucosa (erythroplakia) are much less common than the white lesions. However, at the initial biopsy a far greater number of nonspecific red lesions are found to be malignant.

Squamous cell carcinoma of the oral cavity may spread by local infiltration into surrounding tissues or may metastasize to regional lymph nodes through the lymphatic system. Distant metastasis of oral cancer is rare but does occur. The most common sites for distant metastases are lung, liver, and bone. Lesions of the tongue tend to spread to regional nodes. Lesions of the floor of the mouth and tongue tend to metastasize much earlier than carcinomas of other parts of the oral cavity.

Usually, squamous cell carcinoma is asymptomatic in the early stages. This often leads to a delay in the identification of the lesion and early treatment. Oral cancer can lead to death by (1) local obstruction of the pathway for food and air, (2) infiltration into major vessels of the head and neck resulting in significant blood loss, (3) secondary infections, (4) effects of distant metastases, (5) general wasting of the patient, or (6) complications of therapy.

CLINICAL PRESENTATION
Signs

Squamous cell carcinoma can appear as a white or red patch, an exophytic mass, an ulceration, a granular raised lesion, or combinations of these (Figs. 22-2 to 22-7). Ulcerated lesions often will have raised margins that are indurated on palpation. White lesions with areas of redness tend to have a higher incidence of being cancerous than homogenous white lesions[4] (Fig. 22-8).

Over 90% of the patients with lip cancer present no clinical evidence of regional or distant metastases. In contrast, about 50% of the patients with carcinoma of the tongue have clinical evidence of regional or distant spread of the lesions at the time

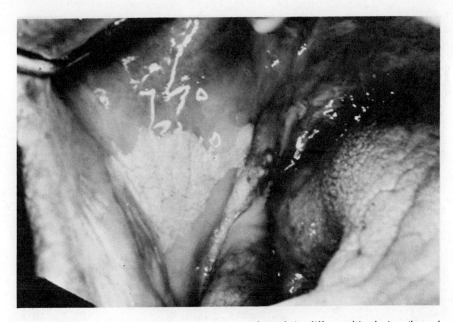

FIG. 22-4. Squamous cell carcinoma appearing as red patch in diffuse white lesion (hyperkeratosis).

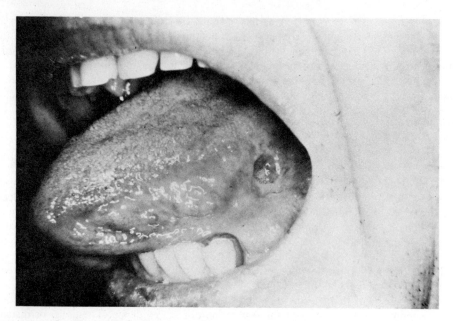

FIG. 22-5. Squamous cell carcinoma appearing as ulcerated lesion with induration and raised margins.

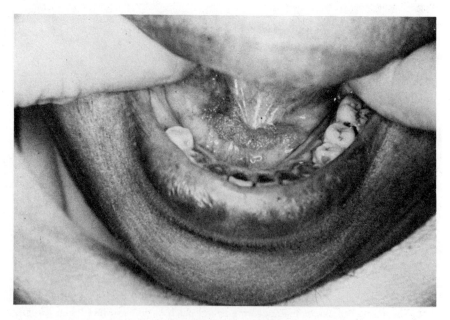

FIG. 22-6. Squamous cell carcinoma appearing as raised, granular lesion.

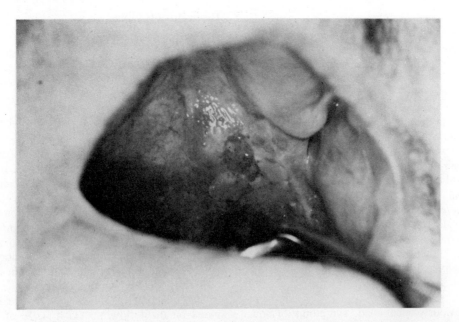

FIG. 22-7. Squamous cell carcinoma appearing as white patch and ulceration.

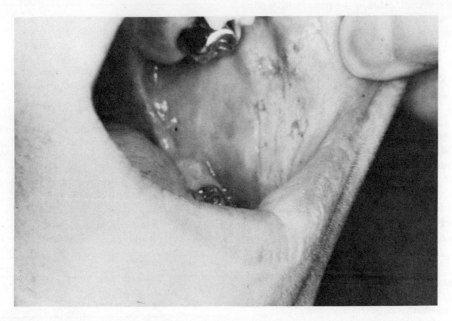

FIG. 22-8. Diffuse white lesion of buccal mucosa with several areas of erythema or redness. Diagnosis: squamous cell carcinoma.

of diagnosis. About 35% to 40% of patients with squamous cell carcinoma of the tongue and the floor of the mouth have no clinical evidence of metastases at the time of treatment but will develop metastatic disease later. In advanced cases of carcinoma of the tongue, the hypoglossal nerve may become involved. The tongue may become atrophic and can develop a tremor on the side of involvement. When the patient sticks his tongue out, the tongue will ''point'' to the side of involvement, i.e., if the right hypoglossal nerve is involved, the tongue will deviate to the right. Carcinomas of the palate can involve the glossopharyngeal and/or vagus nerves, resulting in unilateral paralysis of the soft palate and loss of the gag reflex on the involved side. This can also be found in association with ''hidden'' head and neck tumors the nasopharynx and pharynx.

Symptoms

As previously mentioned, symptoms of squamous cell carcinoma tend to develop late in the course of the disease. In patients with more advanced lesions, pain may become a very significant problem. Large lesions in the posterior portions of the oral cavity may interfere with the passage of food and air. Hence the patient may complain of weight loss and difficulty in breathing. Other symptoms that may be found in association with oral cancer include hoarseness, dysphagia, intractable ulcers, bleeding, numbness, loose teeth, and a change in the fit of a denture.

Location

Tables 22-1 and 22-2 summarize the incidence and location of head and neck cancers and oral cancer. Carcinoma of the upper lip is rare compared to carcinoma of the lower lip. Carcinoma of the dorsum of the tongue is very rare and when found tends to be related to previous treatments, e.g., use of arsenic compounds. Carcinomas that develop next to bone are generally more difficult to manage because of their tendency to infiltrate into the bone. Lesions in the maxillary region have more of a tendency to metastasize than those in the mandibular region. In general, the more posterior the primary lesion is in the oral cavity, the poorer the prognosis.

Laboratory findings

The diagnosis of oral cancer is dependent on a microscopic examination by an oral or general pathologist of tissue taken from the lesion. The more undifferentiated the lesion, the more difficult it is to identify the tissue's origin.

MEDICAL AND SURGICAL MANAGEMENT

If an attempt for a cure or for long-term survival is indicated, the lesion is best treated by surgery or irradiation. At times, a combination of these two techniques may be implemented. In a patient with an advanced lesion for whom there is no chance for a cure or long-term survival, palliation may be gained through radiation therapy or chemotherapy. Some cancer treatment centers use a combination of radiation and chemotherapy for palliation, but it is too soon to determine if significant benefits are provided by combination therapy.[3]

The selection of the method of treatment is based on the following: (1) the size of the carcinoma, (2) the location of the lesion, (3) the pres-

TABLE 22-5. International TNM system of classification of oral carcinoma

T—Size of primary lesion
  TIS—Carcinoma in situ
  T1—Lesion less than 2 cm in diameter
  T2—Lesion 2 to 4 cm in diameter
  T3—Lesion greater than 4 cm in diameter
  T4—Massive lesion with deep invasion

N—Regional lymph node involvement
  N_0—No palpable nodes
  N_1—Single node, homolateral, less than 3 cm
  N_2—Single node, homolateral, 3 to 6 cm or Multiple nodes, homolateral, none over 6 cm
  N_3—Single or multiple homolateral nodes, one greater than 6 cm in diameter or bilateral nodes (stage each side of neck) or contralateral node(s)

M—Distant metastasis
  M_0—No known distant metastasis
  M_1—Distant metastasis located PUL, OSS, HEP, or BRA
    PUL—Pulmonary
    OSS—Osseous
    HEP—Hepatic
    BRA—Brain

ence of regional or distant spread, (4) the general health status of the patient, and (5) the degree of differentiation of the lesion based on histopathologic evaluation. In addition, the functional and cosmetic problems involved in rehabilitation may influence the selection of treatment, as may the acceptance of recommended procedures by the patient.

The international tumor-node-metastases (TNM) system of classification and staging of head and neck lesions is used to evaluate and classify the tumor's status.[1,2,3] This classification helps in the selection of treatment and allows for the comparison of treatment results from one center to another. Tables 22-5 and 22-6 summarize the international TNM system for classification and staging of oral carcinomas. The goal of the management of a patient with oral cancer is to provide maximum length of survival and improved quality of survival. This goal is achieved by the following means: (1) early detection of the primary lesion, (2) sound management of precancerous lesions, (3) use of effective therapeutic measures that will result in the least disabling and disfiguring changes, (4) early application of measures to facilitate full rehabilitation, and (5) selection of effective palliation procedures for the patient who cannot be treated in an attempt for a cure.

The procedures involved in early detection of the primary lesion and the management of the precancerous lesion will be discussed in the section on dental management.

The pretreatment management of the patient with oral carcinoma involves procedures to rule out the presence of distant metastases to liver, lung, bone, brain, etc. The patient's general health status is determined as is his nutritional status. If surgery is indicated, a preoperative evaluation concerning the construction of prosthodontic appliances may be needed. This may include impressions, etc. The method of treatment selected depends on a number of factors, as previously described. Each of the treatment methods will be discussed here in general terms.

Surgery

The prime advantage of the surgical removal of the cancerous lesion is that the margins can be examined to ensure that the lesion has been removed completely. Other advantages are that the treatment is given at a single time and that it usually results in few problems to the patient once healing has occurred.

The major disadvantage of surgery for the treatment of oral cancer occurs when the extent of surgery needed to remove the lesion results in major functional and cosmetic problems to the patient. In addition, surgery carries certain risks in terms of morbidity and mortality.

In general, a patient with a small to moderate sized lesion that shows no evidence of metastases is treated by surgery. Primary closure is performed with small lesions located in movable tissue; secondary healing is allowed to occur with lesions located over bone, such as on the hard palate, as long as there is no evidence of bone involvement by the tumor. Larger lesions may require grafting to manage the surgical defect.[1]

A patient with a small- to moderate-sized lesion that has invaded bone is usually treated by surgical means. A patient with a small- to moderate-sized lesion and regional metastases will be treated by surgical removal of the primary tumor in continuity with a radical neck dissection. A patient with a very large primary lesion for whom no chance of long-term survival is possible is not a candidate for surgery. Also, a patient with bilateral node involvement or distant metastases is not treated by surgical means. In a few selected patients with large lesions, surgery may be used as a palliative measure.

A patient with squamous cell carcinoma of the tongue or floor of the mouth who shows no clinical

TABLE 22-6. International TNM system of staging of oral carcinoma

Stage	Classifications
I	T1, N_0, M_0
II	T2, N_0, M_0
III	T_3, N_0, M_0
	T1, T2, or T_3, N, M_0
IV	T4, N_0, N, M_0
	Any T, N_2, N_3, M_0
	Any T, any N, M

evidence of metastases is often treated by surgical removal of the primary tumor and a ''prophylactic'' neck dissection. The neck dissection also may be done when the primary tumor is treated by radiation techniques. The reason for the ''prophylactic'' neck dissection is that studies indicate that about 30% to 35% of patients who present with no clinical evidence of metastases develop metastases following treatment of the primary tumor. A patient who has had a prophylactic neck dissection under these circumstances has about a 40% chance of one or more lymph nodes being microscopically positive for squamous cell carcinoma. If the primary lesion is treated by radiation, the neck dissection is usually performed about 2 weeks following completion of radiation therapy.[1,3]

Cryosurgery is used in the treatment of oral cancer to a very limited degree.[1] Its selection is based on (1) a lesion located on or adjacent to bone, (2) a patient with extensive cardiopulmonary disease (who is a poor medical risk), and (3) a patient with recurrent tumors or persistent tumor following surgery or radiation treatment.

Radiation

The primary advantage of radiation therapy for treatment of oral cancer is the preservation of normal tissues and function. The disadvantages include the following: (1) treatment is prolonged over several weeks, (2) radiation injury may occur to surrounding normal tissues, and (3) the long-term potential for induction of a new lesion.[3] The larger and deeper the lesion, the more radiation needed to treat the patient.

Squamous cell carcinomas of the lip, buccal mucosa, soft palate, tongue and floor of the mouth are often treated by radiation. Primary lesions of the alveolar ridge and hard palate are less often treated by radiation. A patient with recurrent tumor following surgery is usually treated by radiation. Combination therapy using radiation and surgery is used, but at this time, it is not clear if increased survival is obtained. A patient with advanced oral cancer often is treated by radiation for palliation.[3]

Three methods of radiation therapy are used, (1) interstitial, (2) implantation, and (3) external beam.[1] Implantation techniques are used for small, superficial lesions. Interstitial methods can be used with carcinoma of the tongue or with large primary lesions before treatment with external beam cobalt-60. The most common method of radiation therapy used for oral cancer is external beam techniques (Table 22-7). The superficial lesions are treated through a single field. Larger and/or deeper lesions are usually treated using multiple fields to reduce the amount of radiation to normal tissues and to concentrate a maximum amount of radiation on the tumor site. Cobalt-60 is the most common source used for external beam irradiation for large and/or deep oral cancers. The usual dosage ranges from 5000 to 7000 rad, given in separate doses of 150 to 200 rad over a 6 to 7 week period with 4 or 5 treatment days followed by 2 or 3 nontreatment days.[2] Radiation therapy can be followed by some very significant complications, depending on the normal tissues that are in the path of the radiation beam.

Table 22-8 lists the effects of radiation on different tissues, and Table 22-9 describes the complications that may result. These will be discussed in detail in the section on Dental Management of the Cancer Patient.

TABLE 22-7. Types of external beams used for treatment of oral cancer

Energy level	Terminology	Source	Clinical use
80 to 150 V	Low voltage	X-ray	Superficial lesions
150 to 400 kV	Orthovoltage	X-ray	Skin tumors
500 kV to 8 meV	Supervoltage	Cobalt-60	Deeper lesions
8 to 200 meV	Megavoltage	Linear accelerator	Larger lesions
10 to 15 meV	Electron beam	Electrical	Superficial lesions

From Rothwell, B.R.: The medically compromised patient. In Hooley, J.R., and Daun, L.G.: Hospital dental practice, St. Louis, 1980, The C.V. Mosby Co., p. 265.

Chemotherapy

Chemotherapy is used for palliative care in a patient with advanced squamous cell carcinoma. The agents are given systemically or infused on a local or regional basis. Most chemotherapeutic agents will cause breakdown of the mucous membranes (mucositis), cause bone marrow depression (infection, bleeding, and anemia), produce gastrointestinal changes (diarrhea, malabsorption), and cause cardiac and pulmonary dysfunctions (Table 22-10). The drugs most often used for treatment of advanced squamous cell carcinoma are methotrexate, fluorouracil, and hydroxyurea.[3] Agents that have been used in combination with radiation include hydroxyurea, dactinomycin, bleomycin, and fluorouracil. Several agents have been tried in combination, such as cyclophosphamide (Cytoxan), procarbazine, and methotrexate.[1]

Pretreatment preparation

The larger cancer treatment centers have a team that deals with the patient with head and neck cancer. The head and neck tumor board usually consists of a radiation oncologist, a head and neck surgeon, a dentist, and a medical oncologist. The patient is evaluated, and the most appropriate treatment is recommended to the patient. Alternatives, if available, are discussed with the patient, and the risks and complications of treatment are explained. Once the patient has accepted the recommended treatment, the patient is prepared for receiving treatment. In cases of small, superficial lesions that only require local excision, this step is simple. However, for the patient who needs major surgical resection and reconstruction, thorough counseling becomes much more complex and important.

The patient needing extensive surgery will be sent for consultation with a maxillofacial prosthodontist, dentist, speech pathologist, and psychologist. Presurgical casts will be made, and recommendations as to the types of prostheses that can be constructed and the types of surgical preparation that might be needed are explained to the patient. The patient is told about the problems that will occur with speech, etc., and what steps will be taken after surgery to help overcome these problems. A psychologic evaluation of the patient will be made to serve as a basis for counseling concerning the emotional problems to be faced during rehabilitation.

Following surgery, the psychologist will help the patient deal with psychological problems that are common to major cancer surgery, including the following: (1) concern about recurrence of the tumor, (2) changes in body function and body image, (3) mourning for the lost body part, (4) disfigurement, (5) the tendency to withdraw from friends and family, and (6) the loss of self-esteem.

TABLE 22-8. Radiation effects on normal tissues in path of external beam

Mucosa
　Epithelium—atrophy
　Vascular
　　Internal thickening
　　Stenosis of lumen
　　Obliteration
　　Decreased blood flow

Muscle
　Fibrosis
　Vascular changes

Bone
　Decrease in numbers of osteocytes
　Decrease in numbers of osteoblasts
　Vascular changes—decreased blood flow

Salivary glands
　Atrophy of acini
　Vascular changes
　Fibrosis

Pulp—necrosis (orthovoltage)

TABLE 22-9. Complications of radiation therapy

Nausea and vomiting—early

Mucositis—starts about second week

Xerostomia—starts about third week

Radiation caries—delayed

Muscular dysfunction—delayed

Osteoradionecrosis—delayed
　More common in mandible
　Less common in maxilla

Pulpal pain and necrosis—delayed
　With orthovoltage, not found with cobalt-60

TABLE 22-10. Effects of chemotherapy

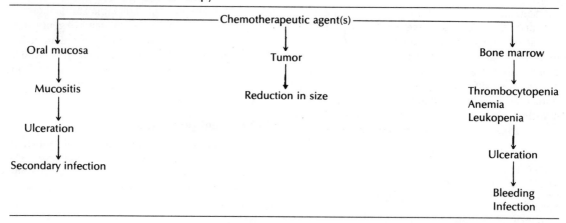

The psychologist will also help the patient cope with the anxiety and/or depression these problems cause.[3]

All members of the treatment team can help the patient during the surgical and postsurgical periods by letting him know that it is acceptable to resent the way he feels and that his feelings are normal and appropriate. Otherwise, the anxiety or depression needs to be acknowledged and legitimized. The patient needs to feel supported and accepted as a person of worth and value. Every attempt should be made to restore function or replace the lost part. Finally, vocational counseling and contact with a social worker may be needed to help the patient return to society as a contributing, worthwhile person.[3]

A patient who needs radiation therapy must be seen by a dentist before the start of treatment. The status of the dentition and the oral hygiene level must be evaluated, necessary extractions performed, and large carious lesions restored. The role of the dentist will be discussed in the next section of this chapter.

Once treatment has been completed, the oral cancer patient must be placed on a recall program. Usually, the patient is seen once every month during the first year, once every 2 months during the second year, once every 4 months during the third year, and once every 6 months during the fourth and fifth years. After 5 years the patient should be examined at least once a year. This recall program

is very important because (1) a patient with one oral cancer tends to develop additional lesions because of the "field" effect[3] (2) latent metastases may develop, (3) the initial lesions may recur, and (4) complications related to therapy can be looked for and managed.

DENTAL MANAGEMENT
General considerations

One of the more important roles the dentist plays in the management of the cancer patient relates to early detection of the lesion. A head and neck examination and an intraoral soft-tissue examination should be performed on each and every dental patient as he enters the practice. This examination should be repeated on a regular basis as often as possible, but at least during recall visits. The examination only takes a few minutes and may save the life of the patient with an "early" cancerous lesion.

The dentist should be aggressive in determining the nature of lesions that cannot be identified by clinical findings. It is impossible to diagnosis nonspecific white epithelial lesions of the oral mucosa without microscopic examination. If the dentist thinks that an oral ulceration or white lesion is traumatic in origin, the source of trauma should be eliminated or modified and the patient asked to return in 7 to 10 days. The traumatic lesion should be healed by the time of the return visit. If the lesion is still present, it must be biopsied. If no clues were found at the initial visit that could explain the cause of the lesion, a biopsy is in order immediately. If the dentist does not perform biopsies, the patient must be referred to an oral surgeon for the biopsy. Small lesions can be excised, and larger lesions can be sampled by one or more incisional biopsies. Large ulcers are best sampled at the margin, as the central portion may be necrotic and of no value in establishing a diagnosis. Diffuse white lesions are best sampled by taking tissue from areas of fissuring and/or erythematous areas that may be within the lesion (see Fig. 22-8). It is not necessary to have normal tissue in these samples, because the pathologist knows what normal tissue looks like. He or she needs tissue from the part(s) of the lesion that will be most diagnostic.

A patient who presents with a lesion that appears clinically to be cancer or a patient who has a less obviously cancerous lesion but has hard, fixed, and/or matted lymph nodes should be referred directly to a cancer treatment center or to a head and neck surgeon in the community (see Fig. 22-1). The patient should be told of the concern that he may have a serious problem and that immediate evaluation by specialists must be done. If the patient seems willing to talk, the concern about cancer should be discussed, with the benefits of prompt diagnosis and treatment strongly emphasized. The patient should be dealt with in a honest and direct manner, and as many of his questions should be answered as possible. The patient should be asked if he has a preference concerning a cancer treatment center; if not, the dentist should be prepared to recommend one. If possible, the dentist should phone the selected center and make an appointment for the patient. This should be followed by a letter to the physician in charge to introduce the patient and describe the findings and clinical impression. If the spouse is present, it is usually advisable to share your findings. In rare cases, it would be best to withhold the clinical diagnosis from the patient and share it with a member of the family.

A patient who has a diffuse white lesion in which multiple sampling has shown no evidence of dyskeratosis (premalignant changes) is managed in one of two ways. If the patient is in poor general health, the lesion is too extensive for complete removal, and/or the patient is available for periodic recall, the lesion should be left and the patient examined every 3 to 6 months, with a biopsy done when any clinical changes are noted in the lesion. Even if the lesion does not change clinically, it would be advisable to sample it every 1 to 2 years for "hidden" histologic findings that may indicate a significant change is taking place.

In a patient with a diffuse lesion in which one or more of the samples show changes that are considered premalignant the lesion should be completely removed whenever possible. This may not be advisable in a patient with serious systemic disease or if the lesion is just too extensive. In these cases, the patient can be managed by an oral surgeon or through a cancer treatment center.

Treatment planning modifications

Dental treatment planning for the patient with oral cancer begins when the lesion has been found and a diagnosis established. Planning involves the pretreatment evaluation and preparation of the patient, the posttreatment management of the patient, and the long-term management of the patient from a dental standpoint.

PRETREATMENT EVALUATION

The dentist needs to be aware of the type of treatment selected for the patient and of whether the lesion stands a good chance of being controlled (Table 22-11). A patient who is going to receive palliative therapy may not want replacement therapy for missing teeth. However, it is important that this patient be free of active dental disease. In contrast, a patient who has an early lesion, with no evidence of regional spread, that will be treated by local excision can be managed for future dental care as a normal patient. An exception is that the dentist will recall the patient for frequent examination for evidence of metastases, recurrence of the lesion, or presence of a new cancer.

Radiation patients. There are several very important dental considerations for the patient with oral cancer who is going to receive radiation therapy. If the beam will pass through the jaw bones and/or major salivary glands, the patient will be subject to osteoradionecrosis and radiation caries. Potential sources of infection to the radiated bone must be treated or removed before the initiation of radiation therapy.

TABLE 22-11. Distribution and relative 5-year survival by subsite and extent of disease*

Location	Number of cases†	Localized		Regional		Distant		Surv. % all stages
		Dist. %	Surv. %	Dist. %	Surv. %	Dist. %	Surv. %	
Lip	2645	90	89	7	57	1	‡	86
Tongue	3414	44	52	40	22	12	7	33
Floor of mouth	2146	44	65	44	31	8	18	45
Other oral cancers	2362	49	61	36	29	11	18	44

From Public Health Service: Management guidelines for head and neck cancer, U.S. Department of Health, Education, and Welfare, Public Health Service, National Institute of Health, Pub. No. 80-2037, 1979.
*Ratio of survival rate to rate expected of individuals in general population with same age group, sex, race, and calendar year of observation.
†White patients only.
‡Number of cases too small to yield reliable data.

TABLE 22-12. Causes of radiation caries

Decreased salivary flow
Change in quality of saliva—decreased buffering capacity
Poor oral hygiene
Changes in oral flora

Before radiation therapy the following recommendations apply. A patient with broken-down teeth that are nonrestorable or a patient who has no interest in saving teeth should have them extracted. Patients with advanced periodontal disease should have the teeth removed. Nonvital teeth should be endodontically treated or extracted. All active carious lesions should be restored. Chronic inflammatory lesions in the jaw bones should be examined and treated if necessary. To allow for adequate wound healing, extractions and other surgical procedures should be performed at least 2 weeks before the start of radiation therapy. The bone at the wound margins should be trimmed to eliminate sharp edges and to allow for primary closure of the wound.

The patient who will be retaining teeth must be informed concerning the problems associated with decreased salivary function, which includes xerostomia and radiation caries[2,3] (Table 22-12). Radiation caries (see Fig. 22-9) can progress very quickly, and if pulpal tissues becomes infected and the infection extends to the surrounding irradiated bone, extensive infection and necrosis can result. The importance of effective hygiene procedures

and the maintenance of good oral hygiene must be emphasized.

Impressions should be made so that custom trays can be constructed using soft, flexible mouthguard material. These trays are used to hold 5 to 10 drops of a 1% to 2% acidulated fluoride gel that should be inserted into the mouth for 5 minutes each day. The fluoride application should follow cleaning with toothbrush and dental floss. When the tray is taken out of the mouth, any excess gel left in the mouth should be spit out. If the 1% to 2% acidulated gel is found to be irritating to the tissues, a equal amount of a 0.5% neutral sodium fluoride gel can be substituted.[2]

Surgical patients. The dental preparation of the oral cancer patient who is going to be treated by surgery is not as critical as for the radiation patient. However, active oral infection should be treated. Teeth that are broken down should be removed. Teeth that may be used for the retention of prosthetic appliances can be restored if indicated. The better the patient's dental health, the lower the risk of dental infection complicating the healing process or causing a serious postoperative infection. When possible, the dentist should be in direct consultation with the maxillofacial prosthodontist so that proper coordination of the patient's dental and tooth-replacement needs can occur during the presurgical and postsurgical phases.

Oral complications

In this section the oral complications associated with the treatment of oral cancer will be considered from the standpoint of what the dentist may offer to minimize the discomfort of the patient and how

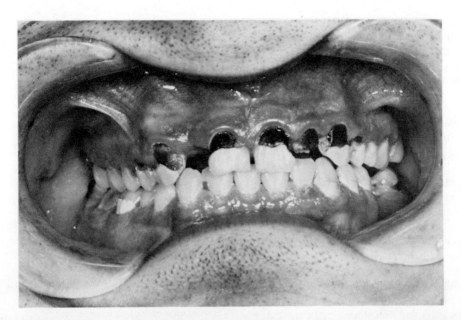

FIG. 22-9. Patient who received radiation therapy for oral cancer. Note extensive cervical caries. (Courtesy R. Gorlin, D.D.S., Minneapolis, Minn.)

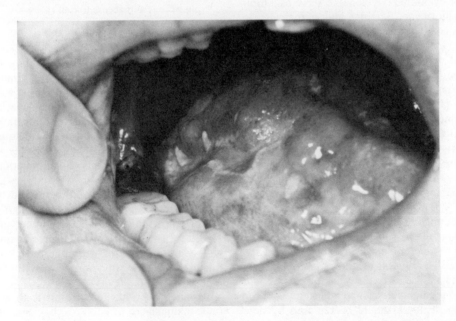

FIG. 22-10. Patient who was receiving radiation therapy. Note extensive mucositis that developed because of radiation effects on oral mucosa. (Courtesy R. Gorlin, D.D.S., Minneapolis, Minn.)

future dental complications related to the altered oral environment can be prevented and/or dealt with when they occur.

The functional and cosmetic problems caused by major surgical procedures can be best managed by presurgical preparation and planning. Prosthetic appliances can be constructed once healing has occurred. Transitional appliances can be fabricated if additional surgical procedures are indicated to prepare the site for the construction of a "final" prosthetic replacement device.

During radiation therapy the patient often will develop a mucositis (Fig. 22-10). The breakdown of the oral mucosa begins about the second week of radiation therapy and usually subsides a few weeks after the completion of treatment. The mucositis results in ulceration, pain, dysphagia, loss of taste, and difficulty in eating. If major salivary glands have been irradiated, xerostomia will follow the initial onset of mucositis. The combination of mucositis and xerostomia make the patient very uncomfortable and make it difficult for him to maintain a proper nutritional intake. During this acute phase, the patient can be managed by: (1) using a bland mouthwash to keep ulcerated areas as clean as possible, (2) using an antihistamine solution or dyclonine (Dyclone) to serve as a topical anesthetic agent, (3) taking milk of magnesia to serve as a coating agent to protect the surfaces of ulcerated areas from local irritation, and (4) applying topical steroids to reduce the inflammatory reaction (see Table 22-13). Vitamin supplementation at therapeutic levels is often indicated during this acute phase, as is bland, high-protein liquid diet. A patient who wears dentures will be much more comfortable if the dentures are not worn during this acute phase.

Once the mucositis has healed, the long-term management of the patient involves dealing with the chronic xerostomia, altered bone, and related problems. The patient should avoid the use of his dentures during the first 6 months, because mild trauma to the altered mucosa can result in ulcerations and necrosis of underlying bone. Once the patient starts wearing his dentures, he must be told to come to the dentist if any sore spots should develop so the dentures can be adjusted.

Ill-fitting dentures should be replaced by new dentures. Salivary flow may be stimulated by sugar-

TABLE 22-13. Management of oral complications of radiation therapy

Mucositis
    Sodium bicarbonate mouthwash
    Elixir of diphenhydramine (Benadryl) or dyclonine (Dyclone)
    Topical steroids
    Milk of magnesia
    Orabase
Xerostomia
    Sugarless lemon drops
    Sorbitol-based chewing gum
    Buffered solution of glycerine and water
    Xero-Lube
Radiation caries
    Oral hygiene procedures
    Topical fluoride gel
    Frequent dental recall
    Restoration of early carious lesions
Osteoradionecrosis
    Avoidance of trauma to mucosa
    Avoidance of extractions
    Irrigation with saline, antibiotics
    Hyperbaric oxygen, tetracycline antibiotics
    Resection
Muscular dysfunction
    Tongue blades to help patient retain maximum opening of jaws and access to oral cavity

less lemon drops or sorbitol-based chewing gum. If the radiation damage to the salivary glands is too extensive, salivary substitutes such as a buffered solution of glycerine and water OraLube, or Xero-Lube can be prescribed. In very severe cases of xerostomia a small amount of petrolatum can be applied to the "mucosal" surface of the denture.

To minimize the effects of the radiation on the muscles around the face and the muscles of mastication, a mouth block should be placed when the patient is receiving external beam irradiation. Then the patient should be given a number of tongue blades to place into the mouth several times each day. These procedures will minimize muscle contracture and allow for more normal function and access to the oral cavity.

A patient who has retained his teeth must continue maintenance of good oral hygiene, which includes a daily brushing and flossing and in some cases the continued use of the daily application of fluoride gel using the custom trays that were constructed before radiation therapy. All carious lesions should be treated when first detected. Frequent recall of the patient is a must for reinforcement of hygiene procedures and detection of oral disease that could involve bone and lead to necrosis. The risk of bone infection and necrosis is much greater with extraction of teeth than with endodontic therapy. Thus if the pulp has become infected, endodontic therapy is the preferred treatment, assuming the tooth is restorable.

The use of prophylactic antibiotics to prevent infection following surgical procedures in patients who have had radiation therapy is suggested. However, the effectiveness of the coverage can be greatly reduced because of the altered blood flow to the affected bone. The reduction in blood flow following radiation therapy is much greater in the mandible than the maxilla because of the limited source and lack of collateral circulation. This accounts for the greater frequency and severity of osteoradionecrosis in the mandible.

Once necrosis occurs, conservative management is usually indicated. The exposed bone can be irrigated with a saline or antibiotic solution. The patient can be directed to use oral irrigating devices to clean the involved area. However, extreme pressures should be avoided when these devices are prescribed. Severe cases may benefit from hyperbaric oxygen treatment, which consists of 2 hours per day with up to 60 sessions in a hyperbaric "chamber." Tetracycline antibiotics also can be prescribed. Cases that do not respond to conservative measures may require surgical resection of the involved bone.[1,2]

A patient receiving chemotherapy for palliation of oral cancer is very susceptible to ulceration of the oral mucosa, infection of surrounding tissues, and excessive bleeding following minor injuries. When mucositis is present, the management would be the same as that previously described for the patient receiving radiation. Antibiotics in large doses are indicated to treat any acute oral infection. When surgical procedures must be performed in the oral cavity, prophylactic antibiotic coverage is indicated. Local measures along with platelet replacement usually can prevent or control excessive bleeding. Before any dental care is rendered, medical consultation is needed to establish the patient's current status and to develop a management plan.

Emergency dental treatment

Treatment of emergency dental problems in a patient who has received radiation or who is receiving chemotherapy must be as conservative as possible. Medical consultation is suggested before the patient is treated. Surgical procedures should be avoided whenever possible. Antibiotic coverage is indicated if invasive or surgical procedures must be used. The platelet status must be determined and supplemented when indicated. The cancer patient who has been treated by surgery and who has healed can be managed as a "normal" patient for any emergency dental treatment.

REFERENCES

1. Archer, W.H.: Oral and maxillofacial surgery, ed. 5, Philadelphia, 1975, W.B. Saunders Co., pp. 1806-1836.
2. Hooley, J.R., and Daun, G.: Hospital dental practice, St. Louis, 1980, The C.V. Mosby Co.
3. Public Health Service: Management guidelines for head and neck cancer, U.S. Department of Health, Education, and Welfare, Public Health Service, National Institute of Health, pub. no. 80-2037, 1979.
4. Shafer, W.G., Hine, M.K., and Levy, B.M.: A textbook of oral pathology, ed. 4, Philadelphia, 1983, W.B. Saunders Co., pp. 92-130.

23

BEHAVIORAL CONSIDERATIONS

Problems may be encountered in dental practice that stem from the dentist's or the patient's behavioral patterns or both rather than from the physical conditions being treated. In addition, some oral disease processes, such as myofascial pain-dysfunction syndrome, may have a significant emotional component in their etiology.

A good dentist-patient relationship will reduce the number of behavioral problems encountered in practice as well as modify the intensity of the emotional reaction to many problems. A positive dentist-patient relationship is based on mutual respect, trust, understanding, cooperation, and empathy. When present, role conflicts between the dentist and patient can be avoided or dealt with effectively, the anxious patient can find support that will minimize the damaging effects of anxiety, and the angry or uncooperative patient can be accepted and encouraged to share the reasons for his feelings and behavior and thus become a more peaceful and cooperative patient. In addition, patients with emotional factors that are contributing to certain oral diseases or symptoms can be better accepted and more effectively managed by the dentist.

In this chapter, the dentist-patient relationship will be considered from a viewpoint of the social roles involved. The reactions of the patient to illness and to the dentist will be discussed. The anxious, depressed, uncooperative, and angry patient will be considered. Finally, patients with psy-chophysiologic and conversion disorders found in the oral region will be described.

PRACTICE MODELS

Three behavioral practice models have been described for medicine and dentistry. These are the active-passive, guidance-cooperation, and participation models.[8] The active-passive model would be appropriate for the emergency patient under general anesthesia who is treated for facial fractures by the oral surgeon.

In the guidance-cooperation model the patient is actively involved, but the dentist is still the dominant active member in the relationship. All directions and basic decisions are made by the dentist, and the patient is expected to follow directions. An appropriate application of this model would be the treatment of a patient with an acute oral infection. The dentist would diagnose the problem and place the patient on a 7- to 10-day course of penicillin therapy. An example of the inappropriate use of the guidance-cooperation model is the mandatory 5-day plaque control program for all patients in a dental practice. Unless certain patients are more involved in the decision-making process, their level of cooperation may be low. Although the procedure may be rational and sound from the dentist's viewpoint, it may not fit the needs and value systems of these patients.

For these patients the participation model may be more appropriate. It is based on an active involvement of the patient in the decision-making process and the patient as an active partner during therapy. This model is most appropriate for the patient who wants to be involved in designing and implementing his own personal oral health program with the help of the dentist.

Problems in patient understanding and cooperation during complex restorations, preventive programs, and orthodontic therapy can develop because of the inappropriate selection and application of a behavioral practice model. Patients who believe that external factors control their lives may be most effectively managed using the guidance-cooperation model. The dentist makes the decisions and directs the program much like a parent-child relationship. On the other hand, a patient who feels that he controls his life would best be managed using the participation model. This patient would be involved with decisions concerning therapy and be provided with alternatives concerning an oral health program from which he could select. This model would be represented by an adult-adult relationship. It should be clear that all patients do not fit any one model. It also should be clear that all dentists, at a given point in their personal development, are not able to function in a true participation model. There are patients with whom some dentists should not become involved if they do not have the maturity and flexibility to adapt a management plan based on the patient's behavioral and dental needs.

DENTIST-PATIENT RELATIONSHIP

The expectations by the patient of the dentist and by the dentist of the patient may be greatly influenced by cultural values.[2] In the "western" culture of the United States the value orientation tends toward the beliefs that man is dominant over nature, man is both good and bad, the future can be influenced, and human behavior is dominated by rational problem solving. This has led to a scientific approach to medicine and dentistry, in which the relations between healer and patient tend to be impersonal, treatment procedures are strange and unfamiliar to the patient, the family and patient take little part in making decisions or conducting treatment, seriously ill persons are hospitalized for treatment, and the treatment procedures are expensive.

In the United States, sick persons are expected to want to get well, to seek the most skilled help, and to cooperate in treatment. Thus the usual patient role in our society is to be taken care of by someone, to take it easy when ill, to try to get well, to obey instructions, not to ask too many questions, etc.[2] The role of the physician or dentist is to be knowledgeable, kind and good. Problems can develop between the patient and dentist when these expected roles are not played or fulfilled. An understanding of this process may be helpful in seeing the nature of certain conflicts between dentist and patient and opening them up for discussion with the goal of developing new expectations that may be more appropriate for the situation and persons involved.

In other cultures the social roles of the doctor and patient may be different than just described. For example, the Spanish-American culture is based on the beliefs that man is either good or bad, the future cannot be influenced, and human behavior is more spontaneous than rational. Thus in Spanish-American folk medicine, a personal relationship develops between healer and patient, treatment procedures are neither strange nor unfamiliar to the patient, the family takes a very active part in deciding on and implementing treatment, seriously ill patients are cared for in the home, and the cost is low.[2]

If the patient comes from one culture and the dentist from another, their expectations of each other's social roles and function may be very different. This can lead to misunderstanding and lack of cooperation. If these expectations cannot be modified by open discussion of the problem between the patient and dentist, it would appear wise that they decide to sever the relationship.

In addition to role conflicts, the dentist-patient relationship may be influenced by the way in which the dentist deals with patients' reactions to an illness. Since the emphasis of this book is the dental management of the medically compromised patient, the reaction of these patients to their medical disease as well as their dental problems must be considered when they are dealt with in the dental office. Ten major behavioral reactions to sickness are listed in Table 23-1.[2]

The patient may believe that it is bad to be sick. This can lead to self-blame and self-rejection. The

TABLE 23-1. Major behavioral reactions to sickness

Depression and self-rejection
Fear
Counterphobia
Anxiety
Frustration and anger
Withdrawal or apathy
Exaggeration of symptoms
Regression
Dependency
Self-centeredness

patient may see the illness as representing a deserved punishment for being an imperfect person. The illness may be viewed as a loss of personal power or loss of personal control. These views may lead to feelings of worthlessness, hopelessness, and guilt.

One of the most intense reactions to illness is fear. This may be a fear that the illness will prevent the patient from achieving his immediate interests and desires, a fear of pain, discomfort, and disability, a fear of the unknown, or a fear of death. It is unfortunate that the American culture tends to inhibit the expression of these fears.

The failure or inability to express fear leads to a counterphobia in some patients. These individuals will demonstrate actions directly opposite to the fear they feel to prove to themselves and others that they are not afraid. For example, this reaction may be seen in the cardiac patient who continues strenuous activities that may endanger his life.

Anxiety is a common response to illness. It occurs in response to the patient's appraisal of what the illness may mean to the patient's life-style and self-esteem at an unconscious level.

The patient may be frustrated by an illness. This may lead to feelings of aggression, which are often expressed as anger. Irritability, crankiness, and loud demands are behaviors that may be expressed by these patients. The patient may develop angry feelings toward the dentist or physician, but there is often a reluctance to express the anger because the role of the patient demands politeness. Thus the anger may be demonstrated by other behaviors,

such as not following orders, not keeping appointments, and being late for appointments.

A sick person often will withdraw and become apathetic. Part of this reaction may be physiologic as a direct result of the illness. However, the frustrated and angry patient who cannot express these feelings because of fear of disapproval may retaliate by withdrawal and become apathetic. In addition, the exaggerated conformance to the role of being a good patient may appear as withdrawal and apathy.

Patients may exaggerate their symptoms to obtain care or to avoid doing things such as attending school or going to work. Often the patient may be unaware of what he is doing. Persons who feel inadequate, who are shy, or who are crafty manipulators are those who most often demonstrate this reaction.

Another important patient response to illness is regression to more childish behavior. When a person is faced with a difficulty that he cannot solve it is not unusual for a regression in behavior to occur. This behavior may be the throwing of things, crying, pouting, sorrowful looks, temper tantrums, and exaggerated helplessness and submission. Such regressive behavior in patients is usually an indication that the patient is having difficulty in coping with the illness and should be viewed by the dentist or physician in that light.

Severe and chronic illnesses require a certain dependency by the patient on others. The more severe the disability, the greater the need for the patient to depend on others. Some individuals cannot accept the fact of their dependency and become anxious and try to deny their need for help. Feelings of resentment, anger, and hostility can develop toward persons in contact with such a patient. Once again, an understanding of this process will allow individuals caring for such a patient to be empathetic and supportive.

Sick people tend to make the world around them very small and develop a preoccupation with their sickness, needs, and fears. They may retreat to highly personal or magical notions about the cause of their illness. For example, cancer patients may believe that their illness is a punishment for swearing at their mother or for "evil" thoughts they have had.

PATIENTS' ATTITUDES TOWARD DENTIST

Childhood experiences and the learned social role of the patient are important factors in the development of the patient's feelings and attitudes toward the dentist. Children learn through the teaching of physicians, dentists, parents, and peers what are the expected roles of the patient and doctor. The attitudes of the patient toward the physician and dentist may be that they are powerful and dangerous. The patient may feel awe, envy, and wonder toward doctors.[1-4]

Past behavior that the patient used to please parents may be transferred or displaced to the doctor in an attempt to please. Other emotions, attitudes, and actions associated with the patient's relationship with his parents also may be transferred to the relationship with the doctor. This type of behavior has nothing to do with who the doctor really is but is displaced to a symbolic power figure who represents the parent in the patient's mind. Transference of socially acceptable behavior such as respect and politeness usually is not destructive to the patient-dentist relationship. However, the transference of a need for unending love, a demand for unceasing attention, the need for protection, a fear of tyranny, and feeling of resentment and hate can be very destructive to the patient-dentist relationship if not understood and dealt with. The patient may place the doctor in a role that is impossible for any person to fulfill. The doctor may be seen as a miracle worker, lordly, powerful, protecting, fatherly, etc. As the patient begins to see the person that the doctor really is, disappointment and anger may result.

The more that dentists reveal of themselves to the patient from the very first contact, the less likely it will be that many of these attitudes and feelings will be directed toward them. Unrealistic expectations and inappropriate behavior should be open for discussion between the dentist and patient if a solid relationship is to be developed and maintained.

DEPRESSION

Depression is described as a feeling of hopelessness, worthlessness, and guilt. Most people have experienced some degree of depression; however, when depression is severe and prolonged it can be extremely debilitating and can lead to self-destruction. The dentist as well as the patient is subject to this reaction. Thus the following material is presented with the intent of being helpful to the reader as well as providing a framework for understanding, recognizing, and dealing with the depressed dental patient.

Individuals who experience themselves as a person only through a role or through someone else tend to be susceptible to significant depression.[6] These types of individuals have their identity wholly associated with their work or social role. These individuals often have a perceived perfect-self that they are trying to live up to and thereby avoid the anxiety that they sense concerning their shortcomings and limitations. The failure to live up to the expectations of the perfect-self leads to a despised self and generates anger and self-hate. The attempts to keep unwanted, terrifying feelings of self-hate, anger, anxiety, and helplessness from emerging leads to depression. Thus depression serves as a numbing process or ''Novocain'' reaction to keep feelings from ''tearing'' one apart with rage and grief. The basic causes of depression are feelings of self-hate, anger, guilt, and helplessness.

The indications of low-grade chronic depression are tiredness even after enough sleep, difficulty getting up in the morning, restlessness, loss of interest in family, work, and sex, being unable to make decisions, being angry and resentful, being a chronic complainer, feeling critical of self, feeling inferior, and day-dreaming excessively.[6]

The following often indicate the presence of severe depression: excessive crying, change in sleeping habits, the thought of food making one sick, weight loss without dieting, strong feelings of guilt, nightmares, thoughts about suicide, feeling unreal or in a ''fog,'' and being unable to concentrate.[6]

Individuals with severe depression should be encouraged to seek professional help. However, until that is sought and available, there are some things that can be done to help the person. Depressed individuals should be encouraged to try to stop feeling guilty about being depressed and should be assured that it is not their fault. They are not depressed because they want to be but because it seems to be the best way to keep themselves together. They should be told not to look on the depression as something that they will be able to recover from immediately, because it will take time. They should be encouraged to remain active. Physical activities such as jogging, tennis, or swimming can be very helpful. If it is too difficult for the patient to talk with people, he should be told that notes can be used to communicate. Friends and family should be encouraged not to scold or criticize. The patient should be reminded that the depression will end. He should be encouraged to eat properly and to find a person who is trusted so that his feelings of anger can be expressed.[6]

PSYCHOLOGIC SIGNIFICANCE OF ORAL CAVITY

The soft tissues of the mouth are an important part of the body from a psychologic viewpoint. The mouth is the area of the body that very early in life is involved with feelings of pleasure and satisfaction during feeding or with frustration and anger if the feeding is late or difficult. The mouth is an area of the body that may be involved with sexual sensations. The mouth is used to show the expression of an emotion that a person is feeling. The mouth is important for speech, appearance, and aesthetics. It is involved, in our society, with the image of health, sex, and youth[3] (Table 23-2).

Dental treatment and manipulation in the mouth may allow the patient to become aware of many of these feelings related to the mouth. For example, if

TABLE 23-2. Psychologic significance of oral cavity

Oral manipulation may activate old feelings associated with feeding as an infant
 If difficulties often occurred—anger and frustration
 If difficulties seldom occurred—pleasure and satisfaction
Oral manipulation may activate sexual sensations
Oral cavity and facial tissues often used to express emotions
Important in our culture for appearance
Image of health, sex, and youth

as an infant the patient was frustrated and angry because of difficulty in feeding, these feelings may be "activated" during a dental visit and expressed as anger toward the dentist. Sexual feelings also may be activated by dental manipulations and, depending on the patient's feelings, a degree of satisfaction regarding sexual needs, affection, or anger may be misdirected to the dentist.

The teeth also have important psychologic significance. They may be symbolic for the expression of aggression, since they were the first weapons of the child. The patient's body image may be reflected in the attitude regarding teeth. To some people the loss of teeth means body destruction. People who have a tendency for "self-destructive" feelings may view a need to lose teeth as a means to gain a degree of satisfaction of these feelings. To some people the loss of teeth may be an important sign of aging prematurely; in others the loss of teeth may be viewed with a loss of sexual potency and youthful optimism.

The dentist may not identify the source of the patient's feelings observed in the dental situation, but the dentist should be aware that the feelings may have important and strong origins having nothing to do with the cavity in a certain tooth.

ANXIETY

Anxiety can be defined as emotional pain or a feeling that all is not well—a feeling of impending disaster. The source of the problem usually is not apparent to the person with anxiety. The feeling is the same as that of the patient with fear, but that person is aware of what the problem is and why he is "fearful."

The physiologic reaction involved with anxiety and fear is the same. It is manifested through the autonomic nervous system. Both the sympathetic and parasympathetic components may be involved. Symptoms of anxiety caused by overactivation of the sympathetic portion include increased heart rate, sweating, dilated pupils, and muscle tension. Symptoms of anxiety resulting from stimulation of the parasympathetic component include urination and diarrhea.

All individuals have an integrating system with which to deal with incoming stimuli. In some this system has been well learned as a child, so that if an overload of stimuli should occur, psychic equilibrium or homeostasis is restored in a short time. In other people a pattern of dealing effectively with these stimuli was not well learned as a child; these persons can be "overloaded" by a smaller input of stimuli, and they take more time to restore equilibrium once overloading has occurred.

Anxiety may occur from an excess of stimuli from the external environment, internal body stimuli, or intrapsychic conflicts. External stimuli include difficulties with job, marriage, interpersonal relationships with other people, loss of loved ones, etc. Some people can handle a number of these kinds of stimuli and still be able to function; others can experience only a few before they become unable to function.

Internal body stimuli include the effect of menopause in a woman, the effect of hyperfunction of the thyroid, etc.

Intrapsychic conflicts may involve frustration with the basic needs of an individual—sexual, aggressive, and dependent. These needs, as described by Freud, are functions of the id. The basic "language" of the id is, "I want it now." For example, if a man saw a beautiful woman or a woman saw a handsome man, the id would express the sexual need by wanting immediate satisfaction. The superego functions as an internal policeman that has been programmed by cultural restraints. The "language" of the superego is "no." In this situation the superego would say "no" to the needs of the id.

This would result in serious internal conflict and must be resolved in some way. The function of the ego is to serve as a mediator between the needs of the id and restraints of the superego. In the preceding example, the ego would say "later" and resolve the immediate conflict.

Most people have learned to develop a good ego function, and they do well in our society. Others have not developed a good ego function and develop symptoms of anxiety resulting from the conflict between the id and the superego.

Signs and symptoms of anxiety

The dentist may detect persons who are anxious by their physical appearance, speech, dress, and presence of certain signs and symptoms.

The anxious person has a look of being over alert, sitting forward in his chair, moving his fingers, arms, or legs, getting up and moving, or pacing around the room. He may always be checking certain parts of his clothing, straightening his tie, etc. On the other hand, he may have sloppy dress habits and other signs that are just the opposite of a concern with having everything perfect. He may show signs of being very watchful of his possessions, always keeping them in sight.

The anxious person may have a very mechanical speech pattern. He may keep talking at a very rapid rate and at times seem to block out thoughts or not to connect thoughts together. When the anxious person is asked a question, often he answers very quickly; in fact, the dentist is often not even allowed to finish the question.

The dentist may see signs of sweating, tension in muscles, increased breathing, and rapid heart rate in the anxious patient. The patient may describe an inability to sleep, or he may wake at an early hour and be unable to go back to sleep. The patient may have diarrhea and increased frequency of urination. In general, he is over alert and tense. He has a feeling of apprehension and of impending diaster, but for no apparent reason. The insomnia, tension, and apprehension lead to fatigue, which makes it even more difficult for him to deal with the anxiety.

Management of the anxious patient

The dentist should talk with the patient and show interest in him as a person. The dentist's verbal and nonverbal communication must be consistent. The dentist should confront the patient with the observation that he appears anxious and then ask the patient if he would like to talk about how he feels. This may include the person's atti-

TABLE 23-3. Management of anxious patient

Show interest in patient

Carry on consistent verbal and nonverbal communication

Confront patient about appearing anxious
  "You seem tense today."
  "Would you like to talk about it?"

Administer sedation

Administer nitrous oxide

tude toward the dentist, etc. During these discussions, tension-free pauses should be allowed to develop between ideas. This will allow a temporary state of regression to occur, which will help the patient to restore a more anxiety-free state. Some patients may respond very well to this approach without ever indicating why they were anxious.

If the patient remains anxious in the dental situation, the dentist may plan to use sedation, nitrous oxide, etc. to better manage the patient during dental treatment (Table 23-3).

PSYCHOPHYSIOLOGIC DISORDERS

Patients who have chronic anxiety may develop organic diseases caused by the overactivity of the autonomic nervous system and its effect on certain target tissues. Examples of such psychophysiologic disorders are peptic ulcers, hypertension, ulcerative colitis, neurodermatitis, and tension headaches.

Oral diseases that are thought to be examples of psychophysiologic disorders include acute necrotizing ulcerative gingivitis, aphthous ulcers, lichen planus, temporomandibular joint dysfunction syndrome, and geographic tongue[5,7] (Figs. 23-1 to 23-3).

In these disorders there is an identifiable lesion with an emotional component to the cause. The pathologic process is potentially dangerous to the patient. The disorder, a peptic ulcer, for example, does not reduce the level of anxiety but rather increases it, and the increased anxiety aggravates the ulcer, even to the point of bleeding and perforation, which of course causes more anxiety.

CONVERSION REACTIONS

A conversion reaction is the result of an unconscious conflict being transformed into a symbolically expressed somatic symptom that reduces the tension and anxiety. In other words, an anxious patient may develop physical symptoms without any evidence of a lesion or pathology present. The basis for the symptoms is an attempt by the patient's psyche to reduce the anxiety "energy" by converting it into a symptom such as pain or paralysis and thus reducing the level of anxiety.

The characteristics of a conversion reaction include the following: no identifiable lesion or pathology can be found, the disorder or reaction has an emotional cause, it is not dangerous to the patient, and it is a defense for the patient in terms of reducing the level of anxiety. The reduction of anxiety by converting it into a symptom is called the primary gain. These patients may also have secondary gains resulting from their condition: because of their symptom they may not be able to work, they may receive increased attention from their family, etc.

The following are examples of symptoms that can be produced by conversion reaction: paralysis, deafness, blindness, strange tastes, and pain. Oral examples of symptoms that can be produced by a conversion reaction include burning tongue, painful tongue, numbness of soft tissue, tingling sensa-

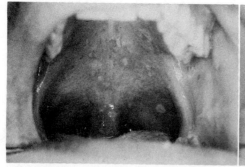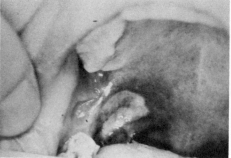

FIG. 23-1. Emotional factors appear to play an important role in some cases of, **A,** aphthous stomatitis and, **B,** periadenitis mucosa necrotica recurrens.

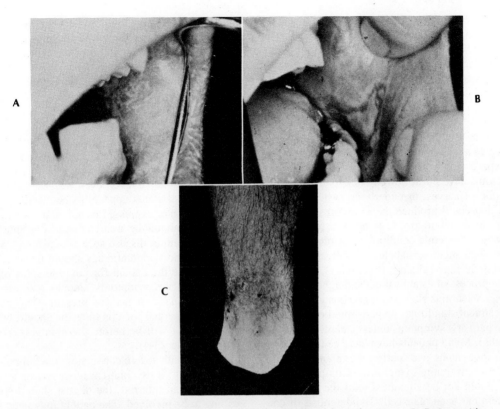

FIG. 23-2. A, Patient with lichen planus involving gingival and buccal mucosa. **B,** Patient with erosive lichen planus involving buccal mucosa. **C,** Patient with skin lesions of lichen planus. Many patients with this disorder have a history of emotional crises occurring just before onset of oral or skin lesions or both.

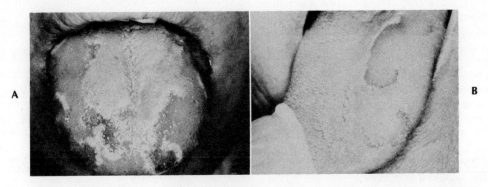

FIG. 23-3. A and B, Geographic tongue. This benign condition is thought to be related to emotional tension and represents an example of a psychophysiologic disorder.

tions of oral tissues, and pain in the facial region.[5,7] To the patient the symptom is very real, and if it is pain, it really hurts.

The diagnosis of a conversion reaction should only be made under the following circumstances; a thorough search from a clinical standpoint has failed to provide any evidence of a disease process that could explain the symptom; the symptoms have been present long enough that if they were related to a disease process it would be reasonable to expect that a lesion would have developed; symptoms have not followed known anatomic distribution of nerves; or underlying systemic conditions that could produce the symptoms have been ruled out by laboratory tests or by a referral to a physician. Systemic conditions that must be ruled out include anemia, diabetes, cancer, and a nutritional deficiency (vitamin B complex).

The process of establishing the diagnosis of conversion reaction is slow and time-consuming. Dental treatment should not be performed on the basis of the patient's symptoms unless a dental cause can be found. Many patients have had needless extractions, root canals, etc. performed in an attempt to correct conversion symptoms. Complex dental care should not be attempted until the conversion problem has been managed. The diagnosis of conversion reaction should not be reached until a thorough search has been made over a period of time for pathology that could explain the symptoms.

After a diagnosis of an oral conversion reaction has been established, the patient can be managed as follows. The findings should be discussed with the patient in the presence of a close relative, husband, wife, etc. During this discussion it should be pointed out that no organic source for the patient's problem could be found, that he does not have oral cancer, and that the pain or symptom is real to the patient.

The possibility of feelings of unhappiness being the source of the symptoms should be pointed out. This will be very difficult for the patient to understand and accept, but it is important "groundwork" to establish. Complex or unnecessary dental procedures should not be performed, even if the patient demands them in the belief that this will cause the symptom to disappear.

The dentist should pay close attention to his or her feelings toward the patient. The symptoms may be viewed as only a device to gain attention and sympathy. This may cause feelings of hostility and anger in the dentist toward the patient, which will not help in the proper management of the patient. The dentist should try to feel empathy toward the patient, try to understand the cause of the problem, and react in a positive manner toward the patient.

An attempt should be made by the dentist to manage the patient with a mild conversion reaction (mild in the sense that the patient is able to function at a reasonable level, even with the symptom, the emotional status appears to be "stable," and he has shown or expressed no suicidal tendencies). The patient should be assured that he does not have a life-threatening disease such as cancer. A series of regular short appointments should be scheduled to reexamine the patient for possible signs of disease, to discuss symptoms, and to reassure him that no tissue changes are present. The patient should be charged for this time, he should be told what this fee will be before the appointments are set up (Table 23-4).

Patients with severe conversion reactions should be referred to a psychiatrist; however, once a patient has been referred, the dentist should still be willing to be involved. The patient may need to be reexamined and the psychiatrist consulted concerning the findings. If the patient feels that the dentist only wants to get rid of him, the suggestion of referral will not be very helpful or effective.

TABLE 23-4. Management of patient with conversion reaction

Mild
  Establish diagnosis
  Talk with relative and patient
  Suggest relation of feelings to problem
  Examine patient to rule out serious disease such as oral cancer
  Do not perform treatment that is not indicated
  Do not become involved in complex treatment
  Recall for support and reexamination
Severe
  Refer to psychiatrist
  Be available to continue to serve role as patient's dentist

---

REFERENCES

1. Adelson, H.: The psychodynamics of the doctor-patient relationship, N.Y. State Dent. J. **36:**95-103, 1970.
2. Bloom, S.W.: The doctor and his patient: a sociological interpretation, New York, 1963, Russel Sage Foundation.
3. Blum, L.H.: Psychological aspects and the dentist-patient relationship. I, N.Y. State Dent. J. **39:**8-10, 1969.
4. Blum, L.H.: Psychological aspects and the dentist-patient relationship. II, N.Y. State Dent. J. **39:**51-55, 1969.
5. Brightman, V.J.: Oral symptoms without apparent physical abnormality. In Lynch, M.A., editor: Burket's oral medicine, diagnosis and treatment, ed. 7, Philadelphia, 1977, J.B. Lippincott Co., pp. 343-369.
6. DeRosin, H.A., and Pellegrino, V.Y.: The book of hope, New York, 1976, The Macmillan Co.
7. Michels, R., and Schoenberg, B.B.: Psychogenic disturbances. In Zegarelli, E.V., editor: Diagnosis of diseases of the mouth and jaws, ed. 2, Philadelphia, 1978, Lea & Febiger, pp. 571-580.
8. Szasz, T.S., and Hollender, M.H.: A contribution to the philosophy of medicine: the basic models of the doctor-patient relationship, Arch. Intern. Med. **97:**585-592, 1956.

INDEX